DEDICATION

To Joy Cordery, OTR, who created the concept of joint protection training, which has helped millions of patients, and whose life-long dedication to giving rehabilitation professionals a voice in the treatment of rheumatic diseases has benefited us all.

TABLE OF CONTENTS

ABOUT THE AUTHORS

Catherine Backman, MS, OT(C), Senior Instructor of Occupational Therapy at the School of Rehabilitation Sciences, The University of British Colombia, Vancouver, BC, is a doctoral candidate in Health Care and Epidemiology.

Michelle L. Boutaugh, BSN, MPH, is Vice President for Patient and Community Services for the Arthritis Foundation National Office in Atlanta, Georgia.

Laurence A. Bradley, PhD, is a Professor of Medicine in the Division of Immunology and Rheumatology at the University of Alabama at Birmingham.

Teresa J. Brady, PhD, LP, OTR, is the Group Vice President, Education at the Arthritis Foundation National Office in Atlanta, Georgia.

Brenda M. Coppard, MS, OTR/L, is an Assistant Professor in the Department of Occupational Therapy, Creighton University, Omaha, Nebraska.

Joy Cordery, OTR, is the former Administrative Director of Rehabilitation Medicine, Cornell Medical Center in New York, New York (retired).

Judith R. Gale, MA, MPH, PT, OCS, is the manager of the Physical Therapy Faculty Practice and is also Assistant Professor of Physical Therapy at Creighton University, Omaha, Nebraska.

Kathleen M. Haralson-Ferrell, MLA, PT, is the Associate Director of the Washington University Regional Arthritis Center, St. Louis, Missouri.

Donna J. Hawley, MN, EdD, RN, is Professor of Nursing, Wichita State University, Wichita, Kansas.

Karen W. Hayes, PhD, PT, is Curriculum Coordinator and Assistant Professor of Physical Therapy at Northwestern University Medical School, Chicago, Illinois.

Gail M. Jensen, PhD, PT, is an Associate Professor, Department of Physical Therapy, School of Pharmacy and Allied Health Professions at Creighton University, Omaha, Nebraska.

Christopher Lorish, PhD, is an Assistant Professor with the Department of Rehabilitation Sciences, UAB School of Health Related Professions, University of Alabama at Birmingham.

William Mann, PhD, OTR, is Professor and Chair of the Occupational Therapy Department at the State University of New York at Buffalo.

Marian A. Minor, PhD, PT, is an Associate Professor of Physical Therapy at the School of Health Related Professions, University of Missouri, Columbia, Missouri.

Carol A. Oatis, PhD, PT, is an Associate Professor of Physical Therapy at Beaver College, Glenside, Pennsylvania.

Cheryl M. Petersen, MS, PT, is an Associate Professor of Physical Therapy at Northwestern University Medical School, Chicago, Illinois.

Mary Rocchi, PT, is the Physical Therapy Supervisor at Ahlbin Centers for Rehabilitation Medicine, Fairfield, Connecticut.

Sue Schuerman, MBA, GCS, PT, is the Assistant Professor at the Division of Physical Therapy Education, University of Nebraska, Omaha, Nebraska.

Judy R. Sotosky, MEd, PT, in private practice in physical therapy in Virginia Beach, Virginia.

A. Joseph Threlkeld, PhD, PT, is the Chairman of the Physical Therapy Department at Creighton University, Omaha, Nebraska.

Rheumatologic Rehabilitation Series

Jeanne L. Melvin, MS, OTR, FAOTA, Series Editor

Volume 1 : Assessment and Management
– *Gail Jensen, PhD, PT, Coeditor*
Volume 2 : Adult Rheumatic Diseases
– *Kathleen Haralson-Ferrell, MLA, PT, Coeditor*
Volume 3 : Pediatric Rheumatic Diseases
– *F. Virginia Wright, BScPT, MSc, Coeditor*
Volume 4 : The Hand: Evaluation, Therapy, and Surgery
– *Edward Nalebuff, MD, Coeditor*
Volume 5 : Surgical Rehabilitation
– *Victoria Gall, MEd, PT, Coeditor*

Each volume is available from

The American Occupational Therapy Association.

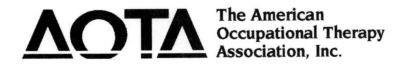

AOTA The American Occupational Therapy Association, Inc.

FOREWORD

This landmark series of five volumes entitled *Rheumatologic Rehabilitation* edited by Jeanne Melvin, MS, OTR, FAOTA, and five distinguished volume coeditors, provides a resource never before available in a single comprehensive publication for clinicians of many disciplines. This compendium is "the authoritative collection" of up-to-date and timely material covering every conceivable aspect of rehabilitation as it applies to rheumatic diseases, as well as related knowledge necessary for the care of these patients by practitioners. The fact that the American Occupational Therapy Association (AOTA) has the foresight to encourage and publish this material, which is pertinent to so many disciplines, gives credence to its dedication to the wide spectrum of care that needs to be provided for patients with rheumatic diseases. There is an emphasis on team care and communication. The series not only provides a primary resource for occupational and physical therapists, but it also is an excellent resource for nurses, psychologists and social workers, psychiatrists, rheumatologists, orthopedists, primary care physicians, and other health care providers.

Jeanne Melvin, for over 25 years, has dedicated her life to transmitting rehabilitation knowledge to the profession and the public. Her unique knowledge of rheumatic illnesses from many perspectives and her active role in several organizations (the AOTA, the Association of Rheumatology Health Professionals [ARHP], the American College of Rheumatology [ACR], and the Arthritis Foundation, to name a few), have led her to know firsthand many of the leaders in this field. She has gathered experts from every area to write definitive chapters relating to each aspect of evaluation and comprehensive treatment of rheumatic diseases. She and her coeditors have carefully reviewed and edited each chapter to assure uniformity, focus, applicability, relevance to a specific audience, excellent writing style, and timeliness. It is because of her editorial abilities and personal relationships with many of the authors that she has been able to create this series.

The series is logically organized into five distinctive volumes. Volume 1: Assessment and Management, Volume 2: Adult Rheumatic Diseases, Volume 3: Pediatric Rheumatic Diseases, Volume 4: The Hand: Evaluation, Therapy, and Surgery, and Volume 5: Surgical Rehabilitation.

While each volume is distinct, the integration is tight. Every important rheumatic disease is discussed. The coverage is wide, including basic rehabilitation information about these illnesses, the bio-psychosocial aspects, and medical and surgical management. Thus, the arthritis specialist will find this compendium readable from cover to cover; the primary care deliverer, be he or she a physician or other health care provider, and the specialists, may use the set as a reference as well. The organization, illustrations, charts, and tables are helpful and extremely well done. Many references are up to the minute.

All in all, I am proud, both to be a part of this important new contribution and to be asked to provide a foreword to the work. It will stand in the forefront of this field as the definitive collection on rehabilitation rheumatology for years to come.

Eric P. Gall, MD, FACP, FACR
Professor and Chairman, Department of Medicine
Chief, Division of Rheumatology
Professor, Department of Microbiology and Immunology
The Chicago Medical School

PREFACE TO THE *RHEUMATOLOGIC REHABILITATION* SERIES

The specialty practice area of rheumatologic rehabilitation has been created in large part by the Association of Rheumatology Health Professionals (ARHP), which was founded to support interdisciplinary communication and education. The impact of the ARHP and its philosophy is manifest in the concept of this series and in the spirit of cooperation shown by the contributing authors, many of whom joined this project specifically because it is an interdisciplinary educational endeavor.

This book is the direct result of the first ARHP Fellowship (1973-4) from the Association of Rheumatology Health Professionals and the Arthritis Foundation, which enabled me to research and write *Rheumatic Disease in the Adult and Child: Occupational Therapy and Rehabilitation*, published in 1977, and then continued into three editions. Although the present series was initially intended to be a revision and expansion of that textbook to include physical therapy, there is now truly little left of the previous text except organizational design, some illustrations, and a few paragraphs in Volumes 2 and 3.

This series focuses on educating physical and occupational therapists because these two professions share knowledge bases in the areas of anatomy, physiology, rheumatology, and rehabilitation to be competent in the physical rehabilitation of people with rheumatic diseases. Also, these professionals must often work together to achieve the desired outcomes for this patient population. Of course, I hope that all professionals interested in the rehabilitation of people with rheumatic diseases will find this series useful.

This series tackles the task of educating therapists about rheumatologic rehabilitation in an unprecedented format. First, the content is divided into five volumes so therapists in adult, pediatric, hand, and orthopedic practice areas can select the volumes most relevant to their interests. The theoretical and research basis for evaluation and treatment is presented in Volume 1 to facilitate the use of this material in OT and PT curriculums. Second, all the disease chapters in Volumes 2 and 3 demonstrate the team approach by being written collaboratively by a rheumatologist, a physical therapist, and an occupational therapist. In Volume 5, *Surgical Rehabilitation*, most chapters are authored by an orthopedic surgeon, OT, PT, and an orthopedic nurse. Third, each chapter in all volumes except Volume 4, has been reviewed from both PT and OT perspectives by the coeditors.

Eighty-six authors from all health professions involved in caring for individuals with rheumatic diseases have contributed to this series, testifying to the editors' commitment to training therapists in the team approach to treatment. The size of this series and the number of contributing authors reflects the growth of rheumatologic rehabilitation in all of the treating disciplines, that is: rheumatology, orthopedic surgery, nursing, patient education, psychology, social work, and pedorthics. Research is occurring in each of these fields that directly affects the practice of occupational and physical therapy. It is no longer sufficient or even possible to learn about rheumatologic rehabilitation as a specialty area in PT or OT from within a single practice area. For PT and OT the new frontiers in rheumatologic rehabilitation during the next 20 years will not necessarily be in advanced interventions unique to each field but, rather, in integrating into practice the research from the areas of patient education, wellness studies, pain management, adherence research, fatigue management, and outcome and functional assessment. In Volume 1 leading researchers and clinicians from all these fields share the latest research and methodologies that are specifically relevant to physical and occupational therapy intervention. Within the fields of PT and OT I have invited both specialists within rheumatologic rehabilitation and those with expertise in assessment or treatment outside of arthritis treatment that could broaden the approach to treatment in rheumatology.

Following is a full preface to Volume 1 and brief prefaces to Volumes 2 through 5.

VOLUME 1 ASSESSMENT AND MANAGEMENT
Coedited by Gail Jensen, PhD, PT

This volume covers the areas of patient management from clinic to community. The authors represent a mix of researchers and clinicians who have focused their writing on bridging theory and practice by applying concepts to specific clinical cases and situations.

One area of patient care that has advanced considerably during the last 10 years is patient education. No longer limited to teaching for compliance of exercises, medications, and joint protection, patient education has expanded to teaching self-management: that is, the skills for maintaining health, slowing disease, optimizing function, coping, communicating, and problem-solving in order to have an active and emotionally satisfying life in the face of a chronic illness. Michelle Boutaugh, RN, and Terry Brady, PhD, OTR, have done an extraordinary job of reviewing a decade of research in this area and outlining the teaching strategies that therapists can use to empower patients along the path of self-management.

Larry Bradley, PhD, a leading research psychologist, reviews the behavioral factors that have been shown to magnify or reduce pain and describes his experience in teaching self-management of pain to people with fibromyalgia and other rheumatic diseases. He clearly demonstrates that pain management for these people now goes far beyond rest, cold packs, and drugs.

In the section on Foundations of Practice, Terry Brady, PhD, OTR, has made a significant contribution to understanding the impact of managed care on people with chronic rheumatic disease and on the rehabilitation process. She brings a special perspective to this task as a rheumatology clinician and as past Director of Chronic Disease Care for a large integrated health-care system.

The hot topic of the decade, clinical outcomes, is addressed in three chapters. Christopher Lorish, PhD, teaches the psychology of evaluation and treatment and how to structure intervention to address psychological issues and maximize patient adherence, which are essential to many outcomes. Donna Hawley, EdD, RN, who conducts and teaches outcome research, describes the issues of achieving and documenting patient outcomes in rheumatology in the most lucid, easy-to-read chapter you will find on this topic. Catherine Backman, MS, OT(C), addresses outcomes research within the framework of functional assessment. Her comprehensive approach to this topic demonstrates how far we have come from using the ADL checklist as our main assessment tool.

In 1965 Joy Cordery, OTR, created the concept of joint-protection training that became a standard intervention throughout the world. In this volume she describes how these concepts have held up over time, the biomechanical basis for the techniques, and the research that has been done so far on this intervention. Most importantly, she defines joint protection for osteoarthritis. Joy Cordery, OTR, and Mary Rocchi, PT, address joint protection for the lower extremities and spine.

Judy Sotosky, MEd, PT, and I teamed up to present a client-centered approach relevant to both PT and OT for the initial interview process that identifies the unique issues of assessing a person with a rheumatic disease.

Therapists need strong musculoskeletal diagnostic skills. To help therapists sharpen their skills in this area, Joseph Threlkeld, PhD, PT, outlines a systematic approach for assessing musculoskeletal function. Karen Hayes, PhD, PT, and Cheryl Petersen, MS, PT, build on these evaluation concepts and provide specific assessment and clinical findings that lead to the differential diagnosis of common joint and soft-tissue disorders.

Impaired ambulation is one of the most common and severe consequences of arthritis; it results from changes at multiple joint sites. Even the simple prescription of walking for exercise can increase lower-extremity and spine problems if basic faults in gait are not identified and corrected. Carol Oatis, PhD, PT, coauthor of *Gait Analysis: Theory and Application* (Mosby, 1995) describes assessment and intervention for common gait problems of people with arthritis.

Once the patient is interviewed, assessed, and treated in the clinic, Marian Minor, PhD, PT, a clinician and researcher on fitness and arthritis, provides the guidelines for teaching patients how to incorporate fitness into their self-management program. With the right exercise program, everyone with inflammatory arthritis, fibromyalgia, and OA can improve their health.

The emphasis on self-management of arthritis during the last 15 years has increased the emphasis on thermal modalities and therapeutic (nonfitness) exercises that patients can do at home and deemphasized clinic-based treatment interventions. Subsequently, fewer advances have occurred in these areas. Sue Schuerman, MBA, GCS, PT, has reviewed and summarized the research done on using thermal modalities and arthritis. This chapter provides a good starting point for therapists wanting to research the efficacy of specific modalities and protocols for treating inflammation. The OT–PT team of Brenda Coppard, MS, OTR/L, Judy Gale, MA, MPH, PT, OCS, and Gail Jensen, PhD, PT, have pulled together state-of-the-art therapeutic exercises, specifically for improving range of motion or correcting physical limitations as opposed to general fitness.

Bill Mann, PhD, OTR, author of *Assistive Technology for Persons with Disabilities, 2nd Ed.* (AOTA, 1995), brings considerable expertise to his chapter on assistive technology. While there are a few new devices that can help people with arthritis, the big news is advances in accessing resources. The Abledata database of more than 20,000 devices and pieces of equipment is now available on the Internet (www.abledata.com) as well as CD-ROM, providing access to thousands of items that are not available in standard ADL catalogues (see chapter 16 and the appendix on footwear selection for examples of what is available on the Abledata website).

For the therapist who says, "I don't have the resources at my facility to teach self-management," Kathleen Haralson-Ferrell, MLA, PT, replies with a chapter that says "look around." There are a host of community organizations and resources, as well as the Internet, available to help patients. Learn how to "source" from this chapter and then share the skill with your patients.

VOLUME 2 ADULT RHEUMATIC DISEASES

Coedited by Kitty Haralson-Ferrell, MLA, PT

It is essential to the successful treatment of people with rheumatic diseases that therapists work closely with the referring physician and integrate therapy with medical management. This requires an understanding of medical management. Volume 2 is designed specifically to help therapists develop this understanding.

This volume contains a chapter on each of the eight major rheumatic diseases: osteoarthritis, fibromyalgia, rheumatoid arthritis, systemic lupus erythematosus, systemic sclerosis, psoriatic arthritis, ankylosing spondylitis, and polymyositis. It also contains a chapter on 19 "less common" diseases. Every chapter is authored by a team consisting of a leading rheumatologist in that disease, a physical therapist, and an occupational therapist. I believe this team approach breaks new ground in the rehabilitation literature. It has taken more work to integrate the material of three authors, but now the roles of the three primary clinicians whose task it is to improve physical function in the patient can all be seen in the same chapter. This should make clear the significance of integrating and coordinating the care given by each team member and can provide an opportunity for each to learn about the others' roles and contributions to the rehabilitation process. This is increasingly important since managed care is forcing a more coordinated approach. When a patient with severe polyarticular RA has only 12 PT and 12 OT visits per year, therapists and doctors must really work together to accomplish all the therapy that is needed. If patients are not on an optimal drug regimen, they may not be able to participate fully in therapy, thus wasting precious visits; if therapists are not aware of the course or prognosis of specific symptoms, therapy can be in vain.

In the section on Foundations of Practice, Betts Carpenter, PhD, MD, an instructor of immunology, explains the process of joint inflammation and puts immunology into a functional context that is accessible for therapists. She has created an original chapter that wonderfully accomplishes this task. John Bland, MD, a renowned clinician and researcher in osteoarthritis, took on the task of explaining the pathophysiology of cartilage and joint structures in a manner that is easy to understand and eminently usable for therapists. This is in stark contrast to most existing chapters on the subject. Eric Gall, MD, who has been a major supporter of rehabilitation for arthritis, explains in lucid language the pro's and con's of the medications currently being used to manage arthritis and how drugs can enhance therapy outcomes. The chapter on Radiographic Imaging is written by Tom Learch, MD, who started his career as an OTR working in rheumatology. He is now a radiologist specializing in musculoskeletal disease and brings a unique focus to the subject of radiographic imaging and what is most important for therapists to know.

VOLUME 3 PEDIATRIC RHEUMATIC DISEASES

Coedited by F. Virginia Wright, BScPT, MSc

This volume truly reflects a Canadian and United States working partnership, with approximately half of the authors from each country. There are four chapters on disease groups emphasizing team treatment: Juvenile Rheumatoid Arthritis by Richard Mier, MD, Virginia Wright, MSc, PT, and Deborah Bolding, CHT, OTR; and Chronic Idiopathic Pain Syndromes, Spondylarthropathies, and Connective Tissue Disorders by Ross Petty, MD, Gay Kuchta, DipOT, and Iris Davidson, BSR (PT).

During the last 10 years we have gained a greater understanding of juvenile arthritis and adult rheumatoid arthritis as separate diseases. Children respond differently to interventions than adults; consequently, interventions need to be different. For children we have learned there is a need for extensive therapy throughout the active course of the disease process, especially considering the potential of cartilage healing in the growing child and long-term or permanent remission.

The disease chapters identify OT and PT interventions applicable to specific clinical problems that are cross-referenced to the separate chapters on physical therapy by Shirley Scull, MS, PT, and occupational therapy by Deborah Bolding, CHT, OTR.

One of the most important advances in pediatric rheumatology is a better understanding of pain in children and how to measure it. This is aptly addressed by Patrick McGrath, PhD, and Anita Unruh, PhD, MSW, OT, authors of *Pain in Children and Adolescents* (Elsevier, 1987).

Recent advances in functional status measures have taken into account both the child's and parent's perspectives. Virginia Wright, MSc, PT, has done an excellent job of bringing all of the issues concerning pediatric outcome assessment into focus.

Michael Rapoff, PhD, a pediatric clinical psychologist with a special interest in adherence, brings together the latest research and clinical strategies for enhancing patient and family adherence to treatment.

Mary Murry-Weir, MBA, PT, NDT, and Jamie Black, OTR, have revised and expanded the chapter on developmental assessment authored by Martha Atwood Sanders, MS, OTR, in *Rheumatic Disease in the Adult and Child, 3rd Ed.*

The impact that arthritis and poor attendance can have on school achievement and the importance of physical, psychosocial, and educational support to prevent problems is addressed by IIona Szer, MD, and Virginia Wright, MSc, PT.

Drs. Bryan Nestor and Mark Figgie, from the Hospital for Special Surgery in New York City, describe the current philosophy and approach to surgical management of arthritis in children.

Finally, the practical application of comprehensive rehabilitation is illustrated by three case studies. Virginia Wright, MSc, PT, describes treatment of a 14-year-old girl with dermatomyositis. Karen Matsurra, PT, describes a young boy with systemic-onset JRA, and Gerri McGirr, OT, describes an adolescent girl with polyarticular JRA.

VOLUME 4 THE HAND: EVALUATION, THERAPY, AND SURGERY

Coedited by Edward Nalebuff, MD

Dr. Nalebuff was the hand surgery consultant on the second and third editions of *Rheumatic Disease in the Adult and Child*. He has a distinguished career as a hand surgeon with a specialty in arthritis and broad experience with disorders such as scleroderma, systemic lupus erythematosus, psoriatic arthritis, rheumatoid arthritis, and osteoarthritis. His superb skills as a clinical photographer make his teachings even more dramatic. This volume continues our 20-year working relationship through coeditorship of Volume 5 and coauthorship of four new chapters on surgery and therapy for rheumatoid arthritis, systemic lupus erythematosus, psoriatic arthritis, and scleroderma.

Andrew Torrono, MD, provides a comprehensive look at the most common hand problem, osteoarthritis, with a special emphasis on treatment of the thumb.

During the last 10 years hand therapy has advanced as a specialty practice area. Two authors have been invited, in part, to bridge the gap and facilitate education between this specialty area and rheumatologic rehabilitation. Judy Colditz, CHT, OTR, who has superb skills in splint fabrication and hand rehabilitation, has integrated and extensively revised the orthotic chapter from *Rheumatic Disease in the Adult and Child, 3rd Ed.* and incorporated the splinting terminology adopted by The American Society of Hand Therapists (ASHT), which uses the term "splint" instead of "orthotic." Terri Wolfe, CHT, OTR, current President of ASHT and owner of a private hand-therapy practice, is on the Advisory Committee for UE Net, the national outcomes database established by ASHT. She and I have extensively revised the chapter on Hand Assessment so that the terminology and recommendations are consistent with ASHT criteria.

Joy Cordery, OTR, expands her original work on joint protection training and examines the biomechanical basis for joint protection of the hand. Bill Mann, PhD, OTR, covers assistive technology specifically to improve function in people with arthritis hand involvement.

Finally, Susan Michlovitz, PhD, PT, CHT, author of *Thermal Agents in Rehabilitation, 3rd Ed.* (FA Davis, 1996) and I describe the effective application of therapeutic exercise and thermal modalities in the management of arthritis of the hand.

VOLUME 5 SURGICAL REHABILITATION

Coedited by Victoria Gall, MEd, PT

This volume contains six chapters, each focusing on surgery and rehabilitation for a specific joint area. Internationally recognized surgeons and therapists from leading hospitals were invited to share their expertise and clinical experience in providing care for patients with severe polyarticular RA as well as monoarticular OA. Susan Kloos, OTR, Bryan Nestor, MD, and Mark Figgie, MD, cover elbow surgery; Thomas Thornhill, MD, Victoria Gall, MEd, PT, Frances Griffin, RN, and Susan Vermette, OTR, cover shoulder surgery; Rick Delamarter, MD, and James Coyle, MD, cover spine surgery; Robert Poss, MD, Scott Martin, MD, Kathy Zavedak, PT, Jill Noaker, CHT, OTR, and Mary Ann Jacobs, MS, RN, cover hip surgery; Thomas Sculco, MD, Sandy Ganz, MS, PT, Jill Noaker, CHT, OTR, and Mary Ann Jacobs, RN, cover knee surgery; and Andrea Cracchiolo, III, MD, teams up with Victoria Gall, MEd, PT, and Denise Janisse, a pedorthist (specialist in prescription footwear and orthotics) who is also President of the National Pedorthic Association, to cover foot and ankle surgery.

Outcome assessments of joint surgery are now based on function and general health status with an emphasis on patient self-report. Several of the more popular functional assessments for the hip, knee, foot, and upper extremities are featured in this volume.

Victoria Gall, MEd, PT, and I review the literature on preoperative education and assessment. It has become increasingly evident that patient education for self-management is the most effective approach because patients have better results when they take an active part in their disease management.

Jeanne Melvin, MS, OTR, FAOTA

Program Manager, Chronic Pain and Fibromyalgia Program
Cedars-Sinai Medical Center, Beverly Hills, California

ACKNOWLEDGMENTS

There are so many people to thank. I am deeply indebted to the five coeditors that made this interdisciplinary series possible: Gail Jensen, PhD, PT, Kitty Haralson-Ferrell, MLA, PT, Virginia Wright, BSPT, MSc, Edward Nalebuff, MD, and Victoria Gall, MEd, PT. They have worked countless hours over the last 2 1/2 years to bring this project to fruition, and they have done a wonderful job. I would also like to thank the 87 contributors, many of whom are among the busiest people in North America, who brought their vast experience to focus on specific topics for our audience. The quality of their contributions has brought tremendous energy to these volumes. I would particularly like to recognize the authors of the multidisciplinary chapters. Writing as a member of a team is difficult; it is hard to cut your material to make room for someone else's. But the multi-authored disease and surgery chapters are unique. Never before has all of this information been integrated into single chapters.

The publishing staff at AOTA have been terrific. Fran McCarrey, Director of Nonperiodical Publications; Maureen Muncaster, Acquisitions Editor; Mary Fisk, Managing Editor; Ethel Anagnoson, Administrative Assistant; and Liz Holcomb, our first Editor, were supportive, helpful, and tolerant of the delays and last-minute changes that tend to be inherent in a project of this size.

A few people have played important roles behind the scenes. Many colleagues were enlisted by authors to review chapters in progress. Their input in helping refine chapters is greatly appreciated. Joy Cordery, OTR, reviewed several chapters for me, including most of the ones I wrote or to which I contributed. Her input and support throughout this project were invaluable. Marian Minor, PhD, PT, was initially involved as a coeditor, and she provided significant suggestions for the outline of the series. Dr. Edward Nalebuff has made an extraordinary contribution to Volume 4, including numerous outstanding photographs. Even the most experienced arthritis hand therapist will learn from his chapters. Tom Learch, MD, also provided an extensive number of excellent x-ray photos for Volume 2. Virginia Wright, MSc, PT, came aboard as a coauthor on two chapters at the last minute and did a terrific job.

I continue to be indebted to the Association of Rheumatology Health Professionals and the Arthritis Foundation for their contribution to my education through the first Allied Health Professions Fellowship (1973), which has made my work possible.

Finally, I would like to thank my husband, Jerry Small, a superb writer who graciously copyedited my contributions and gave me invaluable editorial assistance and support.

PART ONE:
FOUNDATIONS OF PRACTICE

ISSUES AND TRENDS IN RHEUMATOLOGIC REHABILITATION

Jeanne Melvin, MS, OTR, FAOTA

These are turbulent and uncertain times for health care and for the treatment of persons with rheumatic diseases. Our health care system has been going through a major transformation in the last 15 years, and we must try to understand and help steer the new system as it emerges. Do you have a vision for how the rehabilitative care of persons with rheumatic diseases should be delivered in the next century? Do you have a plan for incorporating the bio-psychosocial, patient education, and self-management research outcomes into your practice? If this specialty practice area has any future at all, physical and occupational therapists will have to provide the leadership to create the care delivery programs that they want and that will best serve the needs of patients.

This chapter reviews the social, economic, and policy trends that have shaped the current experience in rheumatologic rehabilitation. This is first defined as a specialty practice area in occupational therapy (OT) and physical therapy (PT). Then, to paint the larger picture, current trends and future directions are identified by leaders in this field and other writers in this volume. As Alvin Toffler (1990) reminded us, "To make sense of today's great changes, to think strategically, we need more than bits, blips, and lists. We need to see how different changes relate to one another."

CHANGE IN THE LAST 15 YEARS

We are now living through what will become historical trends. Imagine that the year is 2030. What will people be saying about rheumatologic rehabilitation in the last part of the 20th century? They are likely to recall how health care costs began spiraling out of control during the inflationary period of the 1970s and how advanced technology and the dominant influence of the market economy turned the helping professions into a health care industry. They will remember that the United States made an attempt to join the ranks of other industrialized nations by creating a national health care plan and that this effort was thwarted by a consortium of insurance companies and other groups. However, it was also a time that finally recognized the civil rights of persons with disabilities with the passage of the Americans with Disabilities Act (ADA) in 1990 to protect persons with disabilities from discrimination in employment, transportation, and public accommodations.

A number of forces converged in the mid-1980s to change the direction of health care and rheumatologic rehabilitation in the United States. "Cost containment" became a national goal and produced Medicare reform in 1983, which encouraged hospitals to focus on acute care and reduce the length of hospitalizations. This reform resulted in empty beds, decreased hospital revenues, the closure or merger of many hospitals, a general downsizing of both hospital-based programs and rehabilitation administration, the closing of inpatient arthritis rehabilitation units, and an expansion of home health care. As a result, some patients with acute rheumatic diseases were discharged more sick than in the past and were treated in outpatient clinics or through home health programs.

The movement of hospitals away from chronic disease care coincided with and ultimately advanced a national trend toward self-management and self-help. The interest in wellness and self-management was reflected in the print and broadcast media with the introduction of health-oriented magazines (including *Arthritis Today* in 1987), health newsletters from major medical universities, and television shows with physicians advising people on how to care for most known illnesses. The Internet gave the average person access to the National Library of Medicine and provided opportunities to interact with others with similar problems. Cyber-patients could scan articles on medical treatment and a wide range of alternative interventions into the Internet for easy downloading by others. The 1980s saw the shift of medical knowledge from the inner circle out to the general populace. The public became smarter and more selective in health care.

Many chose complementary medicines or therapies over allopathic medicine, even though they had to pay out of their own pockets. Holistic, wellness, and mind-body approaches burgeoned in the 1980s and had a profound effect on people with rheumatic diseases. Fitness programs, stress management, relaxation training, cognitive-behavioral strategies, nutritional awareness, and eating plans, all proven to help healthy people, were employed by people with chronic arthritis and pain to help them regain or improve their health. Research during the late 1980s and late 1990s repeatedly demonstrated that physical behavior could influence the mind and that psychological interventions could improve physical functioning of persons with rheumatic diseases.

Rehabilitation for rheumatic diseases began moving from a solely biological model to a bio-psychosocial model. The contribution of psychologists to our understanding of how pain management, cognitive therapy, and behavioral intervention can improve function and quality of life for people with arthritis has been extensive in the 1980s and 1990s. This has given rheumatologic rehabilitation a leg up, but PTs and OTs are not on the horse yet. For the most part, this research is not being applied clinically in therapy programs. This is also true for patient education research on the role of self-management and self-efficacy training (see chapter 3 on adherence, chapter 10 on patient education, and chapter 11 on pain management.)

The interest of therapists in learning mind-body strategies for helping patients with rheumatic diseases continues to grow, with new national conferences specifically for allied health professionals emerging each year.

Fortunately the advances and interest in bio-psychosocial research coincided with the emergence or recognition of fibromyalgia syndrome (FMS) as a "real" disorder. FMS moved from obscurity of an "inorganic" disease (a euphemism for psychosomatic disorder) in the 1970s to being the second most prevalent rheumatic disease following osteoarthritis (OA) in the 1980s. This "promotion" occurred when Dr. Moldofsky and colleagues (Moldofsky, Scarisbrick, England, & Smythe, 1975) were able to associate FMS with a sleep disorder and found that low-dose tricyclic antidepressants helped reduce symptoms. This spurred international interest in improved diagnostic criteria and medical and rehabilitative management. FMS is now estimated to affect 5-9 million persons in the United States alone (Wolfe, 1995). The magnitude of this population has stimulated thousands of therapists outside of rheumatologoic rehabilitation to seek information on treating this disorder more effectively. The current understanding of this disorder as an imbalance of the central neurohormonal system as opposed to a primary muscle disorder (Goldenberg, 1996) mandates that therapists move into a bio-psychosocial model of treatment.

Rheumatologic management also changed in the 1980s. Research documenting that rheumatoid arthritis (RA) patients die an average of 10 years earlier than the general population emphasized that RA was not just a benign chronic condition (Pincus & Callahan, 1986). In addition, early mortality was linked closely to functional disability (Pincus & Callahan). Other studies showed that patients managed on the traditional "pyramid" approach (starting with simple drugs and progressing to more toxic drugs) were showing 60 percent disability after 15 years of RA and 90 percent disability after 30 years. Second-line drugs were not altering long-term outcomes as expected. People with RA were becoming disabled because of joint damage, and most of this damage was occurring in the first few years of disease while patients were being tried on a variety of first- and second-line drugs. In the pyramid drug model, cytotoxic drugs were considered third-line drugs to be used only after second-line drugs such as gold and Plaquenil® had failed. During the 1980s, this philosophy was altered in part when methotrexate, a cytotoxic drug, became a very effective medication for controlling RA and other inflammatory arthritides with minimal toxicity compared to other second-line disease-modifying antirheumatic drugs (DMARDs).

So over the last 10 years the traditional, hierarchical pyramid has been discarded for a more aggressive therapy that consists of treating with immunosuppressive (including cytotoxic) drugs earlier in the course of the disease and combining DMARDs to bring disease under control early, before severe joint destruction occurs. For some patients this means they need less extensive rehabilitation, and for others it means that they need rehabilitation to help them function at work instead of at home.

From the late 1980s to the present, managed care has grown to the point where almost everyone in the U.S. is either in some form of managed care (in its broader sense, including Medicare) or is uninsured. Most are in a total managed-care plan. Managed care has had a profound effect on rheumatologic rehabilitation in a variety of ways, some of which are summarized in Table 1. Its most important impact is the policy requiring all patients to be managed by a primary-care physician who is either a family practitioner or internist. This doctor is the "gatekeeper" who can approve or deny referrals to specialists in rheumatology and to rehabilitation. In most situations, reimbursement by capitation

IMPACT OF MANAGED CARE ON RHEUMATOLOGIC REHABILITATION

MANAGED CARE	POSSIBLE IMPACT ON RHEUMATOLOGIC REHABILITATION
1. Primary care will be provided by internists and family practitioners who function as gatekeepers.	Reduced referrals to PT and OT.
2. Managed care companies rather than clinicians determine services.	They may have limited knowledge of consequences of care or lack of it.
3. Reduced OT and PT coverage.	Less time for treatment and patient education with reduced favorable outcomes.
4. Increased use of technical personnel, i.e., COTA and PTA.	If assistants are asked to do treatment beyond their skill level, patients may not improve and outcomes will decline.
5. Demands for increased productivity and concurrent treatments.	Treatment more rushed, less time for patient education and psychosocial issues (less privacy in treatment).
6. Reduced length of inpatient stays.	Patients with more acute problems will be treated as outpatients.
7. Emphasis on outpatient care.	Closing of inpatient arthritis rehabilitation units.
8. No funding for PT and OT staff at orthopedic, rheumatology, or primary-care clinics at teaching hospitals.	Physicians not trained in arthritis rehabilitation, therefore patients who could benefit from rehabilitation may not be referred and there may be delays in early treatment.
9. Emphasis on the therapist as a generalist rather than a specialist.	Elimination of arthritis clinical positions in rehabilitation. Reduction of research, teaching, and expertise from specialists. Therapists treating may not have sufficient knowledge to provide adequate arthritis treatment.
10. Emphasis on group treatment.	This will reduce the therapeutic options available for physical rehabilitation. It could improve options for wellness training and psychosocial support. Quality of outcome depends on training of group leader. Few therapists trained to run groups.
11. Decreased funding for continuing education.	Fewer opportunities for learning specialized clinical skills.
12. Decreased need for rheumatologists and a decrease in funding for rheumatology training and research.	In the short term, decreased referrals to rehabilitation and opportunities to interact with rheumatologists. In the long term, decreased research and slowing in advances in treatment.

Table 1: Impact of Managed Care on Rheumatologic Rehabilitation

provides an incentive against referrals to specialized care, and in the eyes of managed care this includes rehabilitation (Feinglass et al., 1992). Most primary care physicians have had little formal training in arthritis rehabilitation, and the topic is rarely covered in their literature. The only exceptions are the few primary-care physicians who belong to the American College of Rheumatology and those who receive the *Bulletin on the Rheumatic Diseases*, and now receive the *Arthritis Care and Research*, although new journals such as the *Journal of Clinical Rheumatology* are emerging to help address this need.

Most managed-care plans currently require all patients with OA, fibromyalgia, gout, uncomplicated rheumatoid arthritis (RA), and systemic lupus erythematosus (SLE) to be managed by the primary-care physician. The rheumatologist is designated to manage only severely complicated RA, SLE, spondylarthropathies, and uncommon rheumatic diseases. Rheumatologists also serve on a consultative basis for patients who remain under primary care. Since 1965, therapists working in rheumatologic rehabilitation have aligned themselves with rheumatology and have had scant contact with primary-care physicians. Now therapists need to address this issue by informing those in primary care about their services, offering to do inservice training, writing in the primary-care literature, and lecturing at primary-care conferences. Therapists working in teaching institutions need to become involved in the training programs of primary-care physicians. Otherwise, these gatekeepers will have little understanding of the role OT and PT can play in reducing symptoms and improving the quality of life of people with rheumatic diseases. Therapists also need to serve as patient advocates, promoting the delivery of effective care and improvement of the quality of life.

When managed care becomes fully entrenched, primary care could control the care of 80% or more of patients with rheumatic disease. The issue of educating primary-care physicians about rheumatologic rehabilitation needs to be addressed in the next few years by the Association of Rheumatology Health Professionals and all therapists who are interested in providing care to arthritis patients. The ARHP and the ACR have begun to address this issue with a new book *Clinical Care in Rheumatic Diseases* (Wegner, 1996), written for both primary-care practitioners and rheumatology health professionals. It is an excellent first step in addressing this issue. The ACR has also begun to publish guidelines for treatment of specific rheumatic diseases (1996) or problems like OA of the hip and knee (Hochberg et al., 1995), which include the role of PT and OT and will help guide future practice.

Health care reform to control costs mandates that payers look at the value of what they are paying for. Relman (1988) refers to this as "the era of accountability." So, from the late 1980s to the present a plethora of clinical outcome assessments have been developed to capture that elusive quality of "significant progress," or "improved functioning." In chapter 4, Donna Hawley, MN, EdD, RN, eloquently describes the parameters of the numerous outcome assessments applicable to people with rheumatic diseases.

Eventually outcome studies may be reduced to a few so that wide-based results can be compared. Facilities will likely belong to large databases and will be able to compare their outcomes to other facilities. A current example of this therapy is "UE Net," organized by the American Society of Hand Therapists. Subscribers to UE Net use standardized evaluation and data-reporting methods, submit their outcome data to UE Net, and receive quarterly reports so they can compare their outcomes to other facilities. It is a wake-up call if you find that your department takes 10 sessions to treat a specific condition for which others need only 5 sessions. Outcome data can help practioners improve their performance, but it is still not clear how third party payers will use these databases and who will pay for outcome research.

RHEUMATOLOGIC REHABILITATION AS A PRACTICE SPECIALTY

Rheumatologic rehabilitation has had several peak periods. During the rapid growth of rehabilitation in the early 1960s and before there were many effective medications for RA, arthritis was a major diagnosis in rehabilitation programs. New rehabilitation approaches such as joint-protection training and hand orthotics and greater sophistication in use exercise were developed in the early 1960s; and there was a dramatic increase in the arthritis rehabilitation literature, both in books and journal articles (Cordery, 1965a, 1965b; Hislop & Lamont-Havers, 1964a, 1964b). The Arthritis Foundation (AF) recognized the essential contribution of rehabilitation practitioners in the treatment of patients with arthritis and the need for a multidisciplinary approach. AF sponsored the formation of the Paramedical Section of the Medical Council of the AF in 1965, the precursor to the present Association of Rheumatology Health Professions (ARHP). This organization was totally dedicated to a multidisciplinary approach to treatment of arthritis. (Table 2 contains a time line of events affecting the growth of rheumatologic rehabilitation.)

One month after the Paramedical Section was formed, Medicare was enacted into law. Medicare decentralized health care and greatly expanded access for the elderly. Medicaid was soon to follow. The new laws increased patient access and created a shortage of health care providers. That, in turn, stimulated federal grants to support training of health professionals. The AF and the Paramedical Section benefited from a number of these grants. In 1968 the Paramedical Section became the Allied Health Professions Section. In 1978 it was changed to the Arthritis Health Profession Section, then in 1980 it became the Arthritis Health Professions Association (AHPA) and finally in 1994 it became the Association of Rheumatology Health Professions (ARHP)(Melvin, 1990).

While Medicare was expanding patient demand, orthopedic and hand surgery made dramatic advances. From 1968 to 1972, total joint arthroplasty for hips, knees, and hands became common in the United States, bringing hundreds of rehabilitation health professionals into the field of arthritis rehabilitation. Total hip and knee surgery had such a dramatic impact on arthritis rehabilitation that the 1975 revision of the *Arthritis Foundation Manual for Allied Health Professionals* required that pictures showing patients in wheelchairs be deleted: In 7 years the total joint arthroplasty had eliminated the common association of severe arthritis with the wheelchair.

The Arthritis Act of 1975 resulted in the creation of 24 Multipurpose Arthritis Centers (MACs) funded by the National Institutes of Health throughout the United States between 1977 and 1982. These centers generated considerable research that emphasized the role of rehabilitation professionals and encouraged the inclusion of therapists,

RHEUMATOLOGY AND RHEUMATOLOGIC REHABILITATION: HISTORICAL BENCHMARKS IN THE UNITED STATES

1911	Dr. Joel Goldwaith established one of the first orthopedic arthritis clinics at Carney Hospital in Boston; he encouraged PT as a profession.
1923	Reconstruction Aides returned from WWI to the Robert Brigham Hospital for the Incurable and created the first OT and PT programs for adult RD patients (average length of stay 14 months). The hospital had a teaching relationship with OT and PT schools in Boston.
1926-1938	Doctors began specializing in arthritis, and arthritis clinics for teaching and treatment evolved.
1927	The International Committee Against Rheumatism was formed.
1928	The American Committee for the Control of Rheumatism was created to increase national awareness of the impact of arthritis.
1937	The American Rheumatism Association (ARA) was created; in 1989 the name was changed to the American College of Rheumatology (ACR).
1942	The Arthritis Foundation (AF) was founded.
1949	The National Arthritis and Rheumatism Institute and the National Advisory Arthritis and Rheumatism Council were created.
1950	The National Institute of Arthritis and Metabolic Diseases was created at the National Institutes of Health.
1958	The journal *Arthritis and Rheumatism* was started.
1962	The Arthritis and Rheumatism Foundation funded AOTA and APTA to set up an Advisory Council to the AF.
1965	The ARF and ARA amalgamated. The ARF changed its name to the Arthritis Foundation (AF).
1965	Medicare was enacted, which decentralized health care and improved access for the elderly and disabled.
1966	The first ARHP Scientific Meeting was held.
1966	The current ARHP was formed as the Paramedical Section of the Medical Council of the AF. The first Scientific Meeting was held in Denver in 1967.
1968	Name of the Paramedical Section was changed to the Allied Health Professions Association (AHPA), a section of the AF.
1970	Formation of Arthritis Regional Medical Programs.

Table 2: Rheumatology and Rheumatologic Rehabilitation: Historical Benchmarks in the United States

1971	Rheumatology became a board-certified subspecialty in medicine.
1972	The Allied Health Professions Traineeship Program started. Funded by the U.S. Department of Health and Human Services.
1973	The first AHPA (ARHP) Fellowship was awarded, signifying the commitment of the AF and ARA to educate and train allied health professionals.
1977-1982	National Institutes of Health funded 24 Multipurpose Arthritis Centers throughout the U.S.
1978	The AHPA (ARHP) Grant Program started to fund research.
1980	Regional ARHP conferences were established.
1983	The Arthritis Self-Help Courses were sponsored nationwide by the AF.
1983-1986	Standards of competencies in rheumatology care for PT, OT, and nursing were established in conjunction with national professional organizations.
1988	*Arthritis Care and Research Journal* was initiated as the official journal of the ARHP.
1985	The ACR separated from the AF.
1994	The Arthritis Health Professions Association became the Association of Rheumatology Health Professionals (ARHP), separated from the AF, and joined the ACR.
1996	*Arthritis Care and Research* became the practice journal for the entire ACR, improving communication about rehabilitation and patient care among all rheumatology professionals.

RNs, social workers, and psychologists in staffing and in research projects. This resulted in a great increase in the number of such professionals employed in rheumatologic rehabilitation with an opportunity to participate in research. The MACs were responsible for the great increase in the number of publications by allied health professionals and helped provide the impetus for a specialty journal, *Arthritis Care and Research*. Funding, however, was gradually reduced. By 1995, 14 centers had been re-funded as Multipurpose Arthritis and Musculoskeletal Diseases Centers (MAMDCs) by the National Institute of Arthritis and Musculoskeletal and Skin Diseases (NIAMS). These centers support multidisciplinary research in education, epidemiology, and health services as well a biomedical research (Freeman et al., 1995). They are continuing the work of the MACs.

Coinciding with a trend toward teaching preventive care and self-management to people with chronic illness, in 1983 the Arthritis Foundation began sponsoring the Self-Help Courses for arthritis, lupus, and now fibromyalgia. The self-help and self-management movement actually emerged, in part, because physicians were not referring patients to rehabilitation programs, and it became clear that a lot of the self-care and patient education taught in OT and PT to individuals could be taught in groups at lower cost. Review of medical and patient education outcome research shows that medications offer a 20% to 50% improvement in arthritis symptoms for most patients and that patient education interventions such as the Arthritis Self-Help Courses can reduce symptoms an additional 15% to 30%. The addition of teaching for self-efficacy in these courses further increased quality of life outcomes (Hirano, Laurent, & Lorig, 1994). These outcomes help demonstrate the value of expanding OT and PT treatment to encompass a self-management approach. Outcome measures that document the changes from this type of training are reviewed in chapter 4 on clinical outcomes and in chapter 10 on patient education. Hilliquin and Menkes (1994) found the patient education outcomes so impressive that they flatly stated that patient education programs may be as effective as drug therapy in some cases and can clearly enhance drug treatment.

Leading rheumatologists are now more vocal and visible in their support of rehabilitation for rheumatic disease patients than ever before, ironically at the same time that the majority of RD patients are having their care transferred to physicians who are not familiar with the details of rehabilitation for this population.

THE NEXT 15 YEARS, 1998-2013

It is often said that one can predict the future by looking at the practices of the leaders in a given field and figure that it takes 10-20 years for those practices to become widespread throughout the field. If this theory holds true, then in 15 years or so we might expect that most OTs and PTs treating people with rheumatic diseases will be working within a bio-psychosocial model; they will be influencing the patient's functional status through psychosocial and behavioral approaches as well as through physical ones. Full appreciation of the bio-psychosocial model requires that patients be treated with a team approach.

In addition to teaching patients home exercise programs, therapists will be teaching them self-management strategies, defined as teaching patients skills necessary to carry on an active and emotionally satisfying life in the face of chronic illness (Lorig, 1993). This includes teaching them how a healthy lifestyle can influence their immune system, pain perception, and mood, especially the role of stress management, restorative sleep, fitness exercise, and healthy nutrition. Several centers are now organizing this approach within the framework of "Fatigue Management" (Packer, Brink, & Sauriol, 1994; Tack, 1990). Fatigue is a major symptom that limits function in patients with systemic diseases, FMS, and chronic pain (Bates et al. 1993; Tack, 1990; Wysenbeek et al., 1993). Fatigue-management programs for people with rheumatic diseases that include fitness training along with education create an ideal format for OTs and PTs to work together to improve the patient's functional ability and overall quality of life. Physical and occupational therapists have an advantage in the current health care system in that they are the only health professionals who can get reimbursed for arthritis-patient education and self-management training. Fatigue and self-management programs are very attractive to managed-care plans because they can be delivered in a group format and have been shown to improve quality of life and reduce medical utilization and cost (Hirano, Laurent, & Lorig, 1994). They are attractive to patients because they are focused on symptom reduction and are empowering at a personal level (see chapter 10 on patient education and chapter 12 on joint protection and energy conservation).

Research in pain management has also advanced and documented the value of a number of specific educational strategies including cognitive-behavioral techniques, flare management, and relapse-prevention training (see chapter 11). Pain management training is a major way to improve the patient's self-efficacy, or ability to control symptoms and reduce "learned helplessness." It will be up to therapists to bring this information to patients through self-management training.

Outcome assessment ultimately will become a part of routine practice, and there will be ways of comparing outcomes either to other therapists or other facilities. Therapy by necessity will become more evidence based. Much of the documentation and traditional measures of outcome used in OT and PT have been measures of physical impairment with little emphasis on valid and reliable measures of functional performance or disability. These kinds of assessments will demand collaboration across professions to develop assessments that indicate significant patient outcome (see chapter 4 on clinical outcomes and chapter 8 on functional assessment).

The future in drug management is also very exciting. Increased understanding of the immune system and inflammatory response has led to the ability to identify and develop drugs that are more specific in targeting inflammatory mediators. A new generation of nonsteroidal antiinflammatory drugs (NSAIDs) is on the horizon; they target specific inflammatory mediators and control inflammation without damaging the gastrointestinal system or renal function. This will enable more patients to benefit from NSAIDs and, one hopes, participate more in therapy and fitness programs.

Given the promise of these scenarios, rheumatologic rehabilitation would seem to have good prospects. However, its real future depends on how assertive therapists are in demanding and creating quality care programs, documenting the effectiveness of those programs, and reaching out to educate primary-care physicians, third party payers, and consumers about the value of rehabilitative intervention. The future will also depend upon how supportive they are of national organizations, such as the Association for Rheumatology Health Professionals and the Arthritis Foundation, which lobby for federal funding of rheumatic disease research and training of researchers in rheumatic disease and rheumatologic rehabilitation (see the section on associations at end of chapter 17).

This volume brings to you the perspective and practice of leaders in physical and occupational therapy, psychology, and rheumatologic nursing. Volumes 2 through 5 bring the additional expertise of physicians, surgeons, and orthopedic nurses, with an emphasis on team management. We hope that you discover in their chapters a blueprint for future practice. They are here to help you expand your capacity to help patients with rheumatic diseases regain their health.

REFERENCES

American College of Rheumatology Ad Hoc Committee on Clinical Guidelines. (1996). Guidelines for the management of rheumatoid arthritis. *Arthritis and Rheumatism, 39*(5), 713-722.

Bates, D., Schmitt, W., Buchwald, D., et al. (1993). Prevalence of fatigue and chronic fatigue syndrome in a primary care practice. *Archives of Internal Medicine, 153,* 2756-2765.

Cordery, J. C. (Ed.). (1965a). Rheumatic diseases part I [Special issue]. *American Journal of Occupational Therapy, 19*(3).

Cordery, J. C. (Ed.). (1965b). Rheumatic diseases part II [Special issue]. *American Journal of Occupational Therapy, 19*(5).

Feinglass, J., Schroeder, J. L., Gifford, B., & Manheim, L. M. (1992). Gatekeepers and the medical specialist: The impact of managed care on rheumatologists. *Journal of American Association Preferred Provider Organizations, 2,* 13-17, 34-36.

Freeman, J. B., Blalock, S. J., Holman, H. R., Liang, M. H., & Meenan, R. F. (1995). Advances brought by health services research to patients with arthritis: Summary of the workshop on health services research in arthritis: from research to practice. *Arthritic Care and Research, 9*(2), 142-150.

Goldenberg, D. (1996). What is the future of fibromyalgia? *Rheumatic Disease Clinics of North American, 22,* 2.

Hilliquin, P., & Menkes, C. J. (1994). Evaluation and management: Early and established disease. *Rheumatology.* St. Louis, Mosby.

Hirano, P. C., Laurent, D. D., & Lorig, K. (1994). Arthritis patient education studies, 1987-1991: A review of the literature. *Patient Education Counseling, 24*(1), 9-54.

Hislop, H., & Lamont-Havers, R. (Eds.). (1964a). Arthritis and physical therapy, part 1, [Special issue]. *Journal American Physical Therapy Association, 44*(7).

Hislop, H., & Lamont-Havers, R. (Eds.). (1964b). Arthritis and physical therapy, part 2, [Special issue]. *Journal American Physical Therapy Association, 44*(8).

Hochberg, M. C., Altman, R. D., Brandt, K. D., Clark, B. M., Dieppe, P. A., Griffin, M. R., Moskowitz, R. W., & Schnitzer, T. J. (1995). Guidelines for the medical management of osteoarthritis, Part I: *Osteoarthritis of the Hip 38*(11), 1535-1540 and Part II: *Osteoarthritis of the Knee 38*(11), 1541-1546. *Arthritis and Rheumatism.*

Lorig, K. (1993). Self-management of chronic illness: A model for the future. *Generations,* 11-14.

Melvin, J. L. (1990). Occupational therapy and the AHPA: The last 25 years. *Arthritis Care and Research, 3*(4), 1-3.

Moldofsky, H., Scarisbrick, P., England, R., & Smythe, H. (1975). Musculoskeletal symptoms and non-REM sleep disturbance in patients with "fibrositic sundrome" and healthy subjects. *Psychosomatic Medicine, 37,* 341-351.

Packer, T., Brink, N., & Sauriol, A. (1994). *Managing fatigue.* Tucson, AZ: Therapy Skill Builders.

Pincus, T., & Callahan, L. (1986). Taking mortality in rheumatoid arthritis seriously. Predictive markers, socioeconomic status and comorbidity. *Journal of Rheumatology, 13,* 841-845.

Relman, A. S. (1988). Assessment and accountability: The third revolution in medical care. *New England Journal of Medicine, 319,* 1220-1222.

Tack, B. (1990). Fatigue in rheumatoid arthritis, conditions, strategies and consequences. *Arthritis Care and Research, 3*(2), 65-70.

Toffler, A. (1990). *Powershift.* New York: Bantam Books.

Wegner, S. T. (1996). *Clinical care in the rheumatic diseases.* Atlanta: American College of Rheumatology.

Wolfe, F. (1995). The prevalence and characteristics of fibromyalgia in the general population. *Arthritis and Rheumatism, 38*(5), 19-28.

Wysenbeek, A. J., Leibovici, L., Weinberger, A., & Guedj, D. (1993). Fatigue in systemic lupus erythematosus: Prevalence and relation to disease expression. *British Journal of Rheumatology, 32,* 633-635.

MANAGED CARE IN RHEUMATIC DISEASE: OPPORTUNITY OR OPPRESSION?

Teresa J. Brady, PhD, LP, OTR

INTRODUCTION

Health care is in the midst of an epic transformation in response to market forces. This transition is from arbitrary fee-for-service (FFS) to a capitated, per-member, per-month payment structure, from episodic care for the sick to broadly based population health management, and from fragmented, uncoordinated care to standardized care driven by quality and cost. The transition will no doubt be difficult, but once completed, it has potential advantages for all involved. The current acute care paradigm and its FFS financing system is not well matched to the needs of patients with rheumatic diseases and the professionals who care for them. Some forms of managed care have the potential to improve health outcomes—and consequently the quality of life—of individuals with rheumatic and connective-tissue diseases.

The American Occupational Therapy Association (AOTA), in its managed care sourcebook (AOTA, 1996) defines managed care as "the term used to describe health care systems that integrate financing and delivery of health services" (p. 1). But managed care as a label has ceased to be useful because it has been applied to a heterogeneous group of activities ranging from cost-containment strategies to a fundamental redesign of health care administration, delivery, and financing. Rheumatology professionals and patients alike have collected managed-care horror stories based on their immediate experiences. Many such stories are true, and many managed-care organizations have earned negative reputations, but that is an incomplete picture. Managed care is neither the answer to prayers nor the evil some have portrayed it to be.

Rheumatology health professionals' (RHPs) perspectives on managed care depend on where they reside, both geographically and within their organizations. Perceptions of managed care are similar to the experiment of asking blindfolded participants to describe an elephant based on the part of the animal they can touch. This chapter is designed to move professionals back from the specific part of managed care with which they have had contact to look at the broader picture of the current system of health care delivery and financing, and the opportunities and threats created by managed care.

This chapter is not designed to provide strategies for maximizing FFS reimbursement in the midst of the changing health care environment. There are other resources for that (ACR, 1994; AOTA, 1996). More significantly, although maximizing reimbursement may be important, it is a short-term strategy. Eventually even the term reimbursement will be obsolete. Reimbursement implies payment for a service rendered, which is the essence of FFS financing. As the health care industry moves to prospective payment, shared-risk financing, and population health management, and as rehabilitation departments become cost centers rather than revenue centers, reimbursed services will represent only a minute portion of the business. It is important to restructure care delivery to maximize health outcomes and reduce costs rather than simply maximizing reimbursement.

Managed care offers both strengths and weaknesses for the care of individuals with rheumatic disease. Managed care presents opportunities as well as threats for the future of rheumatology rehabilitation. This chapter will discuss failures of the current health care system to meet the needs of rheumatic disease patients, the dynamics of health care financing and its effect on care delivery, the fundamental underpinnings of various forms of managed care, and the practice changes necessary to survive in the managed-care environment.

FAILURES OF THE ACUTE CARE PARADIGM IN CHRONIC DISEASE MANAGEMENT

The current health care system, policies, institutions, and methods of reimbursement were created in the era of acute illness and are not well suited to meet the challenges of chronic diseases. The current health care system (in reality a "sick-care" system) is based on the acute care paradigm with a strong bias toward treating acute medical problems on an episodic basis rather than multidimensional preventive care over the course of chronic diseases. As described in Table 1, chronic disease problems frequently are due to the interaction of multiple biological, behavioral, and social factors. Chronic disease management is a continuous process that requires a longitudinal, rather than episodic, approach. The aim of intervention in chronic disease is amelioration or management, not cure, and the patient needs to be engaged as an active participant rather than a passive recipient of care (Pawlson, 1994).

The flaws in the current acute care-based FFS health care system are legendary, as Table 2 highlights. Payers and providers alike tend to view health care narrowly and focus on management of the disease processes for a time-limited episode in the specific care setting that they are responsible for delivering or reimbursing. FFS financing provides no incentive to prevent acute episodes, reduce the need for care, or take a longitudinal, multidimensional approach to care. This component-management approach results in frag-

CHALLENGES OF CHRONIC DISEASE

	ACUTE	CHRONIC
CAUSE:	Single agent sufficient	Multiple contributing factors
BASIS OF ILLNESS:	Altered physiology	Biological, psychological, social
TREATMENT AIM:	Cure	Amelioration, management
TIME PERIOD:	Single event	Continuous process
ROLE OF PATIENT:	Passive recipient	Active participant

Table 1: Challenges of Chronic Disease

FLAWS IN THE FEE-FOR-SERVICE HEALTH CARE SYSTEM

- Reinforces a fragmented approach to care *(i.e., payer regulations mandate a reassessment and formulation of a new treatment plan when a patient changes care settings).*

- Emphasizes treatment over prevention, and an episodic approach to care *(i.e., physical therapy covered readily after joint replacement, but limited for early intervention to instruct on exercise and joint protection; will not cover maintenance exercise programs to slow rate of functional decline).*

- Dictates care delivery patterns by setting-centered reimbursement *(i.e., home care occupational therapy not covered unless nursing is also involved; nursing home admissions made to receive services that would be available but not reimbursed in a home or community setting).*

- Provides more extensive coverage for expensive care provided in expensive settings *(i.e., provides coverage for occupational therapy while a patient is hospitalized but limits outpatient or home care coverage for OT).*

- Limits reimbursement for patient education or compliance-inducing strategies *(may cover rehabilitation, but does not cover community-based self-management courses, does not cover telephone follow-up).*

- Emphasizes medical issues, neglects other issues that may affect health outcomes *(i.e., depression, perceptions of helplessness, family stress).*

- Encourages cost shifting *(i.e., early discharge from the hospital without regard for nursing home or home care costs).*

Table 2: Flaws in the Fee-for-Service Health Care System

mented care, absolves providers of responsibility for the recurrence of acute episodes, and financially rewards providers for treating the acute events that occur (Zitter, 1994). The health care system needs a new attitude and a new understanding of health and health care (Selker, 1995). Both the health care delivery and financing systems need to change (Bingewatt, 1996).

To understand more fully the flaws in the FFS system for chronic disease management, it is important to understand the dynamics of FFS financing and how the incentives change with capitation or other shared-risk financing systems.

FINANCIAL DYNAMICS AND THEIR EFFECT ON CARE DELIVERY

FEE FOR SERVICE (FFS)

The FFS payment mechanism facilitated the development of this fragmented, episodic approach to care that emphasizes acute care services provided in expensive settings. In traditional FFS, health care providers are paid a fee for every service they provide. The rate may be based on a fee schedule or some prenegotiated rate per unit of service. Under FFS the provider has no incentive to limit procedures or explore lower cost treatment alternatives. Providers profit in the FFS system by increasing the volumes of procedures they perform. Departments and programs are seen as revenue or profit centers: Increase volumes and revenues will increase. Payers make profits in the FFS system when their income from premiums exceeds their expenses (reimbursement to providers plus administrative costs), and the payer will employ techniques such as prior authorization or preset service limits to reduce costs.

When FFS financing began, there were no incentives for anyone to reduce the costs of health care. As the cost of providing health care services increased, providers increased their service charges and volumes, payers increased premiums to cover their costs, employers did not watch premiums because they paid the premiums out of pretax dollars, and patients had no need to monitor costs because the charges were paid by their insurer. Every participant in the traditional FFS health care system was responding rationally to financial incentives, and health care costs rose exponentially. Managed care grew when health care purchasers (employers and governments) became concerned about the unbridled cost escalation.

To understand the dynamics of FFS financing, it is important to understand the concept of financial risk. With FFS all financial risk is borne by the health plans or payers. If health care expenses exceed the payments received from the purchasers (employers, governments, and private individuals), the payer absorbs that financial loss; if expenses are below income from premiums, the payer pockets the profit. In this system providers have little or no financial risk.

Since payers bear the entire financial risk in FFS, their primary motivation has been to reduce their expenses, and they have done so by denying care, discounting fee schedules, and controlling utilization from the outside. At the same time providers are motivated to increase services, volumes, and charges as much as possible to increase their revenue. These diametrically opposed incentives have produced an adversarial process that has led to rules, regulations, and paperwork.

In the FFS system, hospitals have used specialty arthritis programs to attract patients to the hospital system and "feed the beast" (fill the beds). Even programs that do not produce excess revenues contribute to the hospital profit margin by generating surgical referrals or developing customer loyalty among patients with potentially high medical needs. In effect, arthritis-outpatient and community-education programs are magnets to attract patients and revenue to the hospital system.

Traditional FFS reimbursement does provide freedom of choice: Patients have their choice of providers, and providers have their choice of reimbursable treatment options. FFS allows the use of specialists for arthritis care. However, FFS reimbursement has primarily focused on physical (actually medical) health, does not encourage attention to psychological, social, spiritual, or economic factors that affect health outcomes, does not facilitate coordination of care across providers or settings, and does not financially reward interventions that would reduce the need for health services.

CAPITATION AND OTHER FORMS OF RISK SHARING

Capitation and other forms of shared-risk financing represent a fundamentally different way of paying for health care and require fundamental changes in how care is delivered. With capitation, the provision of health services is a source of cost, not a source of profit. As demonstrated in Table 3, capitation reverses the traditional incentives and financial risks.

With capitation, profits stem from maintaining population health to reduce the need and demand for services rather than increasing the number of admissions, visits, or procedures. Key strategies are to produce the best possible outcomes at the lowest possible cost, to invest in preventive services that will reduce the need for more expensive acute care services, and to provide the right service at the right time and place.

In capitated financing, providers receive a flat fee per member per month (pmpm) to provide whatever care is necessary for that member. Revenue is generated for the health system based on the number of members enrolled and the monthly payment per enrolled member, not by the members' need for services, regardless of whether the member/patient received no health care services this month or spent the entire month in an intensive care unit (ICU). This fixed revenue provides incentives for providers to integrate care and invest in programs to keep members healthy and reduce the need for expensive health care services.

These changed financial incentives will alter the design of the health care delivery system. For example, if data demonstrate that rheumatoid arthritis (RA) patients followed by rheumatologists maintain better health outcomes at lower cost, and some preliminary studies suggest this (Overman, Lewis, Kent, & Uslan, 1995; Yelin, Such, Criswell, & Epstein, 1995), then it makes clinical and financial sense to direct RA patients

COMPARISON OF FEE-FOR-SERVICE VERSUS CAPITATION

FEE-FOR-SERVICE	CAPITATION
Episodic acute care.	Emphasis on primary care and long-term health.
Physicians, hospitals, and health plans are financially independent.	Physicians, hospitals, and health plans are financially interdependent.
Market share based on number of admissions, procedures, or visits.	Market share based on number of covered lives.
Departments and programs are profit centers.	Departments and programs are cost centers.
Higher hospital utilization and more intensive care equals higher system profits.	Lower hospital utilization equals higher system profits.
More patient visits equals higher physician income.	Fewer patient visits equals higher profits.
Practitioner compensation based on volume productivity.	Practitioner compensation based on effectiveness and efficiency of care delivery.
Providers are paid a fee for every service provided.	Providers receive a fixed dollar amount to provide all health services.

Table 3: Comparison of Fee-for-Service Versus Capitation

to rheumatologists as their primary or principal care providers rather than restrict access to specialty care. Similarly, if rehabilitation professionals demonstrate that RA or fibromyalgia patients have better health outcomes when they receive regular, ongoing exercise training from physical therapists, then it will make financial and clinical sense to make exercise training by PTs a part of standard treatment.

Specialty arthritis programs play a different role in risk-sharing plans than they do in FFS. In a capitated environment, every department or specialty program is a cost center, not a revenue center. Revenue comes from overall system enrollment rather than service volumes. There are no incentives in the system to produce services that will attract high volumes of patients, but there are financial incentives to use the services that will reduce global member health care costs over time. Consequently, a specialty program that is a magnet to attract a disproportionate share of expensive patients is counterproductive to the financial health of the system unless the capitation rate is risk-adjusted. Without risk adjustment, the cost of caring for patients who are higher risk or have a history of greater-than-average health care expenses (like rheumatology patients) will exceed the per-member, per-month capitation rate the system is paid.

However, a specialty arthritis program can reduce costs for the health system if it can provide high-quality care for the inevitable enrolled members who have arthritis in a way that reduces the long-term cost of care for these patients. For example, self-management education can reduce the need for more expensive physician visits (Lorig, Lubeck, Kraines, Seleznick, & Holman, 1985). Training in a regular exercise routine may postpone the need for joint replacement or speed recovery after joint replacement. A fibromyalgia management program may reduce doctor shopping or repeated use of ineffective therapies. In a capitated financing system it is not wise to attract expensive patients to the system, but it is wise to have the expertise to take exceptionally good (and cost-effective) care of the individuals in your system who happen to have arthritis.

MANAGED-CARE ORGANIZATIONS (MCOS)

Managed care has taken many forms over the years. Many of the organizations and processes that have been called managed care have made little attempt to manage the processes of care and have focused on managing cost reimbursements and providers. The managed-care movement has evolved from prepaid group practices to a variety of provider arrangements including several forms of health maintenance organizations (HMOs), preferred provider organizations (PPOs), independent practice associations (IPAs), to the emergence of integrated service networks or integrated health systems (IHSs).

The variations among HMOs, PPOs, and IPAs are differentiated by the relationship between the health plan and its affiliated physicians. Whether the organization is an HMO, PPO, or IPA is less important than the underlying financial dynamics and how care is managed. Specifically, it is important to understand what is being managed (costs, providers, or care itself), what strategies are used to "manage" (e.g., does the payer manage through discounts, denials, and prior authorizations, or is it provider-based managed care?), and what are the underlying financial dynamics (e.g., are the financial incentives aligned through risk sharing to reward longitudinal disability prevention, or does the payment structure encourage episodic acute care through FFS or discounted FFS financing?). The following is a brief summary of the alphabet soup of managed care organizations.

PRECURSORS TO MCOS

MCOs were preceded by a small number of prepaid group practices such as the Kaiser Health Plan, formed in the 1930s, and the Group Health Cooperative of Puget Sound, formed in 1947. These original prepaid group practices had historic roots in a moral philosophy of providing accessible, affordable, equitable health care to employee groups such as railroad workers, lumbermen, and miners who did not have access to health care. According to Friedman, these plans stemmed from deeply held values of community and commitment rather than financial interests (Friedman, 1996). Kaiser's beginning is representative of these early prepaid plans. According to Cummings and VandenBos (1981), Kaiser Health Plan began during the Depression when Henry J. Kaiser received a contract to build an aqueduct from Boulder Dam to Los Angeles but had difficulty recruiting and maintaining construction crews due to the lack of medical care. Sydney Garfield, MD, offered to provide all of the services and facilities necessary for comprehensive health care for a charge of 5 cents per employee work hour. Garfield did not ask for any fees for his services, and invested significant effort to prevent illnesses such as sunstroke and heat exhaustion, which were common in the desert. This early Kaiser experience represents the best in managed care. It was based on a fixed dollar amount (or capitated rate) to keep people healthy rather than a fee to treat sick people, emphasized health promotion and prevention, took care of a defined population, and was initiated by the provider not the payer.

HEALTH MAINTENANCE ORGANIZATIONS

In the early 1970s, prepaid group plans were recast into more marketable entities called health maintenance organizations, and their growth was facilitated by the passage of the HMO Act in 1973. The term HMO was coined as a way of making these plans more attractive by highlighting an emphasis on health promotion and prevention. Unfortunately, few HMOs lived up to their promises to maintain health actively, particularly for individuals with chronic diseases. HMOs were designed to attract young, employed individuals without high health risks. In addition to attracting younger, healthier employees, early HMOs contained costs by reducing hospital admissions, decreasing lengths of stay, and eliminating unnecessary procedures. By combining coverage for outpatient and inpatient care into a single premium, HMOs were able to reduce hospital utilization by shifting some services appropriately to less expensive ambulatory care settings. Early HMOs also contracted for lower prices through volume purchasing power (MacLeod, 1993).

HMOs vary in organizational structure (staff, group, network, and IPA models) based on the relationship of physicians to the HMO. Staff-model HMOs have physicians on salary and function similarly to the early prepaid group plans. Group-model (one multispecialty group practice), network model (two or more physician practice groups), and IPA model (multiple solo physicians or group practices) HMOs have physicians under contract to provide care to the HMO's members. Reimbursement is often based on a fee schedule with reduced rates due to volume discounts. The financial risk for the total health care of its members generally resides with the HMO, not the providers, so the HMO employs utilization controls to limit costs.

PREFERRED PROVIDER ORGANIZATIONS AND INDEPENDENT PRACTICE ASSOCIATIONS

PPOs and IPAs are networks of providers formed primarily to negotiate large contracts with payers. PPOs and IPAs involve different arrangements of providers, from closed panels of preferred providers to extended networks of independent practices, but the delivery of care remains focused on acute episodes. PPOs and IPAs control costs by using providers who agree to follow a set of procedures and accept a discounted fee for their services. Patients who are enrolled in some PPO or IPA plans can go outside their provider network but generally have to pay a larger copayment or other financial disincentive. Some PPOs, IPAs, and group-, network-, or IPA-model HMOs are beginning to contract by capitation or other forms of financial risk sharing, which will change the financial dynamics in the future.

In the forms of group- or network-model HMOs, PPOs, and IPAs, managed care is primarily a payer strategy to manage costs and reimbursement by controlling the provider. Cost and reimbursement are managed through contracts, discounts, denials, external case management, and utilization management. This managed reimbursement approach has high administrative costs (e.g., the processing of prior authorizations and utilization monitoring systems) but remains fee-for-service (at a discounted rate), so it reinforces the acute episode approach to health care. It does not provide financial incentives to providers to use a longitudinal, multidimensional approach that would reduce the long-term need for services in chronic disease.

Had MCOs started with chronic diseases in mind, the cost-control strategies they developed might have been different. The original MCOs avoided financial risk and did not learn to manage it. The philosophy of care did not change from episodic acute care. Early MCOs contained cost by attracting a healthy population that did not require expensive services. Early MCOs did not compete for chronic-disease populations; they did not want to attract arthritis patients to their systems, nor did they want to become the health organization of choice for people with chronic diseases.

However, as acute care utilization has been reduced by payer reimbursement management, and as Medicare and Medicaid are moving away from FFS, managed-care organizations can no longer avoid chronic-disease populations. MCOs are learning how to manage, not avoid, financial risk and provide effective care for populations with chronic disease. The initial managed-care strategies of controlling reimbursement to providers will no longer be effective. This is catalyzing the development of the latest generation of managed care, provider-based managed care delivered by integrated health systems that share financial risk. Table 4 compares and contrasts various forms of managed care organizations.

INTEGRATED HEALTH SYSTEMS

As health care markets evolve, a new breed of MCO, an integrated services network, or integrated health system (IHS), is developing. IHSs are networks or partnerships of payers, providers, and members/purchasers responsible for providing the full continuum of health care services (from routine primary care to acute inpatient services) for a defined population for a fixed dollar or capitated amount (Alexander et al., 1995). An IHS represents a fundamental paradigm shift and a true change in philosophy of care and financing, not just a new form of partnership or procedures.

An IHS provides a full array of health care services from primary prevention through residential long-term care. However, it is not enough just to collect the pieces, it is truly mandatory to integrate them. An IHS extends the concepts of integration beyond horizontal consolidation of assets into integration of care, information systems, and financing, and integrates them across time, place, and provider. IHSs are provider driven and put clinical decisions in the hands of those most capable of balancing efficiency and patient care. Table 5 outlines key components and characteristics of integrated health systems.

In an IHS the care philosophy and organization of the delivery system must focus on maintaining the health of the enrolled population rather than providing services to individuals who are sick. This change in philosophy involves moving to more of a public-health concept of care that emphasizes prevention of diseases and disability. Using the local lake or swimming hole as an analogy, a community can either invest in expensive professional lifeguards and highly technical lifesaving procedures, or it can invest in swimming lessons and guardrails to reduce the need for the high-tech lifesaving. The current health care system, dominated by acute care, takes the high-tech lifesaving approach. It invests heavily in professional lifeguards and high-tech lifesaving procedures, but minimally on swimming lessons or self-management. Once the health system is financially responsible for preserving the health of the population, it will have financial incentives to teach prevention and other self-management procedures to reduce the need for acute care services. This change in orientation will be particularly beneficial for individuals with arthritis and other chronic diseases.

Capitation, or other forms of pooled or shared risk financing, are key characteristics of IHSs. In an IHS, all partners share the financial risk. The IHS earns profits by keeping the cost of providing the necessary services lower than the total income from the capitated payment. Consequently capitation provides financial incentives for the longitudinal, multidimensional approach to disease and disability prevention.

Pooled financing also eliminates the benefits of cost shifting. The FFS system encourages providers to shift costs to the next care setting (e.g., discharging patients from the hospital early to save dollars under the diagnosis related group [DRG] without regard to the home-care costs, or postponing tests until a patient is hospitalized, so the costs must be paid through the inpatient benefits rather than the outpatient payer).

COMPARISON OF TYPES OF MANAGED-CARE ORGANIZATIONS

	ORIGINAL STAFF MODEL HMOs	GROUP/NETWORK HMO, PPO, IPA	INTEGRATED HEALTH SYSTEM
PHYSICIANS	Salaried	Contracted	Salaried or risk sharing
WHO BEARS RISK	HMO organization	Payers	All partners in system
FINANCING	Fixed payment per member per month (PMPM)	FFS, discounted FFS	PMPM
FINANCIAL INCENTIVES	Aligned	Conflicting	Aligned
PROFIT STRATEGY	Large enrollment, limited use of services and volume	Payers: decrease utilization; Providers: increase services	Maintain health of enrolled population
COST-CONTROL STRATEGY	Decrease LOS, transfer care to less expensive therapy	Control provider behavior to reduce utilization	Decrease need for and utilization of services
CARE STRATEGY	Enroll healthy individuals, avoid adverse selection	Increase volumes of services to sick individuals	Decrease demand for services, integrate care, health promotion, disability prevention
HOSPITALS	Owned or contracted for services	Independent, increase revenue by increasing market share	Integrated with other providers of care
SPECIALTY PROGRAMS	Minimal, fear of adverse selection	Use to attract patients and increase volumes and revenue	Use to provide cost-effective care to enrollees

Table 4: Comparison of Types of Managed-Care Organizations

KEY COMPONENTS AND CHARACTERISTICS OF INTEGRATED HEALTH SYSTEMS

COMPONENTS

HOSPITALS	Ambulatory care programs
CLINICS	Affiliated physicians
HOME CARE	Outpatient surgery centers
HOSPICE	Home medical equipment
COMMUNITY CARE	Residential long-term care

CHARACTERISTICS

Financial incentives aligned to support longitudinal, multidimensional approach to care over the natural course of the condition.

Full continuum of services provided, including prevention and primary, acute, transitional, community and residential long-term care that is integrated across time, place, and provider.

Integrated care management through interdisciplinary teams, procedures, tools, and practitioners.

Emphasis on self management and disability prevention or delay.

Integrated information services that make it possible to tract clinical, cost, quality, and utilization data across settings and time for individual patients or patient groups.

Allocation of resources to fund most useful and cost-effective interventions regardless of treatment method or setting.

Pooled fixed-dollar or shared-risk financing that provides incentives to utilize common goals and decrease duplication of services, and increases provider flexibility in resource allocation.

Pooled or shared-risk financing resembles a married couple who operate out of a single joint checking account in contrast to a divorced couple operating out of two separate checking accounts. For the couple with the joint checking account, it does not matter who buys the child's school clothes because the expense comes out of their common account. A divorced parent may maximize his or her own finances by maneuvering to have the other parent purchase what the child needs. This protects one parent's finances while shifting the cost to the other parent, but does not reduce the cumulative costs of childraising. Similarly, for true integration and cost savings to occur, all providers who share the population or patient must share the financial risks and rewards of providing care.

A core philosophy of IHSs is to optimize the whole, not just the parts: the whole person, the whole system, and the cumulative costs. Care is organized not around setting or reimbursement strategy but around the problems of the individual, which cross provider settings and extend over the natural course of the condition. Pooled or shared-risk financing provides increased flexibility in resource allocation and rewards collaboration toward common clinical, cost, quality, and utilization goals. Pooled financing provides the opportunity to select treatment options based on what works, not what is reimbursable, and to address other issues that affect health outcomes.

IHSs are beginning to emerge in United States health care markets. Each geographic health care market evolves at its own speed in response to market forces, but all markets follow a predictable pattern. As Table 6 demonstrates, health care markets evolve from unstructured FFS markets to loosely organized markets employing discounted FFS. The market then consolidates and moves into managed competition before evolving into population health management through integrated health systems using shared-risk financing (APM, 1995; Johnson, 1996; Norling & Edwards, 1995).

CHANGES IN PRACTICE AND CONCEPTUALIZATION OF PRACTICE

Success in a risk-sharing (capitated or capitation-like financing) IHS will require changes in professional practice and changes in the way professionals conceptualize practice. Some of these changes will involve integrating cost factors into clinical decision making, gathering outcome data to measure the results of interventions, and using standardized care such as clinical pathways or treatment protocols to achieve the best possible outcomes at the lowest possible costs. These changes will entail role changes, integration of care, alternate delivery mechanisms, and an emphasis on disability prevention and patient self-management.

INTEGRATING COST INTO CLINICAL DECISION MAKING

For many rehabilitation professionals (RHPs), integrating cost factors into clinical decision-making will be a foreign concept, and initially very difficult to implement. Currently there are two barriers to integrating cost into clinical decision making: (a) rehabilitation professionals rarely know the true cost of the services they provide, and (b) professionals have prided themselves on not considering cost or payer source in clinical practice due to a long-standing belief that it is inappropriate to consider cost in treatment planning. RHPs generally avoided awareness of payer until necessity mandated some knowledge of the payer to determine what prior authorization procedures were required.

Making sure patients do not receive differential treatment based on payer source is an admirable goal. However, how smart or admirable is it to be unaware of the cost of services or the comparative costs of different treatment options? Is it a virtue to be unaware that "Works Good" splinting material costs twice as much as "Does the Job Well" splinting material, while both are equally effective for resting splints? Is it a virtue to be unaware that transportation from "Sir Speedy Medivan" is twice as expensive as "Rapid Transit Medivan"? Is it a virtue to be unaware that even though the charge is the same, the actual cost of doing iontophoresis is higher than using ultrasound, and the results are equivalent?

At this time many rheumatology health professionals may know what is charged for a particular service but generally have limited knowledge of what it costs to provide that service. Charges have been set arbitrarily, or based on the community standard, but rarely have they been based on actual cost. To make decisions about cost effectiveness, rheumatology health professionals need to know the true cost, including indirect costs, of providing each service. Rehabilitation professionals will need to develop methods to calculate the unit cost of each service provided.

A key to integrating cost into clinical decision making is to understand the true cost (not charges) of the various treatment alternatives, and to make treatment decisions as if payment for the service were coming from the professional's personal checkbook. Health professionals are already using this kind of discriminant thinking in running their family or household budgets.

Treatment decisions follow similar logic. If a treatment plan of two physical therapy visits per week is likely to achieve the same outcome as three visits per week, the wise clinical and financial decision is to use just two visits per week. However, if evidence demonstrates substantially improved outcomes with four visits per week, then the reasonable treatment plan would be four visits per week. Similarly, if hot packs produce the same benefits as fluidotherapy at less cost, the reasonable treatment plan would start with hot packs. In short, if results are similar, it makes sense to use the less expensive treatment. However, if a more expensive treatment is clearly superior in outcome and will reduce costs in the future, it makes clinical and financial sense to use that more expensive service first.

This type of decision making is based on value (i.e., is a product or service worth what it costs?). Value is calculated as results or outcome divided by cost; value calculations will require knowledge of true costs and measurement of outcomes. Outcome measurement is a second practice change required to succeed in managed-care environments.

MARKET-DRIVEN EVOLUTION OF MANAGED CARE

	UNSTRUCTURED	*LOOSELY ORGANIZED*	*CONSOLIDATIONS*	*MANAGED COMPETITION*	*MANAGING POPULATIONS*
Managed care	Limited managed care (MC)	Little managed care	Heavy MC penetration; Payers and providers begin to align	More than 50% MC penetration; Employer coalitions emerge as purchasers	Extensive MC
Physicians	MDs in private practice, solo or small groups	MDs begin to organize groups, especially primary care physicians	Most PCPs in groups, specialists begin to form groups	Shift in MD supply, MDs not in groups eliminated	MDs integrated into system, share risk
Hospitals	Independent hospitals, overuse of capacity	Consolidation begins; oversupply of beds leads to deep discounts	Increased hospital mergers (horizontal integration)	More pressure to eliminate beds	Vertically integrated systems dominate
Financing	FFS	FFS and discounted FFS	Discounted FFS, some capitation	Managed care payment dominates	Capitation or other full risk sharing
Strategy	Isolated episodes of care, fragmented services	Independent services	Providers develop continua of care	Providers and payers strongly align	Integrated systems manage populations
Examples	Omaha Birmingham Little Rock Newark	Dallas Atlanta Cleveland St. Louis New York City Philadelphia	San Francisco Detroit Denver Boston Seattle Chicago	San Diego Minneapolis Los Angeles Worcester	No markets yet

Table 6: Market-Driven Evolution of Managed Care

OUTCOME MEASUREMENT

Outcome measurement is an essential element of modern health care, particularly managed care. RHPs need outcome data to drive program and treatment decisions, identify best practices, and provide evidence to financial decision makers that rehabilitation services are cost effective and add value.

Outcome measurement has not been a strength of rehabilitation in the past. Much rehabilitation treatment has been guided by best guess rather than best practice, or clinical lore rather than demonstrated outcomes. According to Moncur (1988), many rheumatology rehabilitation treatment recommendations are sacred cows with questionable scientific evidence to support them. These unquestioned sacred cows include treatment recommendations such as the "2-hour pain rule," "10 ROM repetitions on a good day," and "don't substitute activities of daily living for ROM." These clinical pearls may be appropriate, but outcome data are essential to evaluate their usefulness.

Outcome studies need to take place at two levels in rehabilitation practice. Systematic outcome research must be done to evaluate the effectiveness of rehabilitation techniques. These large, controlled studies may best be done at academic centers or large treatment centers. In addition, each professional practice needs to collect outcome data on the effectiveness of their own treatment. These clinical studies do not need to be large, controlled studies but should be a routine part of rehabilitation practice and part of professional quality-improvement programs (Reynolds, 1996). Outcomes of clinical interventions need to be stated in functional terms such as ability to walk unassisted from bed to bathroom, or ability to feed oneself independently. If the increase in ROM measurement or dynamometer reading does not increase functional ability, the intervention may not be perceived as a necessary health care cost (AOTA, 1996). Table 7 identifies sample questions that can be answered through outcomes research and program-specific outcome measurement.

Outcome data may restructure practice, and this is appropriate. Symphony Rehabilitation Services in Cypress, CA, restructured its treatment protocol in response to capitation rates and found no change in outcomes. Total hip patients had been receiving 12-18 OT treatments over as many days for charges of $1,250-$1,800 per patient. After a capitated contract was negotiated at $328 per capita, the OT sessions were reduced to an average of 4.38 OT sessions over 5 days. Staff expected adverse effects, but outcomes for these patients fell within the average range of independence. In addition, a higher percentage of patients were able to go home. The department manager reported that she was unable to make a compelling case for more OT. However, she was able to show that OT services had the greatest impact on safety, and for some diagnoses two treatments per day instead of one produced better outcomes. Similarly, Yasuda gathered 10 years of outcome data on the use of mobile arm supports in the treatment of polymyositis. She was able to demonstrate that arm supports were durable and cost effective over the long term despite a fairly high initial cost (Joe, 1996).

In these situations outcome data restructured practice to reduce costs without a decline in outcomes and were used to demonstrate the value of OT services. Developing

SAMPLE QUESTIONS FOR SYSTEMATIC OUTCOMES RESEARCH AND/OR PROGRAMMATIC OUTCOME MEASUREMENT

Do patients who receive rehabilitation services experience less disability or maintain function and quality of life longer than those who do not?

Do fibromyalgia patients who have worksite evaluations return to work faster or at a higher rate than those who do not receive a worksite evaluation?

What frequency and duration of physical or occupational therapy produces the most effective outcomes at a reasonable cost after total joint replacement?

Are there meaningfully different outcomes with 3 weeks of physical therapy rather than just 2 weeks?

What is the most effective wearing protocol for a specific hand splint?

Table 7: Sample Questions for Systematic Outcomes Research and/or Programmatic Outcome Measurement

systems to measure, record, and analyze outcome data can be difficult at first, but is essential. Outcome data can support the need for and cost-effectiveness of rehabilitation services and can be used to guide the development of best-practice treatment protocols.

BEST-PRACTICE TREATMENT PROTOCOLS OR STANDARDIZED CARE

Treatment guidelines, best-practice protocols, or other forms of standardized care can enhance the effectiveness of rehabilitation services. They also have the potential to make rehabilitation services a routine part of rheumatology care.

Some RHPs have rejected clinical pathways, treatment guidelines, or other forms of standardized care as "cookbook medicine" that does not accommodate the uniqueness of each patient. In reality these forms of standardized or structured care can lead to best possible outcomes at low cost by guiding clinicians to use those treatment strategies that have been demonstrated to produce good outcomes. These guidelines can reduce unnecessary variations in practice that do not add value. For example, a home care agency found a range of 7 to 17 home visits following an uncomplicated total hip replacement. In this case it is reasonable to question how much of this variation is due to patient variables and how much is attributable to variations in therapist practice styles. Variability due to patient circumstances is appropriate and welcome. Variance due to therapist differences in practice style that do not add value may be unwarranted.

The American College of Rheumatology treatment guidelines for management of osteoarthritis include physical therapy, occupational therapy, and the Arthritis Self-Help Course (ASHC) (Hochberg et al., 1995). Outcome studies have demonstrated that ASHC reduces pain, increases self-management behavior, and is appropriate to include in treatment guidelines (Lorig et al., 1985). If outcome data demonstrate that patients who receive early intervention with exercise and joint-protection instruction have better outcomes than those who do not, early rehabilitation intervention will become a routine component of the clinical pathway or treatment guideline. This will enhance referrals and provide patients with the long-term advantage of easy access to these cost-effective services.

ROLE CHANGES: DELEGATION, EXPANSION, AND DIFFUSION

Role changes motivated by managed care include delegation or transfer of responsibility, role expansion, and role diffusion. Delegation or transferring of responsibility to lower-paid health workers is already occurring in medicine. Nurse practitioners and physician's assistants are assuming responsibility for more routine primary-care needs, rather than requiring that higher-paid physicians provide those services. A similar transfer has already happened in rehabilitation with some routine tasks transferred to physical therapy and occupational therapy assistants or aides.

The decisions on which responsibilities to transfer will be made by determining what skill set is required to provide a specific aspect of care. This does not mean turning highly skilled aspects of rehabilitation over to staff who are not trained to perform them well, but determining which parts of care require the skills of the registered or licensed professional and which do not. RHPs need to recognize that not everything in the current scope of practice requires the higher level of skill. Dowel exercises, gait training, or other routine, structured tasks do not require the skills of a licensed or registered professional. Other tasks such as evaluation and complex splinting require a higher level of judgment and skill, and those tasks will need to remain with the licensed or registered professional staff. Transferring appropriate tasks to lower-paid staff will reduce the unit cost and increase the cost effectiveness of rehabilitation services.

The roles of rehabilitation practitioners will expand in several ways in IHS forms of managed care. A key role expansion in provider-based managed care is the inclusion of cost in clinical decision making. A second expansion is expanding clinical assessment and intervention to include a multidimensional view of the patient over a longitudinal time frame. Rather than primarily focusing on the RA patient's physical needs during a particular hospitalization, it may be cost effective over the long term to assess and address the physical, psychological, social, spiritual, and economic factors that affect health outcomes. At times, addressing depression, helplessness, transportation, or economic barriers to compliance may be more cost effective than the immediate focus on gait training or strengthening. Functional outcome at time of hospital discharge is important, but more important is functional outcome at completion of an entire episode of care including hospital, rehabilitation center, and home care. Clinical assessment and intervention need to expand to this multidimensional, longitudinal perspective.

In addition to the transfer of responsibility and role expansion, managed care will catalyze the blurring of professional boundaries. At times, rather than referrals to multiple practitioners who address only their immediate area of expertise, it may be cost effective to reduce the number of professionals involved in a patient's care. For example, if a patient is already receiving physical therapy for lower extremity interventions and also needs intervention for elbow pain, it may be more cost effective to have PT expand their focus rather than make a duplicative referral to OT.

In the past arbitrary distinctions between OT and PT were made, and professionals vigorously defended their roles and turf. This sometimes resulted in duplication of assessment and effort, repetition of information, and fragmented care. Cross-training to equip rheumatology health professionals to cover limited areas of another's discipline will be less disruptive to the patient and more cost effective. This does not mean making every OT into a mini-PT, but identifying tasks traditionally done by one discipline that could be done reasonably well by another professional. Cross-training is not synonymous with the controversial concept of multiskilling (Joe, 1995). Some of this cross-training has already occurred in hand therapy; with appropriate training, physical therapists can assume responsibility for making splints and occupational therapists can use physical modalities. In the future these boundaries may become even more flexible.

INTEGRATED INTERDISCIPLINARY VERSUS MULTIDISCIPLINARY CARE

The terms "interdisciplinary" and "multidisciplinary" are often used interchangeably, but they have different meanings and describe different models of practice. In the multidisciplinary model, disciplines function almost independently of each other, and each discipline performs its own assessment, makes recommendations, and creates a treatment plan. The interdisciplinary model requires collaboration among the disciplines and joint treatment planning. These lead to integrated care, synergistic outcomes, and consistent messages to patient and family.

In true interdisciplinary care, the providers synthesize their findings following assessment, reach agreement on recommendations, and develop a single treatment plan with complementary roles for each professional. Interdisciplinary treatment goals are set in collaboration with the patient, from the patient's, rather than the professionals', perspective, and recognize that the patient is a primary provider of his or her health care. The treatment plan is patient outcome focused, rather than discipline focused, and goal oriented rather than problem focused. Disciplines play distinct roles in meeting the jointly identified treatment goals (Gage, 1994).

An example of an interdisciplinary treatment plan would be the patient goal of learning to relieve and respect pain. Strategies would include learning pain-relief modalities such as use of heat and cold, rest as a pain-relief strategy, and pacing to reduce the occurrence of pain. Physical and occupational therapy providers may each have a distinct role in meeting this combined patient-oriented goal.

A further extension of the single interdisciplinary treatment plan would be an integrated assessment among disciplines, and among professionals of the same discipline in different treatment settings. Rather than the current practice of each discipline in each setting duplicating assessment, the assessment and treatment plan could be done collectively and forwarded to each new treatment setting as the patient is transferred from inpatient or rehabilitation center to the outpatient setting. Both physical and occupational therapists may need to know the number of steps in the house or workplace demands, but each does not need to ask the question. Information gathered by one professional could easily be made available to other professionals involved. The professionals would not need to spend time gathering duplicate data, and the patient would be spared the annoyance of repetition.

ALTERNATIVE DELIVERY MECHANISMS

In current practice the services provided are strongly influenced by what is reimbursable. Provider-based managed care may actually introduce more freedom into treatment planning and provision. Rather than having treatment options limited by what is reimbursable by a specific payer, provider-based managed care may allow providers to substitute alternative delivery mechanisms to achieve the best outcome in a cost-effective way.

Weinberger, Hines, and Tierney (1986) demonstrated improved functional status with the use of telephone support for patients with osteoarthritis (OA). The Arthritis Self-Help Course has demonstrated positive results, yet coverage for education has generally been very limited in an FFS payment system. Kaiser Health Plan of Colorado has been utilizing group visits to physicians for some of their geriatric patients, and are likely to move this form of treatment into rheumatology (Scott, submitted for publication). Kaiser has also used group PT visits for patients with shoulder pain. Others are using group treatment for management of common symptoms such as fatigue. Capitation and provider-based managed care make it clinically and financially wise to use health care dollars to pay for self-management education and other low-cost alternative delivery mechanisms that improve health outcomes.

PREVENTIVE CARE AND SELF-MANAGEMENT

A key alternative delivery mechanism will be preventive care and the facilitation of self-management skills. Preventive care will assume a high priority when capitated financing provides incentives to IHSs to keep individuals as healthy as possible. For individuals with arthritis, the focus will be on disability prevention. Disability prevention will require attention to the whole person, not just the physical aspects of their condition. As health services research identifies other factors such as social support, self-efficacy, and socialization opportunities as contributors to health outcomes, it will become increasingly important to focus interventions on these factors (Sobel, 1995). Some of these factors have received lip service in the current treatment paradigm but have not been adequately addressed or reimbursed.

Research on ASHC has demonstrated the importance of self-efficacy and self-management (Lorig et al., 1989). Professional roles will change as RHPs move from a care-provider to a self-management mindset. RHPs have traditionally focused on the care they are providing; they may neglect to give adequate time and attention to engaging the patient in self responsibility and fostering the development of self-management skills. Physicians have traditionally viewed themselves as quarterbacks of the treatment team; while recognizing that they are not the quarterback, health professionals often perceive themselves to be key players. In reality, both physicians and RHPs are coaches. In day-to-day life with a rheumatic or connective-tissue disease, health professionals can only teach, motivate, and run skill development drills; the patient himself or herself is the one who actually needs to run the plays or provide the care (Brady, 1990).

Rehabilitation professionals are well positioned to help individuals living with rheumatic disease make informed choices to maximize their functional status and quality of life, but this will require a change in professional practice style. Professionals are trained to assess or diagnose the problem and prescribe treatments. As long as health professionals see their role as being responsible for identifying and solving the patient's problems, they will undermine the patient's self-responsibility. Health professionals must realize that regardless of what they do, the person ultimately in charge of managing the condition is the patient. Patient professional interactions should be qualitatively different. Rather than being used to diagnose problems, questions should be used to stimulate patients to a clearer understanding of their problem and help them formulate their own appropriate management plan. The health professional's role is to help patients take effective and appropriate self management of their condition (Coles, 1995).

RHPs should give patients the tools they need to manage their disease from day to day, the information they need to make wise health care decisions, and the support they need to change their behavior and adapt to their changing health status. Provider-based managed care in IHSs will provide the financial incentives to catalyze this transformation to a prevention and self-management mindset to produce high-quality, cost-effective outcomes.

CONCLUSION

At this point in the development of the American health care system, managed care in one form or another appears inevitable due to the need to reduce health care costs. Managed care has the potential, though not the guarantee, to be advantageous to patients with rheumatic disease and to rheumatology professionals, particularly if rehabilitation professionals are able to capitalize on the opportunities managed care presents to streamline operations to those who truly make a difference and to demonstrate that they do make a difference in the functioning of individuals with rheumatic disease. Managed care offers promise for individuals with rheumatic disease, but early forms have not achieved that potential. The IHS approach of leading-edge managed-care organizations changes the financial incentives and has the potential to be well suited to the special health care needs of individuals with rheumatic disease. A summary of the strengths and weaknesses of managed care for rheumatic disease and the opportunities and threats for rheumatology rehabilitation in managed care are presented in Table 8.

This chapter has reviewed the mismatch between the current acute-episode-focused, fee-for-service-financed health care system and the longitudinal, multidimensional care needed by individuals with rheumatic and other chronic diseases. It has outlined the historic roots and multiple forms of managed-care organizations and the interactions between the financing system and the design of the care delivery system. Finally, the chapter highlighted changes in practice and the conceptualization of practice that will be necessary to succeed in provider-based managed care.

Fortunately, the necessary practice changes such as considering cost in clinical decision making, using outcome data to develop best-practice treatment protocols, using integrated, interdisciplinary care and alternative delivery mechanisms to facilitate preventive care and selfmanagement are in the best interest of patients and professionals. These changes will also be economically advantageous for the health care system.

Unfortunately, preparing to meet the challenge of the IHS managed-care environment can seem overwhelming, particularly if managed care has been viewed as an essential evil. Many areas of the country have just begun to explore shared-risk financing; if the environment is still functioning in FFS, the incentives are not yet aligned to facilitate these proposed practice changes. However, change of this magnitude requires adequate preparation, and it is not too early to begin to prepare. Even if the financial dynamics have not yet changed, there are a variety of steps RHPs can take now to begin to prepare for shared-risk, managed care. Examples are outlined in Table 9.

Managed care can be resisted as the devil incarnate, tolerated as a necessary evil, or harnessed to improve health outcomes and quality of life for individuals with rheumatic disease. Meenan (1996) reported that sociologists describe three response options when situations change: loyalty, voice, or exit. Individuals who choose loyalty continue to work within the system as it evolves and adapt to changes as they occur. Some choose voice, resist change, and argue strongly against the new situation. Others choose the exit option and leave the system or reenter the new system in a new role.

Rheumatology rehabilitation and patients with rheumatic and connective-tissue diseases need RHPs to choose loyalty; to use the opportunity managed care presents to make rheumatology rehabilitation an integral component of an integrated health system. According to King (AOTA, 1996), managed care provides an opportunity for the rehabilitation professions to demonstrate once and for all the legitimacy of rehabilitation as an effective method of reducing the overall costs of health care. Rehabilitation professionals have devoted their careers to helping patients adapt to changed circumstances. The time to use that expertise to do the same for the rehabilitation professions has come.

SWOT ANALYSIS—STRENGTHS AND WEAKNESSES OF MANAGED CARE IN RHEUMATIC DISEASE; OPPORTUNITIES AND THREATS FOR REHABILITATION PROFESSIONALS IN MANAGED CARE

STRENGTHS OF MANAGED CARE FOR RHEUMATIC DISEASE

Encourages redesign of care delivery to maximize outcomes and demonstrate cost effectiveness.

Encourages development of alternative delivery mechanisms and increased flexibility in resource allocation.

Encourages integration across settings and professions and over time rather than isolated, fragmented episodes of care.

Emphasizes health promotion and disability prevention, not just disease treatment.

Encourages self-management and responsibility.

Broadens perspective from medical care to health care.

Invests in strategies to reduce the underlying conditions that contribute to poor health (including psychological, social, and environmental factors).

Facilitates treatment selection based on what works rather than what is reimbursable.

Emphasizes functional outcomes.

Reduces cost shifting, and creates incentives to decrease excess or inappropriate utilization.

Decreases cost.

WEAKNESSES OF MANAGED CARE FOR RHEUMATIC DISEASE

Overemphasizes cost containment.

Restricts patient choice of providers, and provider choice of treatment options.

Disrupts preexisting patient-provider relationships.

Increases incentives for underutilization or restriction of benefits.

Introduces uncertainty and chaos into the health care system.

Motivates downsizing and staff restructuring or layoffs.

OPPORTUNITIES

Expand traditional focus on function and outcomes.

Reexamine scope of practice to fit patient need with provider skill level.

Expand disability prevention, delay, or reduction strategies.

Substitute for more expensive providers or care settings.

Expand health promotion activities.

Utilize integrated information systems to track cost and outcomes across time and setting (for individual patients and groups of patients).

Move from multidisciplinary to interdisciplinary care.

Table 8: SWOT Analysis—Strengths and Weaknesses of Managed Care in Rheumatic Disease; Opportunities and Threats for Rehabilitation Professionals in Managed Care

THREATS

Lack of demonstrated outcomes; will become irrelevant if unable to demonstrate value (good functional outcomes at reasonable cost).

Limited information on relative effectiveness, appropriateness, and cost of treatment alternatives.

Limited awareness of cost or integration of cost into clinical decisions.

Preoccupation with turf battles distracts from necessary practice changes.

Energy focused on resisting managed care rather than capitalizing on the opportunities that managed care presents.

Table 8: SWOT Analysis—Strengths and Weaknesses of Managed Care in Rheumatic Disease; Opportunities and Threats for Rehabilitation Professionals in Managed Care (continued)

PRELIMINARY STEPS TO PREPARE FOR RISK-SHARED MANAGED CARE

1. Calculate the true cost of several of the most frequently used treatment strategies and use that information in your treatment planning.

2. Begin to develop an outcome measurement system to identify strategies that lead to the best outcomes.

3. Begin to develop best-practice treatment protocols or clinical pathways. Use outcome data to refine the protocols.

4. Experiment with methods to integrate care among disciplines and across treatment settings.

5. Learn about the financial underpinnings of one of the system's largest at risk contracts (i.e., what care components the system is at risk for) and begin to use that information in your treatment planning.

6. Increase your skills at engaging patient self responsibility and facilitating selfmanagement.

Table 9: Preliminary Steps to Prepare for Risk-Shared Managed Care

References

Alexander, G., Brady, T., Brunnette, M., Burmaster, R., Dickie, B., Ellison, A., Gibson, R., Lally, J., McNamara, L., Meiches, R., Milavitz, B., & Walsh, D. (1995). *The Fairview care model: A work in process.* Unpublished document, Minneapolis, MN: Fairview Health System.

American College of Rheumatology. (1994). *Managed care and the rheumatologist.* Atlanta, GA: Author.

American Occupational Therapy Association. (1996). *Managed care: An occupational therapy sourcebook.* Bethesda, MD: Author.

APM. (1995). How markets evolve. *Hospital and Health Networks, 69*(5), 48.

Brady, T. J. (1990). Point: Patient control of treatment is essential. *Arthritis Care and Research, 3,* 163-166.

Bingewatt, R. (1996). National Chronic Care Consortium statement on Medicare managed care programs. Congressional testimony to House Ways and Means Subcommittee on Health.

Coles, C. (1995). Educating the health care team. *Patient Education and Counseling, 26,* 239-244.

Cummings, N. A., & VandenBos, G. R. (1981). The twenty years Kaiser-Permanente experience with psychotherapy and medical utilization: Implications for national health policy and national health insurance. *Health Policy Quarterly, 1,* 159-175.

Friedman, E. (1996, February). *Why are we doing this? Ethical change and constants.* Presentation to the Fairview Quality Leadership Conference, Minneapolis, MN.

Gage, M. (1994). The patient driven interdisciplinary care plan. *Journal of Nursing Administration, 24,* 26-35.

Hochberg, M. C., Altman, R. D., Brandt, K. D., Clark, B. M., Dieppe, P. A., Griffin, M. R., Moskowitz, R. W., & Schnitzer, T. J. (1995). Guidelines for medical management of osteoarthritis. *Arthritis and Rheumatism, 38,* 1535-1546.

Joe, B. E. (1995). Cross-training, partnerships top Mt. Central conference agenda. *OT Week, 9*(43), 10-11.

Joe, B. E. (1996). Can you justify all those treatments?. *OT Week, 10*(2), 14-16.

Johnson, A. N. (1996, July). Beyond managed care: A new map for the health care industry. *Minnesota Physician,* 1-11

Lorig, K., Lubeck, D., Kraines, R. G., Seleznick, M., & Holman, H. C. (1985). Outcomes of self help education for patients with arthritis. *Arthritis & Rheumatism, 28,* 680-685.

Lorig, K., Seleznick, M., Lubeck, D., Ung, E., Chastain, R. L., & Holman, H. C. (1989). The beneficial outcomes of the arthritis self management course are not adequately explained by behavior change. *Arthritis & Rheumatism, 32,* 91-95.

MacLeod, G. K. (1993). An overview of managed care. In P. R. Kongstvedt (Ed.), *The managed health care handbook* (2nd ed.). Gaithersburg, MD: Aspen Publishers.

Meenan, R. F. (1996). Managed care and the rheumatologist. *Current Opinion in Rheumatology, 6,* 91-95.

Moncur, C. (1988). Attacking the sacred cows. *Arthritis Care and Research, 1,* 116-121.

Norling, R. A., & Edwards, M. C. (1995, September). Fairview's health reform principles. Presentation to Congress.

Overman, S., Lewis, R., Kent, D., & Uslan, D. (1995). Rheumatologists as musculoskeletal managers in Medicare risk programs. *Arthritis and Rheumatism, 38*(9), S269.

Pawlson, L. G. (1994). Chronic illness: Implications of a new paradigm for health care. *Journal of Quality Improvement, 20,* 33-39.

Reynolds, J. P. (1996, March). Outcomes: In the eye of the beholder. *PT Magazine,* 66-72.

Scott, J. Group cooperative health care clinic pilot study results. *Journal of American Geriatrics Society.* Submitted for publication.

Selker, L. G. (1995). Human resources in physical therapy: Opportunities for service in a rapidly changing health system. *Physical Therapy, 75*, 31-37.

Sobel, D. S. (1995). Rethinking medicine: Improving health outcomes with cost effective psychosocial interventions. *Psychosomatic Medicine, 57*, 234-244.

Weinberger, M., Hines, S. L., & Tierney, W. M. (1986). Improving functional status in arthritis: The effects of social support. *Social Science and Medicine, 9*, 899-904.

Yelin, E., Such, C., Criswell, L., & Epstein, W. (1995). Outcomes for persons with RA: Treatment by rheumatologists and non-rheumatologists. *Arthritis and Rheumatism, 38*(9), S187.

Zitter, M. (1994). Disease management: A new approach to health care. *Medical Interface, 7*, 70-76.

3

PSYCHOLOGICAL FACTORS RELATED TO TREATMENT AND ADHERENCE

Christopher Lorish, PhD

INTRODUCTION

Anyone who has tried to follow a medication regimen to completion or to persist with an exercise program to lose weight or stay fit knows the difficulty of starting and maintaining new habits. This is frequently what therapists ask their patients to do, yet therapists often give little thought to the difficulties of adhering to the prescribed treatment. Maintaining function in a person with a chronic musculoskeletal condition usually requires a long-term commitment to self-management that includes splinting, stretching, strengthening, or engaging in a fitness program. Adherence influences both short- and long-term treatments and has an impact on the patient's health.

This chapter will focus on factors that influence patients' adherence to a treatment regimen. These factors are specific and can be assessed and influenced by the therapist. The patient's perspective is emphasized and provides the framework for the chapter since adherence to a home program requires the patient to be the agent for initiating and maintaining the treatment without direct observation by the therapist. This perspective requires that, first, therapists develop interviewing skills that encourage patients to disclose their beliefs about their condition, their fears, other negative feelings, and the important activities that can provide an incentive for doing the treatment. Second, the therapist must use the patient's disclosed beliefs and fears to formulate education efforts and negotiate the most efficacious treatment that the patient is willing to follow consistently. To influence the patient's perspective, the therapist must respect and probe the patient's expertise about the condition and his or her treatment responses to it as well as work to develop a therapeutic alliance with shared responsibility.

A patient's health status depends on four factors: (1) The vagaries of the severity and activity of the musculoskeletal disorder, (2) the efficacy of the prescribed treatment to ameliorate dysfunction beyond natural healing, (3) the patient's adherence to the prescribed treatment for a sufficient length of time, and (4) the patient's involvement in self-management including the patient's use of any self-prescribed therapeutic agents. If a patient does not improve as expected, then treatment decisions must be made after sorting through these four factors and their relationship to lack of improvement. This causal ambiguity is increased by the absence of scientific studies on the dose-response relationship of most treatments and by the unreliability of the patient's reports of adherence to the home program.

ADHERENCE AS A RATE AND A CONCEPT

If patients are adherent to their home programs, does it matter if they do not accurately report what they do? The literature on patient adherence in occupational and physical therapy is scant but suggests that patients have the same difficulty following their therapy regimen as taking their medication consistently. Reports of adherence rates to supervised exercise, the kind typically associated with cardiac rehabilitation programs or other hospital- or clinic-based treatments, ranged from 70% to 94% (Malouin, Potvin, Prevost, Richards, & Wood-Dauphinee, 1992; Pollock et al., 1991), and adherence to unsupervised exercise and splinting home programs ranged from 18% to 57% (Feinberg & Brandt, 1981; Moon, Moon, & Black, 1976; Parker & Bender, 1957; Sluijs, Kok, & Van der Zee, 1993; Taal, Rasker, Seydel, & Weigman, 1993). To understand fully the implications of these findings, the meaning of adherence needs clarification. Meanings and interpretations affect our actions.

Adherence will be used prescriptively to mean therapy-related patient behavior including its frequency, duration, and intensity, that has as its goal the reduction of impairments and the maintenance or improvement of function. It is assumed that the desired behavior is mutually agreed upon by the therapist and the patient. Adherence has both a process meaning (what is done) and an outcome meaning (what are the effects). As a process, adherence means doing things with the patient like negotiating therapeutic goals and solving treatment-barrier problems to increase the likelihood of adherent outcome behavior such as coming to the clinic, correctly completing therapeutic exercises, or modifying the treatment by previously agreed rules. The outcome of these processes is influenced by what occurs between the patient and therapist.

Nonadherent behavior puts the patient at greater risk for worsening the impairment. It can be classified as *unintentional*, for example, forgetting to do the treatment or how to do it correctly, or *intentional*, for example, choosing not to initiate the treatment, doing less or more of it, or doing it differently (Lorish, Richards, & Brown, 1989). If the patient forgets, the therapist can help the patient develop reminder strategies; but if the patient chooses to be nonadherent, the therapist must try to assess the reasons and use education, persuasion, problem solving, and negotiation to influence the patient.

Nonadherence in all its manifestations represents a potential threat to a patient's recovery and function and can limit the length of coverage in Medicare and other managed-care programs that require significant functional improvement to reimburse for services. Adherence requires careful evaluation by the therapist at each follow-up visit.

There are circumstances under which it is appropriate to deviate from the prescribed treatment. Typically, treatment behavior changes occur in response to changes in the condition or the development of treatment side effects. For example, if a joint flares up, strengthening exercises may be temporarily stopped. If patients are to make rational changes in the usual treatment routine, therapists must teach them to distinguish those changes and the appropriate treatment responses to them.

THE PATIENT-THERAPIST RELATIONSHIP

THE PATIENT AS EXPERT

Patients do not come to the clinic with empty minds ready to be filled by the therapist's knowledge and wisdom. Rather they come as "experts" with beliefs and explanations developed over a lifetime about the condition and its treatment. These may be inconsistent with the scientific knowledge or the wisdom of the therapist (Donovan, Blake, & Fleming, 1989; Leventhal & Cameron, 1987; Leventhal, Zimmerman, & Gutmann, 1984). A patient's beliefs about his or her condition are the result of interpreting illness experiences including the effects of any self-prescribed remedies and observations of others with similar conditions. The key beliefs for the therapist to try to understand, because of their influence on adherence, are those concerning etiology, duration, consequences, time frame for healing or reaching goals, and treatability (Leventhal et al., 1984). For example, a patient who believes that arthritis comes with aging and that little can be done for it is expressing an inevitability about the onset and consequences of the disease that would tend to reduce motivation to follow therapy unless convinced otherwise.

The crucial point is that nonadherence can result when the patient must decide between his or her own beliefs and the therapist's knowledge when they do not agree. For example, a patient may not believe it when the therapist says that regular exercise is beneficial if past experience with exercise only made the patient feel worse. Patient education, which is discussed in a later chapter, is the means for changing a patient's knowledge and beliefs. The success of the therapist in modifying the patient's beliefs is tied to the patient's estimation of the therapist's credibility, the quality of the relationship, the therapist's educational efforts, and whether experience with the treatment confirms the therapist's statements.

PATIENT SELF-DISCLOSURE

One of the therapist's responsibilities is rendering his or her best judgment about the most efficacious treatment. Treatment decision making requires accurate, valid information, much of which the patient must choose to reveal to the therapist. Given the short time therapists have with patients in an outpatient clinic, a critical skill is efficiently probing the patient's knowledge, beliefs, feelings, and goals either through direct questioning or questionnaire (Cohen-Cole, 1991). General, open-ended questions are useful for initial assessments of the patient's beliefs, goals, and prior treatments, while specific closed-ended questions are useful for determining what the patient did at home. For example, at the initial visit, answers to open-ended questions about the functional activity the patient most wants to recover or maintain can help establish the treatment's purpose. At a follow-up visit, assessment of the patient's adherence to the home program requires a self-report obtained by closed-ended questions of the frequency, duration, intensity, and correctness with which the activities were completed.

For the therapist to obtain this information, the patient must be willing to self-disclose and have an accurate memory or written record of treatment activities. While a spouse or any other reliable adult can assist with home-treatment data collection and reporting, the best approach is to create conditions that facilitate complete and accurate disclosure by the patient. Self-disclosure is a necessary condition for assessing adherence, and it is crucial for eliciting and working with elements of treatment motivation such as a patient's goals, beliefs, and values. There is evidence that too much disclosure of weaknesses and failings demoralizes a patient, but disclosure of both strengths and weaknesses supports the person's confidence and enhances adherence (DiMatteo & DiNicola, 1982). A patient's self-disclosure may be the light that shines on the path to change, but the therapist's behavior is often critical in turning that light on.

FACILITATIVE THERAPIST BEHAVIOR

Patients are more satisfied and adherent when in a clinic visit the right balance exists between giving and receiving information, sharing emotions, and meeting the patient's goals for the visit (American Psychiatric Association, 1995; Roter, Hall, & Katz, 1987). The amount, accuracy, specificity and thoroughness of the questions asked, and the use of a treatment calendar, diary, or log increase the accuracy of treatment reporting. Use of a self-report record is also a compliance strategy in self-management programs (Dunbar & Agras, 1980; Kanfer, 1980). Therapist behavior that promotes patient self-disclosure includes giving full attention to the patient, asking the patient's opinions, and showing concern, respect, and nonjudgmental empathy (Samuelsson, Ahlmen, & Sullivan, 1993). Tyner (1985) found that focused attention and a posture facing and inclined toward the patient communicates positive feelings of interest. This is important to help overcome the patient's reluctance to ask questions lest he or she seem to challenge the therapist's authority or expertise (Tuckett, Boulton, Olson, & Williams, 1985). Nonjudgmental empathy encourages the patient to feel accepted and safe, and to reveal inadequacies such as not following the home treatment. Therapist behavior that is predominated by advice or information giving and by closed-ended, direct questions tends to inhibit self-disclosure, reduce patient satisfaction, and inhibit teamwork. On the other hand, asking patients questions and soliciting their opinions about past and present conditions and treatments and about treatment goals enhances adherence (Roter, Hall & Katz, 1987).

Since the adherence data suggest that patients will be nonadherent at some time, one strategy for promoting self-disclosure of nonadherence is for the therapist to give the patient permission to admit it by acknowledging that it is difficult even for the therapist to follow a treatment or an exercise program all the time. Then, in the next statement, the therapist can establish the expectation that, even though such "slips" from the program are common and forgivable, the goal is to minimize such slips. Furthermore, to help ensure minimal slips, the patient and therapist can discuss the reasons for the slips and identify ways to reduce adherence barriers or modify the treatment. Assuming that the nonadherence has not been extreme, framing nonadherence as slips and an opportunity to learn ways to minimize them should decrease the patient's guilt (Marlatt & George, 1990).

THERAPIST-PATIENT ALLIANCE

Encouraging patients to disclose their beliefs and feelings is an important step in establishing a therapeutic alliance (Francis, Korsch, & Morris 1969; Heszen-Klemens & Lapinska 1984; Roter, Hall, & Katz, 1987; Walker, 1995) that promotes the patient's sense of control through active involvement in the treatment decision-making process (Schwartz, 1988). The expectation of the patient's active involvement in treatment decisions is established at the first visit between the therapist, patient, and family. The purpose of the alliance is to obtain the patient's active involvement and commitment to achieving the therapeutic goals. Working as a team requires not only patient self-disclosure but also mutual respect for the expertise of each. For this alliance to work, patients must respect therapists' knowledge and skill regarding the assessment and treatment of their specific musculoskeletal problems.

Explicit statements to the patient at the first visit about working as a team to achieve mutually acceptable functional goals and to develop a treatment program to achieve those goals establish the purpose of the relationship and communicate that the therapist respects and cares about the patient's goals (Speedling & Rose, 1985). As part of that teamwork, the patient can also be told that one of the important purposes of each follow-up visit is to review both progress toward functional goals and problems adhering to the treatment. Information is obtained at follow-up visits on problems implementing the treatment and on treatment-goal progress. After discussing possible changes to the treatment or goals, their consequences, and possible problems implementing the changes, agreement on the treatment activities completes the process for that visit.

Promoting a patient's adherence to a treatment involves an ongoing process in which the therapist works to establish a relationship based on caring, respect, and nonjudgmental empathy for the patient while engaged in teamwork to achieve mutually agreed functional goals and to solve the patient's problems by following the home treatment. As this process occurs, the patient's beliefs and ideas about the illness are likely to begin to resemble those of the therapist. The pace of this teamwork process will vary, probably related to whether the patient copes by seeking or avoiding information, with avoiders needing more time (Steptoe, Sutcliffe, Allen, & Coombes, 1991).

INFLUENCING ADHERENCE: THE FOUR DOMAINS

Information must be obtained about the patient's degree of adherence to a home treatment program and about influences that either enhanced or decreased adherence so that the most efficacious treatment program that the patient is willing to follow can be planned jointly. These influences can be classified into four domains that include (1) the patient's emotional responses to the condition, (2) treatment knowledge and skills, (3) motivation, and (4) treatment opportunities. Figure 1 shows these influences as part of a two-directional process mediated by the therapist-patient relationship. Influencing adherence presumes knowing the patient's degree of treatment adherence.

ASSESSING ADHERENCE

Working to influence patients' choices and behavior can follow much the same diagnostic-prescriptive process as treatment. At the first visit, evaluation of barriers and aids to adherence can be accomplished by direct questioning and/or a waiting-room questionnaire. These results are incorporated into a negotiated treatment plan that builds on the strengths or forces that aid adherence while minimizing barriers. The specific treatment behaviors are practiced in the clinic not only for their therapeutic benefit but also to ensure the patient's ability to do them independently at home. This will reveal what the patient is willing to do and serves as the foundation for further negotiations at subsequent visits. Follow-up visits focus on the patient's and therapist's assessment of progress, the patient's report of treatment adherence, and problem-solving discussion of any difficulties the patient had following the treatment. Any of these factors may result in a change of therapeutic goals or treatment. Each clinic visit is an opportunity to influence the patient to maintain high treatment adherence or to influence the patient to choose a more efficacious treatment.

Direct, objective evidence of nonadherence like low blood levels of medication does not exist for physical and occupational therapy regimens. Indirect evidence can be obtained by the patient's oral or written log or diary, the report of a reliable observer of the patient, or the therapist's judgment of the patient's treatment knowledge, behavior, and progress. Given the unreliability of patients' recall or consistent marking of a treatment log, a more realistic measurement expectation is to categorize the patient as "not doing the treatment at all," "doing it some," or "consistently doing it all." No single piece of evidence unambiguously allows the therapist to categorize the patient's adherence. For example, a patient's slow progress may be due to nonadherence, exacerbations of the condition, or poor medication control. Multiple indicators, however, can create a pattern of evidence that makes the inference of nonadherence of some degree more likely to be correct. For example, if the patient is not progressing at the rate the therapist expected, could not state key details of the treatment regimen, and performed one or more of the treatment behaviors in an uncertain or incorrect way, this pattern strongly suggests that the patient has been nonadherent to some degree. Sometimes the evidence is so ambiguous that the only conclusion is that the patient "probably is not" adherent.

In addition to determining if the patient is doing less than prescribed, it may be as important to ask if the patient did more, temporarily stopped, quit, altered, added, or substituted therapeutic activities. When you suspect nonadherence in a patient who is not comfortable revealing nonadherence, it can be helpful to tell the patient that you have a hard time following a treatment plan or doing regular exercise and then ask the patient to describe all the "bad" or "worst things" about the treatment. The answer will likely reveal the reasons for his or her nonadherence. The therapist can approach these reasons in a problem-solving discussion to try to find mutually acceptable alternatives that minimize

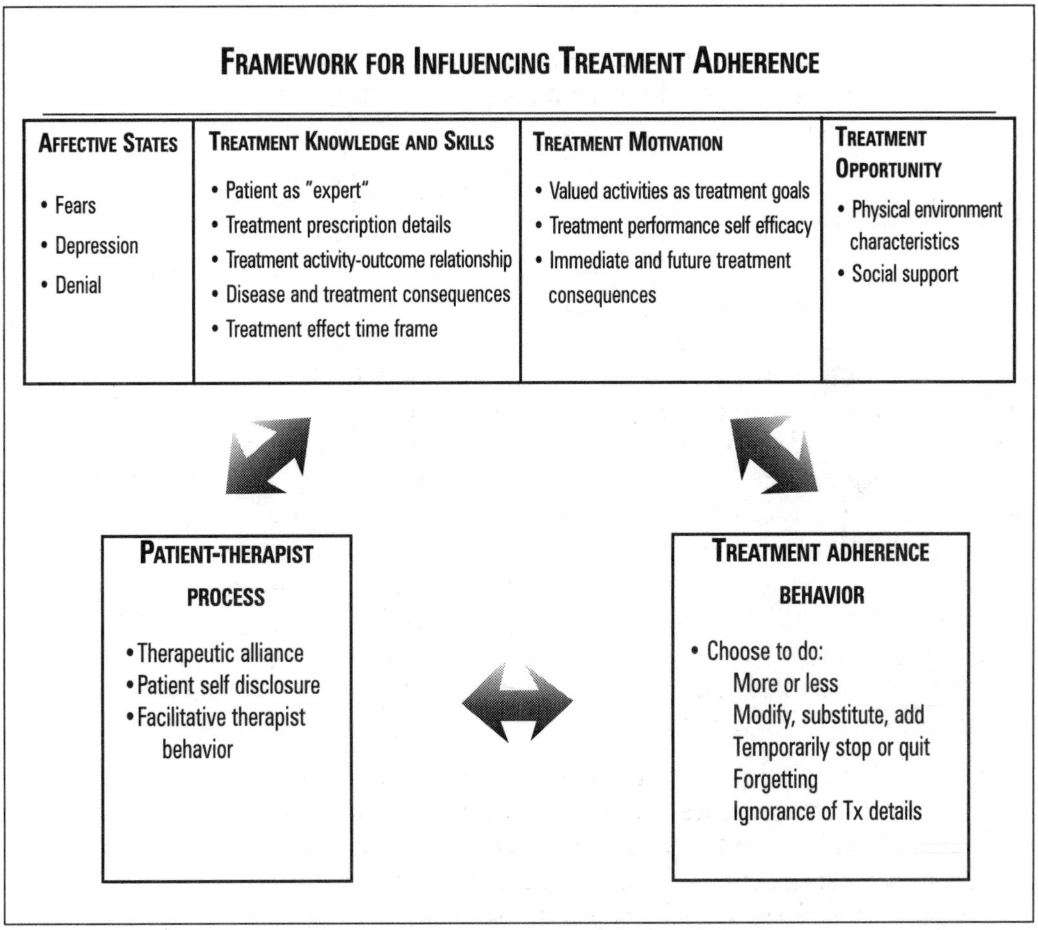

FRAMEWORK FOR INFLUENCING TREATMENT ADHERENCE

AFFECTIVE STATES	TREATMENT KNOWLEDGE AND SKILLS	TREATMENT MOTIVATION	TREATMENT OPPORTUNITY
• Fears • Depression • Denial	• Patient as "expert" • Treatment prescription details • Treatment activity-outcome relationship • Disease and treatment consequences • Treatment effect time frame	• Valued activities as treatment goals • Treatment performance self efficacy • Immediate and future treatment consequences	• Physical environment characteristics • Social support

PATIENT-THERAPIST PROCESS

• Therapeutic alliance
• Patient self disclosure
• Facilitative therapist behavior

TREATMENT ADHERENCE BEHAVIOR

• Choose to do:
   More or less
   Modify, substitute, add
   Temporarily stop or quit
   Forgetting
   Ignorance of Tx details

Figure 1. Framework for Influencing Treatment Adherence; The four domains that influence treatment adherence are shown on the left and the two-directional process on the right.

the stated deterrents. **It is important that the discussion of problems in adhering to the treatment plan occur at each follow-up visit during a review of the treatment activity and progress log and that the expectation for that discussion be established at the first visit.** Table 1 lists methods to reveal nonadherence.

DOMAIN 1: EMOTIONAL RESPONSES TO MUSCULOSKELETAL ILLNESS AND INJURY

Common responses to diagnoses of serious conditions like chronic degenerative diseases and to actual or potential losses attributed to the condition are **fear, depression, and denial. Any of these responses can render the patient unable to attend to therapist-initiated instructional activities and/or unable to initiate independent treatment behavior.** Occasionally, fear can motivate a patient to take action. If any of these responses occur at diagnosis or later, the patient's therapy activities require close supervision by the family or therapist to help ensure their completion. Referral for counseling and/or medication may also be necessary. In addition, the patient can be taught to monitor his or her emotional state and encouraged to initiate appropriate responses including self-refer-

NONADHERENCE ASSESSMENT

1. While the patient is demonstrating an important, specific treatment behavior, ask the patient how many times he or she is supposed to do that movement. This will reveal both whether he or she can correctly perform the treatment behavior and whether he or she knows the correct number of repetitions.

2. Ask the patient or observer how many times in the past week or two the treatment was missed. Cue his or her memory if no log is available by asking him or her to recall each day separately. If missing is admitted, probe the reasons and resolve them or change the program.

3. Assess the patient's progress toward the therapeutic goal and compare it to the expected progress derived from similar patients to determine if he or she is making appropriate progress. If progress is minimal, ask what the worst things are about doing the program. Resolve problems or change the program.

4. Ask the patient how the treatment could be changed to increase or hasten progress.

5. Ask the patient or observer if the patient is doing extra prescribed treatment, has temporarily stopped the treatment, has added a new treatment, or has substituted a treatment for the prescribed treatment. Then ask what effects those changes have had. Discuss risks of the changes and negotiate what is allowed.

Table 1: Nonadherence Assessment

ral to counseling or participation in a support group. Working with a patient's emotional responses requires that the therapist take the time to ask in a caring, respectful, and empathetic way and that the patient feel safe to disclose the emotions.

FEAR

Strain (1979), Pollin and Golant (1994), and Parker and colleagues (1988) summarize the common fears caused by the diagnosis of a chronic illness. These include (a) loss of control, (b) loss of self-image, (c) loss of independence, (d) stigma, (e) abandonment, (f) anger and its expression, (g) isolation, and (h) death. Because of the unpredictability and often destructive effects of inflammatory arthritic conditions on joints and other organs, a patient will be likely to struggle continually with one or more of these issues. Any one of them is capable of producing powerful anticipatory fear reactions, depression, denial, and irrational coping. Temporarily stopping, quitting, or changing the prescribed treatment are likely if the fears are many or strong. Table 2 lists possible ways of inquiring about the patient's fears, specifically the feared consequence, his or her view of the likelihood of it happening, and his or her idea of when the feared consequence will be realized.

Rather than letting the fear take over, the therapist can help the patient take control by encouraging him or her to verbalize what is feared, assess the likelihood of its happening and the actions that can be taken to reduce that likelihood. Many people have a fear of death but do not believe it will occur soon and so are not immobilized by it. However, if a patient fears he or she will become crippled and that the crippling will occur within a month rather than at some time in the distant future, then the proximity of the feared consequence is more likely to be immobilizing unless he or she believes the outcome can be prevented. The responses to the questions in Table 2 become the basis for helping the patient explore the feelings and meanings underlying the fears. This may occur over several visits and can be aided by specific behaviors like listening attentively, reflecting, and clarifying the patient's thoughts and feelings to promote understanding (Egan, 1986).

Once the fear is verbalized, the therapist can provide reassuring, corrective information if the fear is based on incomplete or wrong information. The therapist can promote the patient's reflection by asking why the feared consequence is so bad and if there are other, less negative consequences that are as likely. In addition, the therapist can encourage the patient to make an active response to the fears. The therapist and patient can jointly develop treatment goals, plans, and other activities that prevent or minimize what the patient fears. Encouraging the patient's active response to fear may also involve referral to an appropriate resource such as a psychologist, counselor, or support group whose members face similar fears and are successfully learning to control them. The Arthritis Foundation's Arthritis Self-Help course is one example. Other resources include The Arthritis Foundation's patient educational materials (see chapter 17 on Community Resources; Lorig & Fries, 1990; Pitzele, 1986; Pollin & Golant, 1994). These actions focus on the therapeutic alliance, not on fear, and on the struggle to prevent what is most feared.

ASSESSMENT OF FEAR RESPONSES

1. What have you been told about (the condition) that worries or upsets you the most?
2. What is the worst thing that is likely to happen because of (the condition)?
3. When do you think that will happen?
4. How likely is it to happen?
5. Are there any good things about (the condition)?
6. Do you think (the condition) is controlling you?
7. Do you feel you are not the same person as before?
8. Do you think you have to rely on others too much now?
9. Do you feel different from others and feel judged by others?
10. Do you feel most people don't care about you now?
11. Do you feel so angry that it scares you?
12. Do you feel alone or isolated?
13. Do you think you are going to die soon?

Table 2: Assessment of Fear Responses

DEPRESSION

Depression can immobilize patients to the point that they cannot participate in treatment. Depending on the measurement method and group, the rate of depression can be quite variable. Depression rates of 14% to 80% among persons with rheumatoid arthritis have been reported (Blalock, DeVellis, Brown, & Wallston, 1989; Frank et al., 1988; Katz & Yelin, 1993; Patrick, Morgan, & Charlton, 1986; Revenson, Schiaffino, Majerovitz et al., 1991). Depression can take the form of grief reactions to disease-caused functional losses or role changes, and such grief typically improves without specific treatment (Katz & Yelin). One cause of depression is the psychological response to the prognosis, symptoms, and degenerative joint changes and functional losses often caused by degenerative musculoskeletal diseases (Andersson, Bradley, Young, McDaniel, & Wise, 1985). Other causes of depression include non–disease-related psychosocial stressors linked to financial, work, and relationship changes. Still other causes can be side effects of medication and diseases that precipitate biological changes, like hypothyroidism. All patients, and especially elderly ones with multiple comorbidities and medications, are at greater risk for depression and therefore require close scrutiny at each clinic visit (Rush, 1993).

The severity of depression can be characterized on a continuum ranging from a mild self-limiting sadness in response to normal disappointments and losses to a major depressive disorder characterized by multiple symptoms experienced daily for weeks or longer. Severity is related to the number of symptoms experienced (see Table 3) and the frequency with which the symptoms keep the person from completing routine activities. Any level of depression makes routine activities including doing home treatment more difficult to complete or easier to avoid altogether. Severe depression requires close scrutiny and supervision by the therapist, family, home health personnel, and physician not only because of the patient's likely inability to initiate and maintain the treatment but also, and more importantly, because of the possibility of suicide. Less severe depression may result in sporadic adherence behavior related to the patient's mood and may require increased treatment supervision by the therapist, family, or home health personnel to maintain some level of "treatment habit" until the condition resolves.

Table 3 shows the diagnostic symptoms assessed by observation, direct question, or the use of one of the self-report screening tests (Beck & Steer, 1987; Radloff, 1977; Zung, 1996). According to the American Psychiatric Association (1995), a major depressive disorder is diagnosed when at least one of the first two symptoms exists and five or more of the total symptoms exist simultaneously most of each day for at least 2 weeks. Note that some of these symptoms like weight loss, fatigue, and lethargy can also be an indication of the disease process and not depression (Andersson et al., 1985; Blalock et al., 1989). Therapists should be vigilant for depressive symptoms and ask one or more of the screening questions regularly. If a patient expresses any thoughts of suicide, contact the physician immediately and encourage the patient to see a psychiatrist.

As with the fears associated with a chronic disease diagnosis, therapists can encourage an active response to mild depressive symptoms by listening empathetically, reflecting thoughts and feelings, identifying treatment modifications, increasing supervision during the depression, and reinforcing the value of medication and counseling therapy. Also

DIAGNOSTIC CRITERIA FOR DEPRESSION

- Depressed mood most of the day, e.g., sadness or frequent episodes of crying
- Markedly diminished interest or pleasure in activities, e.g., hobbies, work, sex
- Significant weight gain/loss, e.g., eating significantly more or less than usual
- Insomnia/hypersomnia, e.g., sleeping much more or less than usual
- Psychomotor agitation/retardation, e.g., frequent accidents, lethargy
- Fatigue (loss of energy), e.g., feeling "tired all the time"
- Feelings of worthlessness, e.g., guilt, low self-confidence, loss of interest in appearance
- Impaired concentration, e.g., indecisiveness, confusion
- Recurrent thoughts of death or suicide

Table 3: Criteria Diagnosis of Depression. Source: American Psychiatric Association (1995)

important are encouraging self-management for treatment of depression including activities such as regular exercise, good sleep, stress management, good nutrition, and involvement in community support programs to increase socialization and reduce isolation (see Burns, *The Feeling Good Handbook*, 1989, and Lorig and Fries, *The Arthritis Helpbook*, 1990). Until the immobilizing fears and depression are resolved enough so that the patient can consistently initiate treatment behavior, treatment work should be supervised by the clinic therapist or assistant, a home health worker, or a family member.

DENIAL

Another response to the actual or potential threats of a chronic degenerative disease is denial of its reality, seriousness, or effects. The consequence of this can be that treatment is sporadically followed, stopped, or avoided. For example, a patient for whom a diagnosis of rheumatoid arthritis invokes a vivid picture of being a "crippled, old woman incapable of taking care of herself and in constant pain" may use denial to cope with the thoughts and images and any concomitant anger or depression (Levine, Rudy, & Kerns, 1994) by acting as if such a possibility does not exist, including not following the prescribed treatment. All people use denial to cope with unpleasant or unthinkable thoughts or emotions (Ness & Ende, 1994). Through denial a patient may maintain an unrealistic expectation for a cure so as not to have to contemplate the losses the disease may cause. Also, the therapist or physician may deny the deterioration of the patient's function and thus not change treatment or make referrals.

Denial may be used in different ways. Denial can be an adaptive process that acts like a "rose-colored filter," progressively allowing pieces of grim truth to be processed and accepted while permitting the person to maintain a degree of normalcy and control (Russell, 1993). For others, what a therapist labels as denial may simply be a different view of the situation shaped by the patient's knowledge, cultural and religious beliefs, and

INDICATORS OF PATIENT DENIAL

1. Actively avoiding information, e.g., choosing not to listen, read, or watch disease or treatment information.

2. Selective memory about the illness, e.g., remembering only the least-threatening facts about the illness.

3. Dangerous or bizarre behavior, e.g., continuing work or other activities that risk well-being.

4. Minimizing or negating, e.g., dismissing or excusing signs, symptoms, or consequences of the disease or behavior.

5. Ambivalence, e.g., frequent arguing or "Yes, but . . ." responses to suggestions.

Table 4: Assessing Indications of Patient Denial

values. It may, for example, be a conscious choice not to impose the burden of the patient's problem on others or himself by not changing (Beisser, 1979; Shelp & Perl, 1985). Finally, denial may reflect an underlying ambivalence about the course of action to take (Miller & Rollnick, 1991). Frequent "Yes, but . . ." responses to assessment or treatment suggestions indicate that the patient is in conflict about the diagnosis or treatment.

The importance of how the therapist defines "denial" and judges a patient is that it may determine the patient's response. For example, if the therapist verbally or nonverbally communicates that the patient is in denial because he or she is not agreeing with the therapist's assessment or treatment, then the patient will either accept the judgment and feel guilt for being a "bad" patient or reject the judgment and respond defensively. The former response may lead to acceptance of the therapist's view and commitment to treatment in some patients, but it is hard to predict. The latter often leads to a vicious cycle of therapist "push" and patient "resistance," which only confirms the therapist's label of the patient's denial and the patient's feelings of guilt. Viewing denial as an adaptive process is a positive, potentially more productive approach since it allows the therapist to respond nonjudgmentally and work with the patient to find solutions (Miller & Rollnick 1991; Taleff, 1994). Identifying denial and working with it are important skills if treatment adherence is to be maximized.

Unlike depression, there are no agreed-upon criteria for diagnosing denial or rules for judging its severity. There are behavioral indicators, summarized in Table 4, which suggest that a patient is showing denial, especially if more than one indicator occurs (Ness & Ende, 1994). The interpretation of these behaviors is ambiguous because they could reflect the patient's lack of correct information, honest differences that reflect cultural values or religious beliefs, or fully informed decisions that honestly reflect the patient's values. If the patient's responses cannot be attributed to these alternative explanations with confidence, then the therapist must decide if and how to respond to the denial.

Assuming that there are important negative consequences in not adhering or potential negative consequences in continuing denial of the condition, the patient's best interest is usually served by trying to move the patient toward acceptance of the condition and implementation of the treatment. In addition to the suggestions for responding to the patient's fears, Miller and Rollnick (1991) suggest some other strategies. First, use reflection and interpretation of the patient's statements and emotions to identify discrepancies between the patient's functional or treatment goals and present behavior. Asking the patient to state the negative consequences of the denial behavior and the positive consequences of changing the behavior encourages the patient to confront his or her behavior and its consequences. Second, avoid arguing, accusing, or labeling, since that typically produces defensive behavior. A corollary is that if the therapist senses resistance in the patient, change topics, activities, or the communication process. Third, provide the patient with options, both treatment goals and activities, and allow the patient to select. At the same time, if a patient selects a treatment activity, he or she must be told that it is his or her responsibility to carry it out. If the therapist exudes optimism that it is never too late to start and that there are always options, the patient will not feel hopeless. These behaviors help ensure that the patient remains engaged with the therapist until the conflict or fears diminish or are resolved. Once there is evidence that independent treatment behavior is more likely, working with the patient's knowledge and skills, treatment motivation, and treatment opportunities is appropriate and should be more productive. Until that time, the therapist may have to accept that the patient will do less than is desirable, while remaining vigilant for a reduction in the patient's fear and denial in order to try to move the patient to more desirable treatment behavior.

DOMAIN 2: TREATMENT KNOWLEDGE AND SKILLS

The "patient as expert" section made the point that patients come to a therapist with a set of beliefs about the causes, effects, treatments, and time frame for the condition and treatments. These beliefs can affect the patient's willingness to try or to sustain a prescribed treatment, and they may not be in agreement with the therapist's beliefs. For example, if the patient attributes symptom relief that is quick but short-lived to a "rub," it may be difficult to persuade the patient to adhere to an exercise program that requires more effort and time and whose results may take weeks to be felt by the patient. If a patient believes that the condition is caused by an "evil spirit," then he or she is more likely to accept spiritual or magical treatments than adhere to a medical treatment. If a patient believes that a condition is short-lived, then acceptance of a long-term treatment regimen is less likely until there is acceptance that the condition is chronic. Thus, the educational goal of every clinic visit is to educate the patient to think and make decisions that are more consistent with proven treatments. To elicit the patient's beliefs efficiently, oral or written questions like those in Table 5 can be used to target the specific beliefs that need to be changed. **If time is short, ask the patient about experience with the treatment that is likely to be prescribed and its effects and problems. This can be a useful start for illuminating possible adherence problems and whether the patient believes in the treatment's effectiveness.**

ASSESSING THE PATIENT'S BELIEFS IN THE INITIAL VISIT

1. What do you think you have?
2. What do you think caused your condition?
3. How long do you think it will last?
4. What treatments have you tried, and what results occurred?
5. What treatments have you heard of that work?
6. Have you tried the prescribed treatment? What did it do? Would you be willing to try it again?

Table 5. Assessing the Patient's Beliefs in the Initial Visit

The educational process combines exposure to appropriate health education materials, experiential discovery of what does and does not help, direct instruction by the therapist and other health care professionals, and friends, family, and the mass media, whose accuracy can be problematic. Except for the mass media, the other educational sources can be influenced by the therapist. During the first visit, it may be useful to ask the patient what treatments he or she has already tried and the success of each to determine if there are any competitors to the prescribed treatment. That is, if a patient is convinced that a rub works, the therapist must convince the patient that the rub's effects are not as desirable as the effects of the prescribed treatment. If a patient's beliefs defy changing, one approach is a treatment "experiment" designed to provide "proof" of a treatment's efficacy. After specifying the intensity, duration, and frequency of a treatment and agreeing on the evidence that will count as success, the treatment is applied with the effects noted and then withdrawn with the effects noted.

What knowledge does a patient need to adhere? To be an adherent patient, the patient needs to know a lot. Table 6 summarizes the assessment questions. The patient's understanding of the connection between doing the treatment activities and achieving functional goals will enhance motivation (Bandura, 1986, p. 469). For example, to motivate a patient to do shoulder and elbow range-of-motion and strengthening exercises, explain that these exercises can make it possible to reach into the kitchen cabinets to retrieve objects and resume cooking.

Second, patients must know what they are to do, that is, what, when, how intensely, how often, and where to do their treatment. This minimizes adherence mistakes. This and other treatment information must be committed to memory or at least recorded for easy review. Most therapists provide for this review with take-home sheets of illustrated exercises that specify the details of the treatment.

Third, patients should know the consequences of their disease and treatment (Bandura, 1986). For example, they should know the signs and symptoms of improvement or treatment harm. How is the patient to know that the bodily sensations he or she is feeling are good or bad, dangerous or innocuous, and whether they are caused by the

ASSESSING DISEASE AND TREATMENT KNOWLEDGE

TREATMENT-FUNCTIONAL GOAL CONNECTION
How is this treatment supposed to help you?

TREATMENT DETAILS
What exercises are you supposed to do? When? How many? How often?

TREATMENT-DISEASE CONSEQUENCES
How is your treatment affecting your symptoms and function? How is it supposed to? If you did no treatment, what would the effect be on your condition? On your function? Are these changes important to you? How?

INDICATORS OF TREATMENT OR DISEASE CHANGES
How does your body tell you whether your treatment is working or whether your condition is worsening?

TREATMENT EFFECT TIME FRAME.
When do you expect the changes caused by your treatment to occur?

"WHAT IF . . . ?" RULES
What should you do if your treatment goal is achieved before the next visit? What should you do about your treatment if your condition worsens, gets better, you miss your treatment for a week, or a new symptom develops? When should you increase or decrease the frequency or intensity of your regimen? When should you stop or add other treatment activities?

TREATMENT SKILLS
After practice, please show me how you will do your treatment activities at home.

Table 6: Assessing Disease and Treatment Knowledge

disease, treatment, medication, or something else? If the patient attributes a pain in the big toe to the prescribed leg exercises, there is increased risk that the patient will change the treatment to try to relieve the toe pain. Patients make these decisions based on their experience with how their bodies felt and functioned during and after previous treatments (Pennebaker, 1982). Deviations from that experientially based knowledge are sensed by the patient and often cause the patient to speculate or test why. If the patient concludes that the treatment is causing the pain (a causal attribution), then he or she may decide to wait watchfully or modify the regimen. Signs of improvement can also cause changes to the regimen, as when the patient decides to test the notion of increasing an aspect of the regimen to see if even more improvement will occur.

The consequence of either increasing or decreasing the treatment may delay achieving treatment goals or cause harm to the patient. Having the patient focus on how the body feels during and after each clinic therapy session and expressing or discussing any likely harmful and positive changes and appropriate responses will help the patient make correct causal attributions and respond in a rational way to the change. Writing down the decision rules for modifying or stopping the recommended treatment will help structure the patient's experience and serve as a reference for future decisions.

Patients should know *what* physical changes the disease and the treatments are likely to cause, and they should also know *when* such changes are likely to occur (Bandura, 1986). When a patient modifies or quits a treatment, it is often related not only to the patient's belief of what the treatment is or is not doing but also to the time frame in which the patient believes the change should occur. If, in the patient's mind, he or she has an acute illness (that is, one that will improve in a short time), then the patient may abandon as ineffective a strengthening or stretching regimen that takes 4 or more weeks to produce positive benefits since the condition did not improve as quickly as an infection would have improved. Because every person is different in his or her response to treatment, the therapist can give a range that represents expert opinions on the time needed to respond. A related issue is discussing what the patient should do if the therapeutic goal is achieved before it is expected and before the next clinic visit. The risk is that patients may quit the treatment after proclaiming themselves well, and not realize that maintenance of the improvement depends on continued treatment.

Fourth, patients should know the "what if" rules needed to guide their decisions when changes in disease status or other unexpected changes occur (Bandura, 1986). This knowledge is rooted in the observations of others and in the patient's experience with how the treatment makes his or her body feel. Enough correct repetitions must occur in the clinic so that the patient knows how the activities make the muscles and joints feel during and immediately after the activities. This knowledge serves as the baseline standard against which the patient will compare future treatment activities. That is, if a future application of the activity produces more or less pain, fatigue, soreness, or swelling than previously, then the patient may interpret the symptom as good or bad and take action that is consistent with that judgment. For example, if there are more symptoms than experienced at baseline and the patient judges the change as bad, then he or she may decide to reduce, skip, stop temporarily, or quit the activity. This illustrates the importance of discussing at the first and subsequent visits the "what if" rules for modifying the treatment, that is, when do to more, less, stop, modify the treatment, or call the therapist. Using hypothetical scenarios to apply these rules will develop the patient's ability to make the correct decisions.

Patients must know what to do and why and when not to do something, and they must also be given supervised skill practice to learn how to perform the treatment correctly (Bandura, 1986). Sometimes this is merely learning to apply a source of heat or a splint to a joint; sometimes it involves the correct motions associated with stretching or strengthening exercises. It is not enough that the patient demonstrate correct form. The initiation and continuation of the treatment behavior over time is also related to the patient's confidence in his or her ability to do the behavior independently. This confidence is typically achieved by sufficient supervised practice and feedback until the patient feels confident to do it alone. Providing only unsupervised practice during the training period may allow the patient to practice incorrect form and does not give the patient reinforcement that the movement is correct.

DOMAIN 3: TREATMENT MOTIVATION

When patients do not follow their treatment, many therapists explain the behavior by saying the patient was not motivated. This is not a particularly helpful explanation because it does not provide much guidance on what action the therapist can take to enhance a patient's motivation. Several explanatory theories of motivation have been successfully applied to health behavior, including Bandura's Social Learning Theory (1986), Ajzen and Fishbein's Theory of Reasoned Action (1980), and Becker's Health Belief Model (1978). For this chapter, key concepts from Bandura's Social Learning Theory (1986) are discussed. Questions for assessing these concepts in patients are shown in Table 7.

ASSESSING TREATMENT MOTIVATION

FUNCTIONAL GOAL
What activity is most important for you to maintain or recover? On a 1-10 scale, how important is that activity to you? (This will identify a therapeutic goal and indicate how important it is to the patient. Generally, activities with higher scores will be more motivational than activities with low scores.)

FUNCTIONAL SUBGOALS
In order to reach the functional goal, what other behaviors are necessary to achieve the larger goal? (This helps ensure that the patient knows the connection between treatment activities and achieving the goal.)

SELF-EFFICACY
On a 1-10 scale, how certain are you that you can do your treatment activities at home as well as you did them in the clinic?
Why not? (If less than a 9 or 10, provide more practice and feedback.)

POSITIVE OUTCOME EXPECTATIONS
What are all the good things—physical, social, emotional—that are likely to occur if you follow your treatment and achieve the goal? Which are most important to you?

NEGATIVE-OUTCOME EXPECTATIONS
What are the worst things that will happen if you do this treatment? What are the worst things that will happen if you do not do this treatment? Do the negatives of not doing the treatment outweigh the negatives of doing the treatment? (This permits discussion of the reward/cost balance.)

Table 7: Assessing Patient Motivation for Treatment

A basic assumption of Bandura's theory is that behavior is a function of the interplay between the cognitive and behavioral capabilities of the individual and the physical and social environment in which the behavior occurs. The initiation and maintenance of behavior such as a patient's home treatment is regulated by the thoughts, knowledge, and emotions of the patient and influenced by the performance skills and the physical and social environments in which the behavior occurs. Desired behavior like treatment adherence is more likely if the environment is arranged to support the behavior and if the person has the knowledge, skills, beliefs, and values needed to initiate and sustain the behavior. Therapists can influence the patient's behavior by assisting with ensuring a supportive physical and social environment (see the section on Opportunity) and by encouraging the development and maintenance of the knowledge, skills, and beliefs needed to sustain the behavior. Since knowledge and performance skills were addressed in the previous sections, this section will address the beliefs that are related to the cognitive control of behavior.

GOALS

The first concept is the establishment of a specific, personal goal that influences a wide range of behavior (Bandura, 1986; Locke, Shaw, Saari, & Latham, 1981). Behavior is not random, it is purposive: some goal can usually be ascribed to it. Behavioral goals reflect an intention to bring about some future state, the desirability of which provides the incentive for the behavior. The incentive value of a goal is related to the desirability or importance of the goal. Treatment adherence is more likely if the patient is doing treatment work to achieve a highly valued functional goal, and each patient is likely to value something different. For example, by asking a patient what activity he or she would most like to maintain or recover, or what symptom he or she would most like to control, the response will be the goal to which the patient is most likely to work to achieve and toward which treatment should be directed. Achieving a goal requires a variety of patient self-management tools such as setting a time frame for achieving the goal, specifying subgoals that must be accomplished if the larger goal is to be reached, and defining the evaluative standards and feedback mechanisms for judging progress.

Most therapists understand the concept of staging in treatment planning. They understand that if the patient is to become functional in the kitchen, grip strength, shoulder range of motion, reaching balance, and other tasks need to be mastered first. If a therapist does not explain to the patient the connection between achieving these subgoals and achieving the patient's ultimate goal of working in the kitchen, then the treatment activities designed to achieve the subgoals will lose much or all of their incentive value. For example, most therapists-in-training know that passing each course in school (the subgoal) is a necessary step to graduating and becoming a practitioner (the goal). If a therapist does not understand this connection, the incentive to work to pass a course is very likely diminished. So it is important to discuss the subgoals needed to achieve the patient's functional goal and to list on the patient's treatment log these subgoals, the length of time needed to achieve each, and the indicators of progress. The log not only provides the therapist with adherence information but also helps the patient's self-management (Nelson, 1977). After the first visit in which the treatment plan is developed, subsequent visits with the therapist focus on the patient's progress relative to the plan, discussion and solving of problems the patient encountered in following the plan, and possibly modification of the plan in light of the progress or new problems.

EXISTENTIAL CRISIS

Sometimes patients are unable to identify any goals and exhibit feelings of anger, despair, or hopelessness that suggest having given up. They display no interest in or willingness to do any home treatment. These patients should be evaluated for depression and their physician contacted regarding treatment. Even if treated for depression, some may be experiencing an existential crisis related to their inability to do the activities that gave life meaning and purpose. Clearly these patients represent a great challenge to the therapist, but there are some strategies the therapist can try. One is to refer the patient to a psychologist or pastoral counselor and/or to a community support program until the patient is ready to follow a home treatment. The second is to complete an evaluation to determine the combination of functional improvements and adaptations that are possible that could permit resumption of one or more of the patient's valued activities. Assuming that some functional improvements or adaptations are possible, then the therapist can try to persuade, challenge, or negotiate with the patient to accept the resumption of the activity as the treatment goal with explicit short-term indicators of progress toward the goals. Use of a patient contract and support mechanisms like periodic phone calls from the clinic have proven helpful (Maisiak, Koplon, & Heck, 1989; Weinberger, Tierney, Booker, & Hiner, 1989).

One approach to helping a patient identify a desired activity is to ask the patient to create a detailed mental image of himself or herself doing the activities he or she would most like to do without being constrained by the condition. The imagined activities are shared with the therapist and discussed as to the possibility of recovering enough function to participate in the activity. If the physical damage has been so severe that possibilities for recovering important activities are very limited, then the challenge to identify a meaningful goal is greater. Important resources include encouragement from family and friends, the therapist's empathetic listening and reflection to clarify the patient's thinking, and exposure to other severely limited individuals who have found other ways of identifying meaning and purpose. These may include the patient's realization that his or her family needs him or her, the desire to participate in the maturation process of his or her children, the opportunity to express himself or herself creatively, the need to discover and fulfill a religious purpose, or to serve as a role model for others in a similar situation by organizing ways of helping others. Such redefinitions of a patient's purpose can provide the incentive for any treatment activities. These transformations may take more than just a few visits; but by taking the time to ask and listen to the patient, the therapist can suggest ideas or make referrals to other health professionals or self-help programs to facilitate an eventual transformation. The Arthritis Foundation's Self-Help course has demonstrated success in decreasing pain, depression, and physician visits for up to 20 months (Radloff, 1977; see chapter 10 on Patient Education and chapter 17 on Community Resources).

SELF-EFFICACY

A second important concept is self-efficacy, which is a patient's confidence in his or her ability to perform the specific tasks needed to achieve a goal. This includes confidence in his or her ability to regulate thoughts, emotions, and physical and social environments in order to perform the specific behaviors needed to attain a goal (Bandura, 1986). Persons with high confidence in their ability to perform their treatment are more likely to initiate it and persist in the face of obstacles, while persons with low confidence are less likely to initiate the behavior or persist as long (Strecher, DeVellis, Becker, & Rosenstock, 1986). This makes intuitive sense to anyone who has tried to learn a new skill such as a sport and struggled with the inevitable feelings of uncertainty before achieving mastery. Those who quit before mastery often do so because they lack confidence in their ability to master the treatment behavior. Many people, for example, will stop an aerobics program before learning to do it correctly because they are not confident that they can master the routine.

The therapist's task is to develop the patient's confidence in his or her ability to do the treatment at home under the physical, social, and emotional constraints of the home environment. While clinic practice is the most powerful way to make the patient feel confident about doing the behavior in the clinic, that confidence does not necessarily generalize to the home. To develop this confidence, practice opportunities need to be offered that reflect the constraints imposed by the home environment, if possible. Many therapists will teach exercises to patients not using the clinic equipment but the materials the patient will actually use at home. Ideally, the choice of equipment should be adapted to the patient's home, physical, and social environments. The idea is to develop the patient's confidence in the ability to do the treatment regimen under conditions that mimic those at home as much as possible. In addition to practice opportunities, patients develop self-efficacy beliefs by observing others like themselves and performing similar behaviors or by receiving positive appraisals of their ability from others deemed credible by the patient like, for example, the therapist or a successful, experienced patient. Thus, watching and talking to other successful patients who have mastered the behavior can both increase the patient's confidence and enhance his or her belief in the value of the treatment for reaching the goal.

EXPECTED AND IMMEDIATE CONSEQUENCES

While self-efficacy refers to the person's beliefs about his or her ability to perform a behavior, outcome expectancies refer to the person's beliefs about the immediate or long-term positive and negative consequences of the behavior (Bandura, 1986). The goal provides incentive, and the power of the goal to motivate behavior is enhanced or diminished by the positive and negative consequences of the behavior needed to achieve the goal. For example, if the patient believes that the negative consequences (costs) of achieving the goal are greater than the positive outcomes (benefits), a person may give up, concluding that "it just isn't worth it." The therapist needs to work to try to minimize the negative consequences of doing the treatment while maximizing the positive consequences. One way of discussing this with the patient is to ask the patient to write down all the likely positive and negative consequences of doing a home treatment. Typical negative consequences are pain or other side effects, no treatment benefit, the time it takes, discomfort, expense, inconvenience, boredom, slow progress, or giving up another valued activity like watching television (Sluijs et al., 1993; Taal et al., 1993). Positive consequences may be reduced pain, resumption of valued activities, reduced use of medication, attention and approval from family or friends, improved function, and positive feelings of accomplishment. Once these likely positive and negative consequences are expressed, the therapist and patient can identify ways to reduce the negative consequences and increase the positive ones. The motivational principle is to try to maintain the balance in favor of the positive consequences. The therapist must be vigilant for shifts in the consequences, that is, what was initially a positive consequence, like feeling energized after exercise, might become a negative one in the future. For example, the patient may have trouble sleeping because of being energized by the exercise. If adherence is a problem, the therapist may want to review the positive and negative consequences discussed at the previous visit to see if they have changed value.

In addition, the patient's motivation can be enhanced and the desired behavior increased by adding rewards such as attention and praise from the therapist or spouse, money or other material objects, being able to do valued activities in response to doing the treatment, or accomplishing functional subgoals (Kirshenbaum & Flannery, 1983). These motivational rewards can be built into the treatment plan. At the next visit, the success of the rewards for encouraging adherence behavior is discussed with the possibility of their modification. The discussion of the positive and negative consequences will be ongoing, since people change as do their physical and social surroundings. For example, daily quadriceps exercises are likely to become sufficiently boring and cause the patient to quit. Thus, minimizing the negative consequences can be achieved by introducing variety, regimen changes, or distractions. Even if the patient is motivated, the resources to support implementing the home program must exist.

DOMAIN 4: TREATMENT OPPORTUNITY

The final domain is the opportunity to carry out the regimen. Patients cannot follow a regimen for which they do not have the resources or if the treatment is opposed by others. While this is the last domain to be discussed, it is one that always should be evaluated at the first visit. Just as it is a mistake for a physician to prescribe a medication that the patient cannot afford, a therapist must not ask a patient to do home treatments for which he or she does not have the resources. Table 8 summarizes assessment questions for determining the existence of the resources needed to do the treatment. Treatment opportunity involves such resources as having time to do the regimen, availability and affordability of any equipment like comfortable walking shoes or weights, availability of space or the convenience of the location at which the treatment occurs, and other aspects of the physical environment like temperature, noise, and accessibility to people with handicaps. In addition, supportive people must be available for some treatments that require the participation of another person. This information can be obtained at the first visit. The potential barriers should be discussed with the patient to identify and select solutions, including modifying the treatment. While this may mean that the treatment is not optimal, at least it will be possible.

ASSESSING TREATMENT OPPORTUNITY

TIME	When during the day or evening could you most easily fit in your treatment activities?
EQUIPMENT	Do you have the needed equipment? What difficulties would you have obtaining them?
SPACE	What kind of space do you have for doing your treatment? Are there problems using it, such as scheduling, distractions, or distance?
SUPPORTIVE OTHERS	Will anyone be around to help you in case you need it?

Table 8: Assessing Factors that Influence Treatment Adherence

SUMMARY

Patients do more or less of their home treatment, stop temporarily, substitute, or quit because they choose to or because they make mistakes. Mistakes can be the result of forgetting, ignorance, or incomplete knowledge of what to do. Patients choose not to adhere because they are not sufficiently motivated and knowledgeable, they are overwhelmed by psychological distress such as depression, fear, and denial, or they knew about the treatment and how to do it but lacked the resources needed to fulfill the treatment opportunity. In addition, both mistakes and choices to adhere can be influenced for good or ill by the patient's relationships with the therapist, family, or other persons important to the patient.

While it is impossible to specify from research or theory which of these reasons is most influential generally, much less for a specific patient, the approach for working with patients that is consistent with therapists' training is to assume that any one or combination of these reasons can promote either adherence or nonadherence. A therapist must probe the patient's perspective to determine the most salient reasons for both adherence and nonadherence. Education, problem solving, persuasion, and negotiation are used to decrease the reasons for nonadherence while increasing the reasons for adherence.

Identifying functional activities that the patient wants to maintain or recover and educating the patient about how the treatment will help achieve necessary functional goals provide powerful incentives for adherence. One frequently powerful goal is the desire of most adults to maintain their independence so as not to burden others. By exploring with the patient which daily tasks are critical for maintaining independence, one or more activities will emerge that can be used as therapy goals.

In addition, attention to minimizing the negative consequences of the treatment while trying to maximize the positive consequences, including rewards, will strengthen adherence motivation. The point is that only by working with the patient's perspective in an ongoing process of assessment and problem solving focused on specific adherence influences can therapists improve the likelihood that patients will follow their home treatment. Change is difficult, but it does occur, and that keeps hope alive.

REFERENCES

Ajzen, I., & Fishbein, M. (1980). *Understanding attitudes and predicting social behavior.* Englewood Cliffs, NJ: Prentice-Hall.

American Psychiatric Association. (1995). *Diagnostic and statistical manual of mental disorders* (4th ed.). Washington, DC: American Psychiatric Press.

Andersson, K., Bradley, L., Young, L. D., McDaniel, L. K., & Wise, C. M. (1985). Rheumatoid arthritis: Review of psychological factors related to etiology, effects, and treatment. *Psychology Bulletin, 98,* 358-387.

Bandura, A. (1986). *Social foundations of thought and action: A social cognitive theory.* Englewood Cliffs, NJ: Prentice-Hall.

Beck, A., & Steer, R. (1987). *Manual for the revised Beck Depression Inventory.* San Antonio, TX: Psychological Corporation.

Becker, M. H. (1978). The health belief model and sick role behavior. *Nursing Digest,* 35-40.

Beisser, A. R. (1979). Denial and affirmation in illness and health. *American Journal of Psychiatry, 136,* 1026-1030.

Blalock, S., DeVellis, R., Brown, G. K., & Wallston, K. A. (1989). Validity of the Center For Epidemiological Studies Depression Scale in arthritis opulations. *Arthritis and Rheumatism, 32,* 991-997.

Blalock, S., & DeVellis, R. (1993). Rheumatoid arthritis and depression: An overview. *Bulletin of Rheumatic Diseases, 41,* 6-8.

Burns, D. (1989). *The feeling good handbook.* New York: William Morrow.

Cohen-Cole, S. (1991). *The medical interviews: The three-function approach.* St. Louis, MO: Mosby-Year Book.

DiMatteo, M. R., & DiNicola, D. D. (1982). *Achieving patient compliance: The psychology of the medical practitioners role.* New York: Pergamon Press.

Donovan, J., Blake, D., & Fleming, W. (1989). The patient is not a blank sheet: Lay beliefs and their relevance to patient education. *British Journal of Rheumatology, 28,* 58-61.

Dunbar, J., & Agras, W. (1980). Compliance with medical instructions. In J. M. Ferguson & C. B. Taylor (Eds.), *Comprehensive handbook of behavioral medicine.* New York: Spectrum.

Egan, G. (1986). *The skilled helper: A systematic approach to effective helping* (3rd ed.). Pacific Grove, CA: Brooks/Cole Publishing.

Feinberg, J., & Brandt, K. D. (1981). Use of resting splints by patients with rheumatoid arthritis. *American Journal of Occupational Therapy, 35,* 173-178.

Francis, V., Korsch, B., & Morris, M. (1969). Gaps in doctor-patient communication: Patients' response to medical advice. *The New England Journal of Medicine, 280,* 535-540.

Frank, R., Beck, N. C., Parker, J. C., Kashani, J., Elliot, T., Haut, A., Smith, E., Artwood, C., Brownlee-Duffeck, M., & Kay, D. (1988). Depression in rheumatoid arthritis. *Journal of Rheumatology, 15,* 920-925.

Heszen-Klemens, I., & Lapinska, E. (1984). Doctor-patient interactions: Patients' health behavior, and effects on treatment. *Social Science & Medicine, 19,* 217-221.

Kanfer, F. H. (1980). Self-management methods. In F. H. Kanfer & A. P. Goldstein (Eds.), *Helping people change: A textbook of methods* (pp. 334-389). New York: Pergamon Press.

Katz, P., & Yelin, E. (1993). Prevalence and correlates of depressive symptoms among persons with rheumatoid arthritis. *Journal of Rheumatology, 20,* 790-796.

Kirshenbaum, D., & Flannery, R. (1983). Behavioral contracting: Outcomes and elements. In M. Hersen, R. Eisler, & P. Miller (Eds.), *Progress in behavior modification.* New York: Academic Press.

Leventhal, H., & Cameron, L. (1987). Behavioral theories and the problem of compliance. *Patient Education and Counseling, 10,* 117-138.

Leventhal, H., Zimmerman, R., & Gutmann, M. (1984). Compliance: self-regulation perspective. In W. D. Gentry (Ed.), *Handbook of behavioral medicine* (pp. 369-436). New York: The Guilford Press.

Levine, J., Rudy, T., & Kerns, R. (1994). A two factor model of denial of illness: A confirmatory factor analysis. *Journal of Psychosomatic Research, 38*(2), 99-110.

Locke, E., Shaw, K., Saari, L., & Latham, G. (1981). Goal setting and task performance: 1969-1980. *Psychology Bulletin, 90,* 125-152.

Lorig, K., & Fries, J. (1990). *The arthritis helpbook* (3rd ed.). Reading, MA: Addison-Wesley.

Lorish, C. D., Richards, B., & Brown, S. A. (1989). Missed medication doses in rheumatic arthritis patients: Intentional and unintentional reasons. *Arthritis Care and Research, 2*(1), 3-10.

Maisiak, R., Koplon, S., & Heck, L. (1989). Subsequent behavior of users of an arthritis information telephone service. *Arthritis and Rheumatism, 33,* 212-218.

Malouin, F., Potvin, M., Prevost, J., Richards, C., & Wood-Dauphinee, S. (1992). Use of an intensive task-oriented gait training program In a series of patients with acute cerebrovascular accidents. *Physical Therapy, 72,* 781-793.

Marlatt, G. A., & George, W. H. (1990). Relapse prevention and the maintenance of optimal health. In S. A. Shumaker, E. B. Schron, & J. B. Ockene (Eds.), *The handbook of health behavior change* (pp. 44-63). New York: Springer Publishing Company.

Miller, W., & Rollnick, S. (1991). *Motivational interviewing: Preparing people to change addictive behavior.* New York: The Guilford Press.

Moon, M. H., Moon, B. A., & Black, W. A. (1976). Compliance in splint-wearing behavior of patients with rheumatoid arthritis. *New Zealand Medical Journal, 83,* 360-365.

Nelson, R. (1977). Assessment and therapeutic functions of self-monitoring. In M. Hersen, R. Eisler, & P. Miller (Eds.), *Progress in behavior modification.* New York: Academic Press.

Ness, D., & Ende, J. (1994). Denial in the medical interview: Recognition and management. *Journal of the American Medical Association, 272,* 1777-1782.

Parker, J. C., McRae, C., Smarr, K., Beck, N. C., Frank, R., & Anderson, S. (1988). Coping strategies in rheumatoid arthritis. *Journal of Rheumatology, 15,* 1376-1383.

Parker, L. B., & Bender, L. (1957). Problem of home treatment in arthritis. *Archives of Physical Medicine and Rehabilitation, 38,* 392-394.

Patrick, D., Morgan, M., & Charlton, J. (1986). Psychosocial support and change in health status of physically disabled people. *Social Science & Medicine, 22,* 1347-1354.

Pennebaker, J. (1982). *The psychology of physical symptoms.* New York: Springer-Verlag.

Pitzele, S. (1986). *We are not alone: Learning to live with chronic illness.* New York: Workman Publishing.

Pollin, I., & Golant, S. (1994). *Taking charge: Overcoming the challenges of long-term illness.* New York: Times Books.

Pollock, M. L., Carroll, J. F., Graves, J. E., Leggett, S. H., Braith, R. W., Limacher, M., & Hagberg, J. M. (1991). Injuries and adherence to walk/jog and resistance training programs in the elderly. *Medicine & Science in Sports & Exercise, 23,* 1194-1200.

Radloff, L. (1977). The CES-D Scale: A self report depression scale for research with the general population. *Applied Psychological Measurement, 1,* 385-401.

Revenson, T. A., Schiaffino, K., Majerovitz, S., & et.al. (1991). Social support as a double-edged sword: The relation of positive and problematic support to depression among rheumatoid arthritis patients. *Social Science & Medicine, 33,* 807-813.

Roter, D., Hall, J., & Katz, N. (1987). Relations between physicians' behaviors and analogue patient's satisfaction, recall, and impressions. *Medical Care, 25,* 437-451.

Rush, A. (1993). *Depression in primary care: Detection, diagnosis, and treatment.* (93-0552 ed.). Silver Spring, MD: Agency for Health Care Policy and Research.

Russell, G. C. (1993). The role of denial in clinical practice. *Journal of Advanced Nursing, 18,* 938-940.

Samuelsson, A., Ahlmen, M., & Sullivan, M. (1993). The rheumatic patient's early needs and expectations. *Patient Education and Counseling, 20.*

Schwartz, L. (1988). A biopsychosocial approach to the management of the diabetic patient. *Primary Care, 15*, 409-421.

Shelp, E. E., & Perl, M. (1985). Denial in clinical medicine: A reexamination of the concept and its significance. *Archives of Internal Medicine, 145*, 697-699.

Sluijs, E. M., Kok, G. J., & Van der Zee, J. (1993). Correlates of exercise compliance in physical therapy. *Physical Therapy, 73*, 771-786.

Speedling, E., & Rose, D. (1985). Building an effective doctor-patient relationship: From patient satisfaction to patient participation. *Social Science & Medicine, 21*, 115-120.

Steptoe, A., Sutcliffe, I., Allen, B., & Coombes, C. (1991). Satisfaction with communication, medical knowledge, and coping style in patients with metastatic cancer. *Social Science & Medicine, 32*, 627-632.

Strain, J. (1979). Psychological reactions to chronic medical illness. *Psychiatric Quarterly, 51*, 173-183.

Strecher, V., DeVellis, B., Becker, M., & Rosenstock, I. (1986). The role of self-efficacy in achieving health behavior change. *Health Education Quarterly, 13*, 73-92.

Taal, E., Rasker, J., Seydel, E., & Wiegman, O. (1993). Health status, adherence with health recommendations, self-efficacy and social support in patients with rheumatoid arthritis. *Patient Education and Counseling, 20*, 63-76.

Taleff, M. (1994). The well deserved death of denial: Is it time to let go of this cherished concept. *Behavioral Health Management, 14*, 51-53.

Tuckett, D., Boulton, M., Olson, C., & Williams, A. (1985). *Meetings between experts.* New York: Tavistock Publications.

Tyner, R. (1985). Elements of empathic care for dying patients and their families. *Nursing Clinics of North America, 20*, 393-401.

Walker, A. (1995). Patient compliance and the placebo effect. *Physiotherapy, 81*(3), 120-126.

Weinberger, M., Tierney, W., Booker, P., & Hiner, S. (1989). Can the provision of information to patients with osteoarthritis improve functional status? A randomized, controlled trial. *Arthritis and Rheumatism, 32*, 1577-1583.

Zung, W. W. K. (1996). Self-rating depression scale (SRDS). Indianapolis, IN: Eli Lilley.

4 CLINICAL OUTCOMES: ISSUES AND MEASUREMENT

Donna J. Hawley, MN, EdD, RN

INTRODUCTION

Historically, health care has been offered by a variety of practitioners whose methods and interventions were unquestioned and treatment outcomes unchallenged. The very early connections with religious groups allowed health care practitioners to practice in a safe and cloistered environment. Even in the 20th century, when health care practices came under the scrutiny of the scientific community, practitioners remained apart from outside economic and even political pressures. Practitioners were considered altruistic and health care was "sacred." However, within the last 25 years health care has moved to the business world and faces contemporary economic realities (Hegyvary, 1991).

Relman, in an editorial in the *New England Journal of Medicine* in the late 1980s, described three stages of medical care: expansion, cost containment, and accountability (Relman, 1988). The age of expansion began soon after the close of World War Two and continued to the late 1960s. This era saw growth in all types of services, new and bigger hospitals, almost unlimited third party payments, passage of Medicare and Medicaid laws, and increased specialization among physicians. In the early 1970s, inflation as well as 20 years of rapid growth in the health care system ushered in the inevitable questions related to cost containment. The 1980s saw the development and growth of prospective payment, managed care, diagnosis related groups, and health maintenance organizations (HMOs). Closely tied to cost containment is the third stage, the era of assessment and accountability. This stage involves determining what Relman calls the successes and failures of medical care. Expanding this concept to the full range of health care services, the era of identifying, defining, and assessing the effectiveness (i.e., outcomes) of various health care services is upon us.

Policy makers, third party payers, consumer-patients, and professionals are all questioning health care delivery. Although each group may look at health care services from a slightly different perspective, each pursues evidence documenting the effectiveness of services rendered. Professionals desire data that identify the interventions that are the most beneficial for patients. Consumers want the best care for themselves and their families, often without regard to cost. Third party payers and public policy makers demand effective care delivered at the least possible cost. The common thread from each of these perspectives is effectiveness of care. Effectiveness in any field including health care is determined by looking at the results of what is done. Outcomes are the end result of care and interventions, the clinical changes that have an impact on the incidence and natural course of disease.

OUTCOMES AND QUALITY

Outcomes naturally relate to the quality of the care provided; however, quality of care must be viewed in a broader context than just the outcome of disease or even the outcomes of specific treatments. In Donabedian's classic paper (Donabedian, 1966), which was expanded in the late 1980s (Donabedian, 1988), he described the relationship between outcomes and quality of care. He discussed three areas that could be used to assess medical care quality. Again assuming that medical care includes all health care services, his model illustrates how clinical outcomes fit into the total evaluation of health care services. Outcome is only one aspect of quality care; the other components that contribute to quality are structure and process.

Structure includes the various settings for health care delivery. Material resources (e.g., equipment, physical facilities, and finances) and human resources (i.e., personnel including types, numbers, and qualifications) are major structural components. Also included is the organizational structure or the procedures and policies that permit the utilization of the material and human resources (Donabedian, 1988).

Process is the actual provision of care. Donabedian emphasizes that the process includes not only the services of health care practitioners but also efforts provided by the patient and his or her family. Community or societal resources that permit access to care are included in this category. The efforts of patient, family, and community as well as practitioners affect the clinical outcome (Donabedian, 1988).

The final category is outcome, or the effects of care on the health of individuals and populations (Donabedian, 1988). The quality of the total structure including human and material resources, the efforts by those asking for and receiving care, and the support of the society and community are all important in the eventual outcome. In the final analysis, the ultimate outcome for health care services, from preventive care to complex medical interventions, is the improvement in health or health-related quality of life for individuals and for the population. In this chapter the author discusses only the measurement and evaluation of the outcomes of care, and she fully recognizes that quality care is a complex interaction of structure and process as well as outcomes.

DEFINITIONS

Before reviewing the measurement of outcomes, the major terms used in discussing outcomes need to be defined. Quality of life, health-related quality of life (HRQL), health status, and functional status all have been considered in defining the effects of dis-

OUTCOMES OF DISEASE AND TREATMENT
DEFINITION OF TERMS

QUALITY OF LIFE
A comprehensive term describing total well-being. Various elements unrelated to an individual's health such as sewage treatment, water purification, adequate housing, crime, and educational opportunities influence quality of life. Each person defines quality of life in terms of personal priorities and preferences (Gill & Feinstein, 1994).

HEALTH-RELATED QUALITY OF LIFE (HRQL)
The degree to which one meets the World Health Organization's definition of health: "A state of complete physical, mental, and social well-being and not merely the absence of disease or infirmity" (World Health Organization, 1958). In clinical practice and research, the term is the aggregate effects of disease on the individual's life (Liang, 1987).

FUNCTIONAL STATUS
Functional status is the ability to do the usual daily self-care activities including both basic activities of daily living (ADL) and instrumental activities of daily living (IADL).

HEALTH STATUS
Essentially the same as HRQL. The two terms are frequently used interchangeably. Health status (or HRQL) includes both functional status plus other aspects of health such as emotions and mood, symptoms (e.g., pain, sleep disturbance, fatigue), cognitive abilities, and social activities and roles (Froberg & Kane, 1989).

Table 1: Outcomes of Disease and Treatment: Definition of Terms

ease and its treatment. Each is considered a major or even global outcome of disease and treatments. Table 1 provides definition of the terms. In this chapter, health status and HRQL are considered to be synonymous, and health status will be used.

ISSUES IN MEASUREMENT OF OUTCOMES

When measuring outcomes of interventions, five issues are prominent. These issues include levels of measurement, timing of measurement, cause and effect linkages, variables to be measured, and selection of appropriate measurement instruments.

LEVELS OF MEASUREMENT: INDIVIDUAL VERSUS SOCIETY

Outcome may be studied from several levels ranging from large societal outcome studies to the effects of specific treatments for individuals and groups. Studies at the societal level examine major public-health problems and look at outcomes such as mortality, functional status, well-being, direct costs of providing required health care services, and disability. Emphasis is placed on costs, both as direct disability payments and the more indirect costs incurred from losses in productivity. The medical outcome study (MOS) is an example of a study at the societal level. Described by Stewart and colleagues, this study compared ". . . physicians' practice styles and patients' outcomes in competing systems of care" (Stewart et al., 1989). Both cross-sectional and longitudinal data are available from this study of 22,462 participants.

Another example of large outcome studies is the patient outcomes research team (PORT). PORTs are federally funded outcome research centers started in 1989 by the Agency for Health Policy Research. They examine outcomes for common health problems that are costly both in human and economic terms. The original 14 teams included studies ranging from low birth weight to schizophrenia to back pain, knee replacements, and hip fractures (Anonymous, 1996). Additional studies were funded in 1993. The second phase was designed to examine outcomes as a result of alternative therapies. Diverse areas of study ranged from breast cancer to depression care (Anonymous, 1996).

In addition to these major studies, clinical trials of medications, new medical devices, or psychoeducational interventions look at the group and individual levels of outcome. Multicenter studies of second-line medications or nonsteroidal antiinflammatory drugs (NSAIDs) have provided information about treatment outcomes for individuals with rheumatoid arthritis (Bombardier & Raboud, 1991; Felson, Anderson, & Meenan, 1992). Long-term outcome studies have provided information about work and functional disability in a variety of rheumatic disorders (Wolfe, 1995a).

Individual clinicians may keep outcome data about their patients. A therapist may compare changes in pain following the use of a particular splint or look at functional outcomes following physical therapy. Investigators may examine length of stay and functional ability following joint-replacement surgery at either a single hospital or several different facilities.

Outcomes may be examined at the societal, group, and individual levels. In the rheumatic disorders, long-term outcome studies may examine functional status and work disability for individuals and groups of patients. The annual use of medical care services (hospitalizations, surgeries, medical visits) and mortality after many years of disease are important at the societal level (Pincus, Brooks, & Callahan, 1994; Wolfe et al., 1994). Each level of investigation provides important information about treatment outcomes that collectively will provide the basis for major health care policy as well as for clinical decisions.

TIMING OF THE MEASUREMENT

Determination of the end point or the time for measuring the outcome varies with the question under consideration. For example, the outcome for joint-replacement surgery may be evaluated at several different times depending on the specific outcome of interest. The outcome related to improvement in pain may be determined in the recovery room. The effects of physical therapy may be evaluated as changes in mobility and function of the operated joint at hospital discharge or a few weeks after. Changes in overall functional ability may best be evaluated several months following surgery.

Another example will illustrate this same point. When evaluating psychoeducational interventions, outcomes such as increase in knowledge, changes in pain or depression, or improvement in self-efficacy may be assessed immediately after the interventions. Maintenance of improvements in knowledge, pain, depression, and self-efficacy is also necessary in determining the effectiveness of these interventions. Long-term outcome measurement is as important as, or perhaps more important than, outcomes assessed immediately following an intervention. Lorig and colleagues have demonstrated that important effects on health status may be maintained for several months or even years following these types of interventions (Lorig, Mazonson, & Holman, 1993). Such studies validate that psychoeducational interventions are effective for the long term and not just for an immediate and temporary period. Convincing third party payers to participate in such interventions is enhanced with long-term outcome studies.

The time for measuring the outcome of any treatment is very different for acute compared to chronic diseases. Donabedian (1988) presents a model for looking at the outcome of acute, self-limited disease based on the treatment. As shown in Figure 1-A, in an acute, self-limited disease, individuals return to their preillness health status with or without treatment. The purpose of treatment, then, is either to return the person to normal health in a shorter time than would occur with the natural course of disease, or to reduce the seriousness of the illness. Outcome measurements look at disease severity and duration of illness in relationship to the return to the individual's preillness status.

In a progressive, chronic disease such as rheumatoid arthritis, the aim of treatment is to decrease disease severity to prevent, or at least delay, a decline in health. Return to full health may be feasible during the course of the disease; however, over time the goal is minimizing the decline. Figure 1-B illustrates this point. For example, in rheumatoid arthritis, although the disease trajectory is uncertain, functional health declines over time with or without treatment. Interventions occur along the normal course of the disease and are designed to improve health, often temporarily, and to slow the decline. An intervention such as a cane or specially designed eating utensil may improve or stabilize function for a time, although the pathophysiological damage remains unchanged or may increase. Certain medications such as methotrexate may actually alter pathology. Psychoeducational interventions reduce pain and depression and improve self-efficacy but do not have a major effect on function (Hawley, 1995). Joint replacements improve function and control pain even while the disease may continue to progress in other joints or systemically. For these reasons, measurement of outcome in chronic diseases must occur at several points along the disease continuum. Determination of the time to measure the outcome of a specific intervention is difficult and remains a major issue in ongoing outcomes research.

CAUSE AND EFFECT LINKAGES: ATTRIBUTION OF OUTCOMES TO INTERVENTIONS

Closely related to the appropriate timing of outcome measurement are causal linkages between treatment and the outcomes (Hegyvary, 1991). Attribution of outcome is more than the timing of measurement. It also involves isolating the effects of interven-

MODEL DEPICTING OUTCOME FOR AN ACUTE, SELF-LIMITING DISEASE

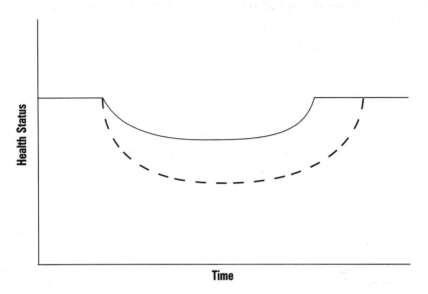

Figure 1-A. This graph depicts the course of an acute, self-limited disease with and without intervention. The dotted line depicts the outcome of such a disease if untreated. The solid line depicts the outcome for the same disease if treatment is provided. In both situations full health status is achieved; however, with treatment the time to full health status is shorter and the disease is less severe. Adapted from Donabedian (1988). Reprinted with permission.

MODEL DEPICTING OUTCOME FOR A CHRONIC, PROGRESSIVE DISEASE SUCH AS RHEUMATOID ARTHRITIS

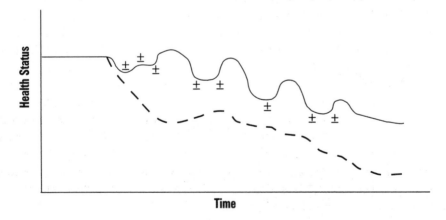

Figure 1-B. This graph depicts the course of a chronic, progressive disease such as rheumatoid arthritis, with and without intervention. The dotted line depicts the outcome of such a disease if untreated: Health continues to decline. The solid line depicts the outcome for the same disease if treatment is provided at various times. In both situations health continues to decline; however, with treatment the decline is slowed, and health even improves at various times following treatments. The plus symbols indicate hypothetical interventions that improve and slow the decline in health status. Outcome measurement should be done at appropriate times following interventions in order to demonstrate the effectiveness of interventions.

tions from other factors that are important in determining outcomes. Two areas are particularly important.

First, numerous factors other than an intervention can affect the outcome, including individual motivation, socioeconomic factors, and demographic characteristics. Family and community support have an important impact on disease outcome. In clinical trials, random assignment to treatment and control groups controls for these individual differences. Comprehensive studies with sample sizes sufficient to permit statistical controls for such differences may be used in long-term observational studies where randomization is not possible. Even with sophisticated statistical analyses, the interaction among individual characteristics, social support, and interventions presents major considerations in outcome research.

The second area relates to the independent effect or causal links between treatments and outcome, especially for those interventions separate from surgery or medications. The issue is particularly appropriate for consideration by nonphysician health care providers. Improvement in pain and function following joint-replacement surgery has a strong causal link. Clinical trials and long-term observational studies have confirmed that second-line medications are causally linked to improvement for rheumatoid arthritis patients. However, the causal links and contributing effects of professional-patient interaction, psychoeducational interventions, the team or multidisciplinary approach, nursing care, and certain physical therapy interventions to health status changes are more difficult to verify, and validation studies are limited. Two examples related to psychoeducational interventions and multidisciplinary care exemplify this issue.

In clinical trials of various psychoeducational interventions, participants have shown improvement in outcome variables such as pain, psychological well-being, and knowledge, and limited changes in behavior such as adherence with exercise, joint protection, and relaxation (Daltroy, 1992; Daltroy & Liang, 1991; Daltroy & Liang, 1993; Holman & Lorig, 1987). However, the magnitude of improvement is small (Hawley, 1995; Mullen, Laville, Biddle, & Lorig, 1987). Interventions are not standardized. Skill and personality of those conducting programs may be strongly related to the study result. It is not clear what component of a complex psychoeducational intervention contributes to the outcome. Medical interventions occurring simultaneously with the psychoeducational intervention are a major factor that is often not evaluated (Hawley, 1995). Likewise, when evaluating a medical intervention, the contributions of educational programs are not considered in the analyses. Although well-received and valued by patients and professionals alike, additional research is needed to document the causal, independent links of psychoeducational interventions and outcome.

The multidisciplinary approach to delivery of care for persons with rheumatic disorders is another illustration of the importance of the attribution of outcome to intervention. Yelin (1991, p. 1648) pointed out that health professionals have not appropriately evaluated multidisciplinary care or, in his words, determined "what is inside the team care box." While the multidisciplinary approach and improvement in outcome for patients with rheumatoid arthritis have been shown to be related, the relationship remains unclear (Ahlmen, Bjelle, & Sullivan, 1991; Raspe, Deck, & Mattussek, 1992; Vlieland,

Zwinderman, Vandenbroucke, Breedveld, & Hazes, 1995). Is outcome changed by individual activities, the combination of activities, the attention effect, or the gestalt of the multidisciplinary approach (Yelin, 1991)? Recent threats to team care, both in the United States and Europe (Anderson, Needleman, Gatter, Andrews, & Scarola, 1988; Lambert et al., 1994; Scott, Long, & Silman, 1995) indicate that a systematic analysis (Boyle & Decoufle, 1990) of multidisciplinary care is still most relevant.

VARIABLES TO BE MEASURED

To measure health status, the term must be divided into subcomponents and the subcomponents operationally defined. Fries has developed a model that is one logical and useful way to categorize clinical outcomes (Fries & Spitz, 1990). He calls the model a hierarchy of outcomes. The model begins with the global outcome and becomes more specific as one moves down the hierarchy to the various subdimensions that constitute health status. Fries identifies five components to global outcome including mortality, disability, discomfort or symptoms, iatrogenic problems, and economic issues. As shown in Figure 2, these areas are consistent with various definitions of health status and also reflect the areas that are important to patients. As described by Fries, surveys and interviews indicate that in the long term, people ". . . desire to be alive as long as possible; to function normally, to be free of pain and other physical and psychological or social symptoms; to be free of iatrogenic problems from the treatment regimen, and remain solvent" (Fries & Spitz, 1990, p. 26).

Each subdimension, with the exception of mortality, may be further subdivided into specific components. In Figure 2, subcomponents have been added to reflect important areas within the chronic rheumatic disorders. Again, the model is one way for organizing and planning the measurement of outcomes. Clinicians and investigators may select specific outcomes under each subdimension, depending on the purpose of the measurement. For example, in a clinical trial of a hand splint for a patient with rheumatoid arthritis, the outcome measure may be pain, hand function, costs, and patient satisfaction. On the other hand, long-term outcome studies of patients with rheumatoid arthritis may measure mortality, work and functional disability, pain, depression, medical visits per year, and drug side-effects. According to Fries, the goal is to do comprehensive assessment and in longitudinal studies to look at "cumulative assessment of treatment impact" (Fries & Spitz, 1990, p. 28)

SELECTION OF APPROPRIATE MEASUREMENT INSTRUMENTS

Assessment of outcome supplements the standard examination methods that include health history, physical examination, laboratory tests, and radiography. These standard assessments provide information about the current disease status and thus in one sense they may be indicators of outcome. The erythrocyte sedimentation rate (ESR), tender joint counts, and X-rays provide evidence about the pathology. The ESR and tender joint counts provide indications of outcomes in short-term medical situations and in clinical trials. X-rays demonstrate joint damage as a result of disease progression. These approaches

A HIERARCHICAL MODEL FOR OUTCOMES

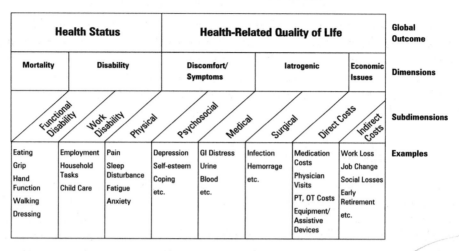

Figure 2. This figure illustrates the subdimensions of health status or health-related quality of life. There are five major subdimensions that comprise health status. These major categories may be further divided. As one moves down the hierarchy, outcomes become more specific and measurable. In comprehensive assessment of outcomes, each major category is measured; however, the specific aspect of each category varies with the clinical situation or the research questions. This model is adapted from the work of Fries and Spitz (1990).

give little indication of how the disease is affecting the patient from his or her own point of view and provide little evidence about daily functioning. Health status assessments go beyond demonstrating the pathological progress of the disease. Instead, they should describe the effects of the chronic disease from the patient's perspective and give clues about mortality, disability, discomfort, iatrogenic problems, and economic issues.

Several methods are available to address the various subdimensions of health status. Direct observation, clinician estimation of functioning, and questionnaires have been used. The first two methods are the most common and are important in clinical practice. They contribute some indications of functional ability but provide limited opportunity for input from the patient. Questionnaires using interviewers, surrogate responders, and, most commonly, written patient self-reports have become the major approach to the assessment of outcome in a variety of chronic diseases including the rheumatic disorders (Fries & Spitz, 1990; Guyatt, Feeny, & Patrick, 1993; Jette, 1993; Stewart et al., 1989). Questionnaires are inexpensive, may be administered quickly in clinical and research centers, and provide the important outcome information as viewed by the person managing the disease. Each of these methods is discussed below.

DIRECT OBSERVATION AND CLINICIAN ASSESSMENTS

Standardized observational methods for hand function, hand and arm strength (grip strength), lower-extremity movement, and range of motion (Keitel Index) are available for looking at specific physical aspects of functional status. These methods are described in detail in Table 2. None comprehensively assesses functional status; however, these types of assessment are important in demonstrating the outcomes from specific types of therapies and may be used routinely in clinical settings. With the exception of the time to walk 50 feet test (Anderson, Felson, Meenan, & Williams, 1989; Decker et al., 1982), the measures described in Table 2 are sensitive to change and are valid methods for evaluating the component of functional status listed. The Keitel Index takes about 10 minutes to complete and requires the time of a health care professional. These factors may limit its usefulness in daily practice. The button test and the timed-stands test require purchase of special equipment, although the costs are low. Grip strength is a common outcome measure in clinical trials and has been shown to be sensitive to improvement in inflammation as well as function for a person with rheumatoid arthritis (Anderson et al., 1989). Measurement can be done quickly in a busy outpatient clinic (Hawley, 1996).

Clinicians may be asked to evaluate an outcome using their professional judgment. For example, physician global assessment is based on the collective evaluation of the patient's health status, considering the presenting symptoms, apparent functioning, and various diagnostic tests. The global assessment requires the physician to estimate the patient's total disease activity on a 0 to 4 scale, with 0 being none, 1 mild, 2 moderate, 3 severe, and 4 very severe (Decker et al., 1982). Other clinicians might adapt such an assessment technique; however, caution is in order. While the physician global assessment has been shown to be sensitive to short-term change during clinical trials (Anderson et al., 1989), in practice settings results are not impressive (Kivela, 1984; Kwoh et al., 1992). Physicians may even overestimate physical limitations compared to patients' perceptions (Kwoh et al.). Other clinicians might indeed experience the same difficulties as physicians. Asking the patient seems a more useful approach to a global assessment of functioning, pain, and general health status.

The American College of Rheumatology Revised Criteria for Classification of Functional Status in Rheumatoid Arthritis may be used as a "rapid, global assessment of functional status by health professionals" (Hochberg et al., 1992, p. 499). These criteria may be used to classify patients for determination of eligibility for research or to describe a group of patients seen in a particular clinic; however, these criteria are not sensitive enough to changes in function over time to be used in daily clinical practice (Hochberg et al., 1992; Stucki, Stoll, Bruhlmann, & Michel, 1995). More detailed assessments are needed to determine important clinical change over time (Hawley, 1996).

SELF-REPORT QUESTIONNAIRES OF HEALTH STATUS IN RHEUMATOLOGY

A number of questionnaires have been developed during the last quarter of a century to measure the various subdimensions and components of health status. These questionnaires vary from measuring a single subdimension (such as ability to do basic daily activities, pain, or fatigue) to comprehensive ones having several subscales to measure numerous aspects of health status.

Health questionnaires may be classified as generic and disease-specific. Generic instruments, as the name implies, look at general categories of outcome variables (e.g., ADL, pain, fatigue, depressive symptoms, general perceptions of health) that are impor-

STANDARDIZED MEASURES FOR EVALUATING PHYSICAL FUNCTIONING IN CHRONIC RHEUMATIC DISORDERS USING DIRECT OBSERVATION

MEASURE
PURPOSE
MEASUREMENT METHOD
COMMENTS

GRIP STRENGTH (DECKER ET AL., 1982)
Measurement of hand, wrist and forearm strength

A sphygmomanometer with a mercury column is used. The patient squeezes the cuff inflated to 30 mm/Hg as hard as possible. The highest level on the mercury column of three attempts is recorded.

Motivation, handedness, pain threshold, and muscle weakness will affect score as well as involvement of any joint from the elbow to the hand (Decker et al., 1982). Grip strength has been shown to be sensitive to change in clinical trials (Anderson et al., 1989).

TIME TO WALK 50 FEET (DECKER ET AL., 1982)
Measurement of lower extremity function

Individual walks 50 feet on a flat surface using any aids or assistive devices. Time is recorded in the nearest 0.1 second.

Patient motivation is influential (Decker et al., 1982). Low reliability and insensitive to changes in disease (Anderson et al., 1989).

BUTTON TEST (PINCUS & CALLAHAN, 1992)
Measurement of hand function

Standard board with 5 buttons. Patients are timed while they unbutton and button with both right and left hand separately. Two scores are meaned.

Motivation is an important factor. Useful in disorders with direct effect on hand function (e.g., rheumatoid arthritis).

TIMED-STANDS TEST (NEWCOMER, KRUG, & MAHOWALD, 1993)
Measurement of lower-extremity function

Number of seconds used in standing up and down 10 times from a chair using only the lower extremities.

Motivation, age, and nonmusculoskeletal comorbid conditions may affect scores. Sensitivity to change has not been determined (Newcomer et al., 1993).

KEITEL INDEX (DECKER ET AL., 1982; SULLIVAN, AHLMEN, BJELLE, & KARLSSON, 1993)
Upper- and lower-extremity function with emphasis on range of motion

Measures 24 standard tasks of peripheral and axial joint motion performed by patients. Evaluation is by trained observer. Time: 10-15 minutes (Decker et al., 1982).

Motivation may be a factor. Time and personnel to observe and score tasks are a factor in its use. Scale is sensitive to short-term change (Kalla, Smith, Brown, Meyers, & Chalton, 1995).

Table 2: Standardized Measures for Evaluating Physical Functioning in Chronic Rheumatic Disorders Using Direct Observation. Reproduced from Hawley (1996).

tant in a variety of diseases. They are important in studies that compare across diseases or compare healthy populations with various disease states (Stewart et al., 1989). Clinically they may be used when looking at broad outcomes of a particular unit such as an entire occupational or physical therapy department, a hospital, or even a group of people enrolled in a specific health care insurance plan. Generic instruments give general information related to health.

The generic instruments are often too broad and too insensitive to important clinical changes for use when looking at a single disorder or when evaluating specific treatments. For evaluating outcomes of a disease or an intervention, a disease-specific instrument is often the appropriate choice. For example, pain is a very important outcome variable in the rheumatic diseases but has minimal importance when studying the outcomes of chronic hypertension. An instrument that does not assess pain is of little use for patients with rheumatoid arthritis, fibromyalgia, or osteoarthritis. Even within the rheumatic diseases, specificity becomes important. Following knee-replacement surgery, lower-extremity function is especially important; however, in systemic lupus erythematosus (SLE) fatigue may be a major factor but ambulatory ability is not (Liang et al., 1984). The disease-specific instruments focus on problems or symptoms that are unique or important to the particular condition under consideration. Clinicians and researchers need to investigate the available instruments to determine which one is most suitable for their practice or their research.

The generic and disease-specific instruments commonly used in rheumatology practice and research and their respective subscales are listed on Table 3. Each of these instruments has data readily available concerning reliability, validity, and sensitivity to change (Anderson, Aaronson, & Wilkin, 1993; Wolfe, 1995b). Each instrument is described below.

GENERIC HEALTH STATUS INSTRUMENTS

The Nottingham Health Profile (NHP) was designed to measure "distress relating to severe or potentially disabling conditions" (Anderson, Aaronson, & Wilkin, 1993). Developed in England, it has been translated and tested in several languages including French, Swedish, Spanish, Dutch, and Italian. The NHP includes 38 true-false questions evaluating physical abilities, pain, sleep, social isolation, emotional reactions, and energy level (Hunt et al., 1981). The instrument may be self-administered or completed by an interviewer; completion by self-report takes about 10 minutes. Comparisons of the subscales with analogous subscales from Arthritis Impact Measurement Scales (AIMS) and the Health Assessment Questionnaire (HAQ) produced equivalent results, although the NHP may be less sensitive to change than the rheumatic disease-specific AIMS and HAQ (Fitzpatrick, Ziebland, Jenkinson, & Mowat, 1992, 1993). The instrument is best used to measure major disabling conditions rather than minor disorders or minor degrees of physical limitations (Anderson et al., 1993). NHP has been widely used internationally but has had limited use in the United States.

The Sickness Impact Profile (SIP), developed in 1976, has been tested with numerous chronic diseases including the rheumatic disorders, and it has been used as part of clinical studies in several European countries (Anderson et al., 1993). The instrument

DOMAINS OF HEALTH STATUS QUESTIONNAIRES

DOMAIN	F-HAQ	HAQ	CLINHAQ	MHAQ	FSI	AIMS	AIMS2	WOMAC	SF-36	SIP	NHP	FIQ
FUNCTIONAL DISABILITY	X	X	X	X	X	X	X	X	X		X	X
EATING										X		
BODY CARE					X					X		
MOBILITY					X	O	O			X		
DEXTERITY						O	O					
ADL AND SELF CARE						O	O					
ARM FUNCTION					X							
PHYSICAL FUNCTION						O	O					
PAIN	X	X	X	X		X	X	X	X	X	X	X
SOCIAL ACTIVITIES & ROLES					X	X	X	X	X	X	X	X
SOCIAL ROLES & FUNCTION						O	O		O			
HOME MANAGEMENT					X					X		
SOCIAL ACTIVITIES						O	O		O			
RECREATION & PASTIMES										X		
SOCIAL INTERACTION VS. ISOLATION										X	O	
SOCIAL SUPPORT										X		
COMMUNICATION	X		X							X		
WORK AND DISABILITY	X								X	X		X

Note: F-HAQ = Complete HAQ; HAQ = Health Assessment Questionnaire; CLINHAQ = Clinical HAQ; MHAQ = Modified HAQ; FSI = Functional Status Index; AIMS = Arthritis Impact Measurement Scales, Original Version; AIMS2 = Arthritis Impact Measurement Scales, Version 2; WOMAC = Western Ontario and MacMaster University Osteoarthritis Index; SF-36 = MOS 36-Item Short Form Health Survey; SIP = Sickness Impact Profile; NIP + Nottingham Health Profile; FIQ = Fibromyalgia Impact Questionnaire; X = A major section or scale of the instrument; 0 = Subsection or subscale of the instrument.

Table 3: Domains of Health Status Questionnaires. Modified from Wolfe (1995b). Reprinted with permission.

DOMAINS OF HEALTH STATUS QUESTIONNAIRES

DOMAIN	F-HAQ	HAQ	CLINHAQ	MHAQ	FSI	AIMS	AIMS2	WOMAC	SF-36	SIP	NHP	FIQ
SYMPTOMS												
SLEEP AND REST			X							X	X	X
STIFFNESS				X				X				X
FATIGUE AND ENERGY			X	X					X		X	X
GI PROBLEMS			X	X								
ALERTNESS AND COGNITION										X		
ADVERSE DRUG REACTIONS	X		X									
GLOBAL MEASURES												
GLOBAL DISEASE SEVERITY	X	X	X	X								
GLOBAL HEALTH & WELL-BEING			X	X					X		X	
SATISFACTION			X	X			X					
EMOTIONS AND MOOD			X	X		X	X		X	X	X	X
DEPRESSION			O			O	O					O
ANXIETY			O			O	O					O
HELPLESSNESS & ATTITUDE				O								
FINANCIAL ASPECTS	X											
INDIRECT COSTS	O											
DIRECT COSTS	O											

Note: F-HAQ = Complete HAQ; HAQ = Health Assessment Questionnaire; CLINHAQ = Clinical HAQ; MHAQ = Modified HAQ; FSI Functional Status Index; AIMS = Arthritis Impact Measurement Scales, Original Version; AIMS2 = Arthritis Impact Measurement Scales, Version 2; WOMAC = Western Ontario and MacMaster University Osteoarthritis Index; SF-36 = MOS 36-Item Short Form Health Survey; SIP = Sickness Impact Profile; NIP + Nottingham Health Profile; FIQ = Fibromyalgia Impact Questionnaire; X= A major section or scale of the instrument; 0 = Subsection or subscale of the instrument

Table 3: Domains of Health Status Questionnaires (continued). Modified from Wolfe (1995b). Reprinted with permission.

may be self-administered or completed by a trained interviewer. It contains 136 Yes or No items within 12 dimensions of physical and psychosocial functioning. Twenty to 30 minutes are required for administration. Specific sections include sleep and rest, eating, work, home management, recreation and pastimes, ambulating, mobility, body care and movement, social interaction, alertness behavior, emotional behavior, and communication (Bergner, Bobbitt, Carter, & Gilson, 1981). Since the SIP does not have a pain sub-scale, a supplemental instrument to evaluate pain is essential when studying outcomes in the rheumatic disorders. The SIP is the most comprehensive of the generic, multidimensional health-status questionnaires (Wolfe, 1995b) and is suitable for clinical research. The length of time needed for administration limits its usefulness in clinical settings.

The Medical Outcome Study Short Form 36 (SF-36) (Ware & Sherbourne, 1992) was developed in the United States as part of the Medical Outcomes Study, a comprehensive study of physicians' practice styles and patients' outcomes in competing systems of care (Stewart et al., 1989). The SF-36 contains eight areas of health status including limitation in physical activities because of health problems, limitation in social activities because of health problems, limitation of social activities because of physical or emotional problems, limitation in usual role because of health problems, bodily pain, general mental health (psychological distress and well-being), vitality (energy and fatigue), and general health perceptions. Approximately 10 minutes are needed to complete it, and scoring may be done in even less time. Its brevity, both in items and completion time, as well as its ease in scoring makes it an appropriate outcome measure for clinical practice, research, health policy studies, and population surveys. The SF-36 has been tested in large populations, and normative information is available (Mchorney, Ware, Lu, & Sherbourne, 1994). Questions concerning sensitivity of the pain scale and functioning scales in severely ill or impaired populations have been raised (Anderson et al., 1993). The SF-36 is an important instrument due to its use as an outcome measure for health policy research in the United States and the major ongoing efforts to translate and validate the instrument in at least 15 other countries (Anderson et al., 1993; Hawley, 1996).

DISEASE-SPECIFIC HEALTH STATUS QUESTIONNAIRES

Several instruments have been developed and validated for use across the rheumatic disorders. Even among these instruments, varying specificity exists. The Health Assessment Questionnaire (HAQ) and its modifications, the Arthritis Impact Measurement Scales (AIMS) and its revision, and the Functional Status Index (FSI) are the more general of the disease-specific instruments. On the other hand, the Western Ontario MacMaster Universities Osteoarthritis Index (WOMAC) and the Fibromyalgia Impact Questionnaire (FIQ) are examples of instruments that are focused on particular disorders and are more specific than the AIMS or HAQ. The WOMAC and the FIQ evaluate osteoarthritis of the hip and knee and fibromyalgia, respectively. Each of these instruments is briefly described below, and the domains included in each instrument are listed in Table 3.

The Health Assessment Questionnaire has several versions and has been modified by researchers interested in adapting it for use in clinical practice and research studies. The full HAQ, the HAQ, the CLINHAQ and the Modified Health Assessment Questions, known generally as the M-HAQ, are based on the measurement of outcomes conceptualized by Fries (Fries, 1983; Fries, Spitz, & Kraines, 1980; Fries, Spitz, & Young, 1982). The full HAQ is a detailed questionnaire assessing economic costs, medications and their side effects, use of all types of health care services, comorbidities as well as functional disability, pain, and global disease severity. The full HAQ is long (over 20 pages) and has been used in long-term outcome studies of rheumatic diseases, but the complete version has not been published. The instrument is modified occasionally to remain concordant with changing health care delivery practices. The full HAQ is not suitable for use in clinical practice due to its length (Wolfe, 1995b).

The HAQ, as cited repeatedly in the literature and used widely in clinical studies, refers to the short functional disability scale (24 questions) from the full HAQ. This instrument asks about eight activities of daily living that include dressing, arising, eating, walking, hygiene, reach, grip, and general activities (e.g., running errands, getting in and out of a car) (Fries et al., 1980). Scores range from 0 (able to perform all activities without difficulty) to 3 (unable to do activities even with help). In addition to the functional disability scale, visual analogue scales measuring severity of pain during the last week (0 = no pain, 100 = severe pain) and global disease severity (0 = doing very well, 100 = doing very poorly) are frequently included as part of the HAQ (see Figure 3 for examples on visual analogue scales). Unlike the full HAQ, this brief instrument may be completed and scored in less than 5 minutes and is very suitable for use in both research and clinical settings. The HAQ functional disability scale has been translated into several languages and is used throughout the world (Ramey, Raynauld, & Fries, 1992). The instrument is sensitive to changes in clinical trials and in long-term outcome studies. It has been shown to predict mortality and future disabilities, and it has been used in studies across the spectrum of rheumatic diseases (Ramey et al.). Modifications have been made for use with children (Singh, Athreya, Fries, & Goldsmith, 1994) and patients with ankylosing spondylitis (Daltroy, Larson, Roberts, & Liang, 1990), systemic sclerosis (Poole & Steen, 1991), and psoriatic arthritis (Husted, Gladman, Long, & Farewell, 1995).

The Modified Health Assessment Questionnaire (MHAQ) is an adaptation of the HAQ (24-item scale) by Pincus and colleagues. The authors wanted an instrument that, in addition to functional status, would assess additional areas of health (e.g., patient satisfaction, stress, and learned helplessness) and yet would also be brief enough for use in routine clinical practice (Pincus, Summey, Soraci, Wallston, & Hummon, 1983). To accomplish this goal, they shortened the HAQ from 24 to 8 items and added scales related to patient satisfaction with function and patient interpretation of his or her change in ability to perform routine activities during the previous 6 months. The MHAQ has been used extensively in clinical trials, in long-term observational studies, and as a vital part of routine outpatient care. Revisions have taken place since its original publication. The MHAQ covers two double-sided pages and includes the shortened functional disability scale plus questions related to activity levels (walking, running, climbing stairs), sleep, stress, depression, anxiety, and stiffness, visual analogue scales for pain, gastrointestinal distress, and fatigue, the Learned Helplessness Scale, and items related to comorbidity, medication side effects, and demographics (Wolfe & Pincus, 1995).

The CLINHAQ was adapted by Wolfe (1994) from the original HAQ. He wanted an instrument that could be used daily in a large outpatient rheumatic disease clinic to assess several dimensions of health status. The CLINHAQ is a "derivative" instrument integrating several scales and subscales from established instruments as well as including new ones (Wolfe, 1995b). It contains the HAQ functional disability scale, five visual analogue scales (pain, global disease severity, sleep disturbance, gastrointestinal distress, and fatigue), a pain diagram, and the anxiety and depression subscales from the original AIMS (see below). This instrument has been used for numerous reports of long-term outcome across a variety of rheumatic diseases as well as part of an ongoing clinical practice (Hawley & Wolfe, 1993; Wolfe, 1994; Wolfe et al., 1994).

The Arthritis Impact Measurement Scales have been published in two versions, the original AIMS and its revision, AIMS2. Both are detailed and comprehensive rheumatic disease health-status instruments. The original AIMS, published at about the same time as the HAQ functional disability scale, included more scales than the HAQ and went well beyond assessment of functional status. The instrument evaluated the outcome or impact of arthritis in terms of both physical function (scales for mobility, physical activity, dexterity, and activities of daily living) and psychosocial aspects of chronic arthritis (subscales for social role, social activities, pain, depression, and anxiety) (Meenan, Gertman, & Mason, 1980). The instrument has been extensively validated and has been shown to be sensitive to clinical changes. It has been used in a large number of clinical trials and in long- and short-term observational studies. Translations are available in several languages (Meenan, Mason, Anderson, Guccione, & Kazis, 1992). The length (over 20 minutes to complete) and complexity of scoring have limited its use in routine clinical practice.

AIMS2, published in early 1992, added new subscales and revised the existing scales where appropriate. New subscales evaluate patient satisfaction, patient preference or priority areas for health-status improvement, and attribution of symptoms or problems to arthritis (Meenan et al., 1992). The AIMS2 contains renamed and new domains of mobility level, walking and bending, hand and finger function, self-care, household tasks, social activities, support from family and friends, arthritis pain, work, level of tension, and mood (Meenan et al., 1992). The instrument is the most comprehensive of all disease-specific health-status instruments. In clinical research on the rheumatic disorders it is the instrument of choice when a comprehensive assessment is required and there is sufficient time for study participants to complete the scale. Its length precludes its use for busy clinical practices.

The Functional Status Index (FSI) evaluates activities of daily living and instrumental activities of daily living including gross mobility (walking inside, climbing stairs, and chair transfer), personal care (hygiene and dressing), hand activities (opening jars and writing), home chores (laundry, reaching, yard work and vacuuming), and social or role activities (driving and performing one's job). A total of 18 items are included. Respondents are asked to rate the amount of help they need, ranging from "able to do independently" to "unable to do." They also rate the degree of difficulty and the pain involved in each activity (Jette, 1987). The instrument has been used in clinical trials, as a program evaluation instrument, and within routine clinical practice (Jette, 1987).

The Western Ontario and MacMaster Universities Osteoarthritis Index (WOMAC) is self-administered and was developed to assess outcomes in clinical trials of osteoarthritis (Bellamy, Buchanan, Goldsmith, Campbell, & Stitt, 1988a, 1988b). Specifically, it measures pain when walking, climbing stairs, and lying in bed, stiffness after awakening and after resting during the day, and difficulty with physical function activities including descending stairs, rising from a chair, bending, lying in bed, and getting on and off the toilet (Bellamy et al., 1988a). The instrument has been shown to respond to clinical changes in nonsteroidal antiinflammatory drugs in clinical trials (Bellamy et al., 1988a, Bellamy, Kean, Buchanan, Gerecz-Simon, & Campbell, 1992), after hip and knee arthroplasty (Bellamy et al., 1988a), and following a physical therapy intervention (Young et al., 1991). The WOMAC can be completed by the patient in 10 minutes and scored in a short time. A Likert scale format is available, in which patients respond to each item on a five-point scale consisting of none, slight, moderate, severe, and extreme. A visual-analogue format in which patients respond by marking a visual-analogue scale is also available. This instrument could be used in a practice setting when caring primarily for people with osteoarthritis.

The Fibromyalgia Impact Questionnaire (FIQ) is a brief, 10-item questionnaire assessing the impact of fibromyalgia. It includes items related to physical function, work status, depression, anxiety, sleep, pain, stiffness, fatigue, and well-being (Burckhardt, Clark, & Bennett, 1991). The instrument has been used in studies of fibromyalgia; however, its very narrow focus limits its use in studies and in clinical practice.

FUNCTIONAL STATUS IN CHILDREN

Instruments to evaluate the health status of children with rheumatic disorders are limited in number and scope. The American College of Rheumatology (ACR) Functional Class and the Chronic Activity Limitations Scale (CALS) have been used; however, neither scale appropriately describes the disabilities of children with juvenile rheumatoid arthritis (JRA). Using either instrument, over 85% of the disabilities of children with JRA fall into the categories of none or only minor (Lovell, 1992). Recently, age-appropriate instruments that assess pain and functional ability have been tested (Tucker, DeNardo, Abetz, Landgraf, & Schaller, 1995). The Juvenile Arthritis Functional Assessment Scale (JAFAS), the Juvenile Arthritis Functional Assessment Report (JAFASR), and the Child HAQ (C-HAQ) are three such scales.

Designed for children over 7 years of age, the JAFAS evaluates 10 activities of daily living (e.g., buttoning a shirt or blouse, cutting food, walking, and bending) via observation by a health professional (Lovell et al., 1989). The Juvenile Arthritis Functional Assessment Report (JAFASR) may be self-administered. There are two versions, one to be completed by the child (JAFASP-C) or a health professional and the other by the child's parent (JAFAS-P). Responsiveness to clinical changes has not been determined. In addition, the age at which a child is capable of completing the questionnaire independently or when a surrogate is needed has not been determined (Howe et al., 1991).

The Child HAQ (C-HAQ), adapted from the functional status scale of the HAQ, assesses functional status, pain, and global severity. Items related to each of the functional areas on the original HAQ (e.g., dressing, eating, arising) were added so that there is at least one item for each functional area that could be completed by children of all ages. For example, "able to remove socks" was added to the dressing and grooming area since a healthy 1-year-old child can perform this activity but could not accomplish the other listed activities, specifically tying shoelaces and shampooing hair. The child or parent may complete the scale (Singh et al., 1994). As with the other scales, responsiveness to clinical changes has not been validated.

ASSESSMENT AS PART OF CLINICAL PRACTICE

As described above, a number of health-status instruments are available for clinical studies and for use in practice settings (Deyo & Carter, 1992; Greenfield & Nelson, 1992; Wolfe & Pincus, 1995). The HAQ functional status scale, the MHAQ, and the CLIN-HAQ are the most feasible for use in ambulatory rheumatology clinical practice settings. They are brief, easily completed by most patients while waiting to see the health care professional, and may be scored quickly. The routine of a clinic is not disrupted by the questionnaires and a minimum of staff and patient time is required (Wolfe & Pincus). The MHAQ and the CLINHAQ measure important aspects of health status in addition to functional ability (i.e., pain, psychological distress, fatigue, and satisfaction).

In settings where time limitations are not as restrictive as outpatient clinics, the AIMS or AIMS2 provides very complete information. If one is studying outcome in osteoarthritis following orthopedic surgery, the WOMAC is an excellent choice. It can be completed and scored quickly. In primary care clinics where a variety of chronic health problems are seen and time is limited, the SF-36 may be the instrument of choice. It can be completed quickly and inexpensively, yet it provides valuable information for comparisons among chronic diseases. In all settings, a balance between administration costs and comprehensive information must be achieved.

Another alternative exists for the clinician who wants to evaluate outcomes from the patients' point of view but has very limited time or finds the adoption of an entire self-report questionnaire impossible for any number of administrative or bureaucratic reasons. The visual analogue scale (VAS) is one method for measuring outcomes of care that can be quickly adapted by a single practitioner (see Figure 3). A VAS is a double-anchored line, usually 10 cm in length, that represents the continuum of a phenomenon (McDowell & Newell, 1987). VAS scales may be horizontal or vertical. These scales have been used most frequently to measure pain intensity, but they may be adapted for use in evaluating a variety of subjective symptoms. For example, these scales can measure quality of sleep, the amount of fatigue, the degrees of stiffness, the amount of difficulty performing various tasks, or quality of mood. Visual analogue scales have been shown to be reliable, valid, and sensitive to change (Bellamy et al., 1988a; 1988b; Gaston-Johansson

VISUAL ANALOGUE SCALES

NO PAIN_____PAIN IS AS BAD AS IT COULD BE

NO PAIN_____SEVERE PAIN

DOING
VERY WELL_____DOING VERY POORLY

FATIGUE IS   FATIGUE IS A
NO PROBLEM_____MAJOR PROBLEM

SLEEP IS   SLEEP IS A
NO PROBLEM_____MAJOR PROBLEM

Figure 3. Examples of Visual Analogue scales commonly used in outcome studies in the rheumatic disorder.

& Gustafsson, 1990; Huskisson, 1974; Joos, Peretz, Beguin, & Famaey, 1991; Lee, Hicks, & Nino-Murcia, 1991).

SUMMARY

The time has arrived when clinicians must begin to measure the outcomes of their practices systematically with valid and reliable instruments. They must join researchers in measuring the effects of their interventions and in sharing the findings with colleagues. Patients as well as third party payers and health policy makers demand evidence that our practice improves the health status of the patients we serve. Health status encompasses the effects of disease on the individual's physical, psychological, and social functioning and is the goal and the comprehensive outcome measure for health care services. Valid, reliable, sensitive methods and instruments are available for looking at health status. Incorporation of outcome evaluation into routine practice is not only necessary for economic and other pragmatic reasons, but it is also appropriate from a professional point of view. Understanding how interventions affect the health status of patients is essential to quality patient care.

REFERENCES

Anonymous. (1996). Status of the patient outcomes research teams (PORTs): An interview with Richard J. Greene, MD, PhD. *Medical Outcomes Trust Bulletin, 4*, 3.

Ahlmen, M., Bjelle, A., & Sullivan, M. (1991). Prediction of team care effects in outpatients with rheumatoid arthritis. *Journal of Rheumatology 18*, 1655-1661.

Anderson, J. J., Felson, D. T., Meenan, R. F., & Williams, H. J. (1989). Which traditional measures should be used in rheumatoid arthritis clinical trials. *Arthritis and Rheumatism, 32*, 1093-1099.

Anderson, R. B., Needleman, R. D., Gatter, R. A., Andrews, R. P., & Scarola, J. A. (1988). Patient outcome following inpatient vs. outpatient treatment of rheumatoid arthritis. *Journal of Rheumatology, 15*, 556-560.

Anderson, R. T., Aaronson, N. K., & Wilkin, D. (1993). Critical review of the international assessments of health-related quality of life. *Quality of Life Research, 2*, 369-395.

Bellamy, N., Buchanan, W. W., Goldsmith, C. H., Campbell, J., & Stitt, L. (1988a). Validation study of the WOMAC: A health status instrument for measuring clinically important patient-relevant outcomes following total hip or knee arthroplasty in osteoarthritis. *Journal of Orthopedic Rheumatology, 1*, 95-108.

Bellamy, N., Buchanan, W. W., Goldsmith, C. H., Campbell, J., & Stitt, L. W. (1988b). Validation study of WOMAC: A health status instrument for measuring clinically important patient-relevant outcomes to antirheumatic drug therapy in patients with osteoarthritis of the hip or knee. *Journal of Rheumatology, 15*, 1833-1840.

Bellamy, N., Kean, W. F., Buchanan, W. W., Gerecz-Simon, E., & Campbell, J. (1992). Double-blind, randomized, controlled trial of sodium meclofenamate (Meclomen) and diclofenac sodium (Voltaren): Post validation reapplication of the WOMAC Osteoarthritis Index. *Journal of Rheumatology , 19*, 153-159.

Bergner, M., Bobbitt, R. A., Carter, W. B., & Gilson, B. S. (1981). The Sickness Impact Profile: Development and final revision of a health status measure. *Medical Care, 19*, 787-805.

Bombardier, C. & Raboud, J. (1991). A comparison of health-related quality-of-life measures for rheumatoid arthritis research. The Auranofin Cooperating Group. *Control Clinical Trials, 12*, 243S-256S.

Boyle, C. A., & Decoufle, P. (1990). National sources of vital status information: Extent of coverage and possible selectivity in reporting. *American Journal of Epidemiology, 131*, 160-168.

Burckhardt, C. S., Clark, S. R., & Bennett, R. M. (1991). The fibromyalgia impact questionnaire: Development and validation. *Journal of Rheumatology, 18*, 728-733.

Daltroy, L. H. (1992). Arthritis patient education. *Bulletin of Rheumatic Disease, 41*, 2-4.

Daltroy, L. H., Larson, M. G., Roberts, W. N., & Liang, M. H. (1990). A modification of the Health Assessment Questionnaire for the spondyloarthropathies. *Journal of Rheumatology, 17*, 946-950.

Daltroy, L. H., & Liang, M. H. (1991). Advances in patient education in rheumatic disease. *Annals of Rheumatic Disease, 50 Suppl 3*, 415-417.

Daltroy, L. H., & Liang, M. H. (1993). Arthritis education: Opportunities and state of the art. *Health Education Quarterly, 20*, 3-16.

Decker, J. L., McShane, D. J., Esdaile, J .M., Hathaway, D. E., Levinson, J. E., Liang, M. H., Medsger, T. A., Jr., Meenan, R. F., Mills, J. A., Roth, S. H. & Wolfe, F. (1982). *Dictionary of the rheumatic diseases: Volume I: Signs and symptoms.* New York: Contact Associates International, Ltd.

Deyo, R. A., & Carter, W. B. (1992). Strategies for improving and expanding the application of health status measures in clinical settings: A researcher developer viewpoint. *Medical Care, 30*, MS176-MS186.

Donabedian, A. (1966). Evaluating the quality of medical care. *Milbank Quarterly, 3*, 166-206.

Donabedian, A. (1988). The quality of care: Can it be assessed? *Journal of the American Medical Association, 260,* 743-748.

Felson, D. T., Anderson, J. J., & Meenan, R. F. (1992). Use of short-term efficacy/toxicity tradeoffs to select 2nd-line drugs in rheumatoid arthritis — a meta-analysis of published clinical trials. *Arthritis and Rheumatism, 35,* 1117-1125.

Fitzpatrick, R., Ziebland, S., Jenkinson, C., & Mowat, A. (1992). A generic health status instrument in the assessment of rheumatoid arthritis. *British Journal of Rheumatology, 31,* 87-90.

Fitzpatrick, R., Ziebland, S., Jenkinson, C., & Mowat, A. (1993). A comparison of the sensitivity to change of several health status instruments in rheumatoid arthritis. *Journal of Rheumatology, 20,* 429-436.

Fries, J. F. (1983). Toward an understanding of patient outcome measurement. *Arthritis and Rheumatism 26,* 697-704.

Fries, J. F., & Spitz, P. W. (1990). The hierarchy of patient outcomes. In B. Spilker (Ed.), *Quality of life: Assessments in clinical trials* (pp. 25-35). New York: Raven Press Ltd.

Fries, J. F., Spitz, P. W., & Kraines, R. G. (1980). Measurement of patient outcome in arthritis. *Arthritis and Rheumatism, 23,* 137-145.

Fries, J. F., Spitz, P. W., & Young, D. Y. (1982). The dimensions of health outcomes: The health assessment questionnaire, disability and pain scales. *Journal of Rheumatology, 9,* 789-793.

Froberg, D. G., & Kane, R. L. (1989). Methodology for measuring health-state preferences— I: Measurement strategies. *Journal of Clinical Epidemiology, 42,* 345-354.

Gaston-Johansson, F., & Gustafsson, M. (1990). Rheumatoid arthritis: Determination of pain characteristics and comparison of RAI and VAS in its measurement. *Pain, 41,* 35-40.

Gill, T. M., & Feinstein, A. R. (1994). A critical appraisal of the quality of quality-of-life measurements. *Journal of the American Medical Association, 272,* 619-626.

Greenfield, S., & Nelson, E.C. (1992). Recent development and future issues in the use of health status assessment measures in clinical settings. *Medical Care, 30,* MS23-MS41.

Guyatt, G. H., Feeny, D. H., & Patrick, D. L. (1993). Measuring health-related quality of life. *Annals of Internal Medicine, 118,* 622-629.

Hawley, D. J. (1995). Psycho-educational interventions in the treatment of arthritis. *Bailliere Clinical Rheumatology, 9,* 803-823.

Hawley, D. J. (1996). Health status assessment. In S.T. Wegner, B. Belza, & E. P. Gall (Eds.), *Clinical care in the rheumatic disease.* Atlanta, GA: American College of Rheumatology.

Hawley, D. J., & Wolfe, F. (1993). Depression is not more common in rheumatoid arthritis: A 10 year longitudinal study of 6,608 rheumatic disease patients. *Journal of Rheumatology, 20,* 2025-2031.

Hegyvary, S. T. (1991). Issues in outcomes research. *Journal of Nursing Quality Assurance, 5,* 1-6.

Hochberg, M. C., Chang, R. W., Dwosh, I., Lindsey, S., Pincus, T., & Wolfe, F. (1992). The American College of Rheumatology 1991 revised criteria for the classification of global functional status in rheumatoid arthritis. *Arthritis and Rheumatism, 35,* 498-502.

Holman, H., & Lorig, K. (1987). Patient education in the rheumatic diseases—pros and cons. *Bulletin of Rheumatic Disease, 37,* 1-8.

Howe, S., Levinson, J., Shear, E., Hartner, S., McGirr, G., Schulte, M., & Lovell, D. (1991). Development of a disability measurement tool for juvenile rheumatoid arthritis: The juvenile arthritis functional assessment report for children and their parents. *Arthritis and Rheumatism, 34,* 873-880.

Hunt, S. M., McKenna, S. P., McEwen, J., Backett, E. M., Williams, J., & Papp, E. (1981). The Nottingham Health Profile: Subjective health status and medical consultations. *Social Science Medicine, 15A,* 221-229.

Huskisson, E. C. (1974). Measurement of pain. *Lancet, 2,* 1127-1131.

Husted, J. A., Gladman, D. D., Long, J. A., & Farewell, V. T. (1995). A modified version of the health assessment questionnaire (HAQ) for psoriatic arthritis. *Clinical and Experimental Rheumatology, 13*, 439-443.

Jette, A. M. (1987). The functional status index: Reliability and validity of a self-report functional disability measure. *Journal of Rheumatology, (suppl. 15) 14*, 15-19.

Jette, A. M. (1993). Using health-related quality of life measures in physical therapy outcomes research. *Physical Therapy, 73*, 528-537.

Joos, E., Peretz, A., Beguin, S., & Famaey, J.P. (1991). Reliability and reproducibility of visual analogue scale and numeric rating scale for therapeutic evaluation of pain in rheumatic patients. *Journal of Rheumatology, 18*, 1269-1270.

Kalla, A. A., Smith, P. R., Brown, G. M. M., Meyers, O. L., & Chalton, D. (1995). Responsiveness of Keitel functional index compared with laboratory measures of disease activity in rheumatoid arthritis. *British Journal of Rheumatology, 34*, 141-149.

Kivela, S. L. (1984). Measuring disability — do self-ratings and service provider ratings compare? *Journal of Chronic Disease, 37*, 115-123.

Kwoh, C. K., O'Connor, G. T., Regansmith, M. G., Olmstead, E. M., Brown, L. A., Burnett, J. B., Hochman, R. F., King, K., & Morgan, G. J. (1992). Concordance between clinician and patient assessment of physical and mental health status. *Journal of Rheumatology, 19*, 1031-1037.

Lambert, C. M., Hurst, N. P., McGregor, K., Hunter, M., Forbes, J., & Lochhead, A. (1994). A pilot study of the economic cost and clinical outcome of day patient vs. inpatient management of active rheumatoid arthritis. *British Journal of Rheumatology, 33*, 383-388.

Lee, K. A., Hicks, G., & Nino-Murcia, G. (1991). Validity and reliability of a scale to assess fatigue. *Psychiatry Research, 36*, 291-298.

Liang, M. H. (1987). The historical and conceptual framework for functional assessment in rheumatic disease. *Journal of Rheumatology, (suppl. 15) 14*, 2-5.

Liang, M. H., Rogers, M., Larson, M., Eaton, H. M., Murawski, B. J., Taylor, J. E., Swafford, J., & Schur, P. H. (1984). The psychosocial impact of systemic lupus erythematosus and rheumatoid arthritis. *Arthritis and Rheumatism, 27*, 13-19.

Lorig, K. R., Mazonson, P. D., & Holman, H. R. (1993). Evidence suggesting that health education for self management in patients with chronic arthritis has sustained health benefits while reducing health care costs. *Arthritis and Rheumatism, 36*, 439-446.

Lovell, D. J. (1992). Newer functional outcome measurements in juvenile rheumatoid arthritis: A progress report. *Journal of Rheumatology Supplement 33*, 28-31.

Lovell, D. J., Howe, S., Shear, E., Hartner, S., McGirr, G., Schulte, M., & Levinson, J. (1989). Development of a disability measurement tool for juvenile rheumatoid arthritis: The Juvenile Arthritis Functional Assessment Scale. *Arthritis and Rheumatism, 32*, 1390-1395.

McDowell, I., & Newell, C. (1987). *Measuring health: A guide to rating scales and questionnaires.* New York: Oxford University Press.

Mchorney, C. A., Ware, J. E., Lu, J. F. R., & Sherbourne, C. D. (1994). The MOS 36-Item Short-Form Health Survey (SF-36).3. Tests of data quality, scaling assumptions, and reliability across diverse patient groups. *Medical Care, 32*, 40-66.

Meenan, R. F., Gertman, P. M., & Mason, J. H. (1980). Measuring health status in arthritis: The arthritis impact measurement scales. *Arthritis and Rheumatism, 23*, 146-152.

Meenan, R. F., Mason, J. H., Anderson, J. J., Guccione, A. A., & Kazis, L. E. (1992). AIMS2. The content and properties of a revised and expanded Arthritis Impact Measurement Scales Health Status Questionnaire. *Arthritis and Rheumatism, 35*, 1-10.

Mullen, P. D., Laville, E. A., Biddle, A. K., & Lorig, K. (1987). Efficacy of psychoeducational interventions on pain, depression, and disability in people with arthritis: A meta-analysis. *Journal of Rheumatology, 14*, 33-39.

Newcomer, K. L., Krug, H. E., & Mahowald, M. L. (1993). Validity and reliability of the timed-stands test for patients with rheumatoid arthritis and other chronic diseases. *Journal of Rheumatology, 20,* 21-27.

Pincus, T., Brooks, R. H., & Callahan, L. F. (1994). Prediction of long-term mortality in patients with rheumatoid arthritis according to simple questionnaire and joint count measures. *Annals of Internal Medicine, 120,* 26-34.

Pincus, T., & Callahan, L. F. (1992). Rheumatology function tests: Grip strength, walking time, button test and questionnaires document and predict long term morbidity and mortality in rheumatoid arthritis. *Journal of Rheumatology, 19,* 1051-1057.

Pincus, T., Summey, J. A., Soraci, S. A., Jr., Wallston, K. A., & Hummon, N. P. (1983). Assessment of patient satisfaction in activities of daily living using a modified Stanford Health Assessment Questionnaire. *Arthritis and Rheumatism, 26,* 1346-1353.

Poole, J. L., & Steen, V. D. (1991). The use of the health assessment questionnaire (HAQ) to determine physical disability in systemic sclerosis. *Arthritis Care Research, 4,* 27-31.

Ramey, D. R., Raynauld, J., & Fries, J. F. (1992). The health assessment questionnaire 1992. *Arthritis Care Research, 5,* 119-129.

Raspe, H. H., Deck, R., & Mattussek, S. (1992). The outcome of traditional or comprehensive outpatient care for rheumatoid arthritis (RA): Results of an open, nonrandomized, 2-year prospective study. *Z Rheumatology, 51,* 61-66.

Relman, A. S. (1988). Assessment and accountability: The third revolution in medical care. *New England Journal of Medicine, 319,* 1220-1222.

Scott, D. L., Long, A. F., & Silman, A. (1995). Disease outcomes in rheumatology. *British Journal of Rheumatology, 34,* 704-706.

Singh, G., Athreya, B. H., Fries, J. F., & Goldsmith, D. P. (1994). Measurement of health status in children with juvenile rheumatoid arthritis. *Arthritis and Rheumatism, 37,* 1761-1769.

Stewart, A. L., Greenfield, S., Hays, R. D., Wells, K., Rogers, W. H., Berry, S. D., McGlynn, E. A., & Ware, J. E., Jr. (1989). Functional status and well-being of patients with chronic conditions. Results from the Medical Outcomes Study. *Journal of the American Medical Association, 262,* 907-913.

Stucki, G., Stoll, T., Bruhlmann, P., & Michel, B. A. (1995). Construct validation of the ACR 1991 revised criteria for global functional status in rheumatoid arthritis. *Clinical and Experimental Rheumatology, 13,* 349-352.

Sullivan, M., Ahlmen, M., Bjelle, A., & Karlsson, J. (1993). Health status assessment in rheumatoid arthritis. II. Evaluation of a modified Shorter Sickness Impact Profile. *Journal of Rheumatology, 20,* 1500-1507.

Tucker, L. B., DeNardo, B. A., Abetz, L. N., Landgraf, J. M., & Schaller, J. G. (1995). The childhood arthritis health profile (CHAP): Validity and reliability of the condition-specific scales. *Arthritis and Rheumatism (Suppl.), 38,* S183(abstract).

Vlieland, T. P. M. V., Zwinderman, A. H., Vandenbroucke, J. P., Breedveld, F. C., & Hazes, J. M. W. (1995). In-patient treatment for active rheumatoid arthritis: Clinical course and predictors of improvement. *British Journal of Rheumatology, 34,* 847-853.

Ware, J. E. & Sherbourne, C. D. (1992). The MOS 36-item short-form health survey (SF-36). *Medical Care, 30,* 473-483 (abstract).

Wolfe, F. (1994). Data collection and utilization: A methodology for clinical practice and clinical research. In F. Wolfe & T. Pincus (Eds.), *Rheumatoid arthritis: pathogenesis, assessment, outcome, and treatment* (pp. 463-514). New York: Marcel Dekker.

Wolfe, F. (1995a). A database for rheumatoid arthritis. *Rheumatic Disease Clinics of North America, 21,* 481-500.

Wolfe, F. (1995b). Health status questionnaires. *Rheumatic Disease Clinics of North America, 21,* 445-464.

Wolfe, F., & Pincus, T. (1995). Data collection in the clinic. *Rheumatic Disease Clinics of North America, 21,* 321-358.

Wolfe, F., Mitchell, D. M., Sibley, J. T., Fries, J. F., Bloch, D. A., Williams, C. A., Spitz, P. W., Haga, M., Kleinheksel, S. M., & Cathey, M. A. (1994). The mortality of rheumatoid arthritis. *Arthritis and Rheumatism, 37,* 481-494.

World Health Organization. (1958). *World Health Organization: The first 10 years of the World Health Organization.* Geneva, Switzerland: Author.

Yelin, E. H. (1991). What's inside the team care box? Is it the parts, the connections, the attention, or the gestalt. *Journal of Rheumatology, 18,* 1647-1648.

Young, S. L., Woodbury, M. G., Fryday-Field, K., Donovan, T., Bellamy, N., & Haddar, R. (1991). Efficacy of the interferrential current stimulation alone for pain reduction in patients with osteoarthritis of the Knee: A randomized placebo controlled clinical trial. [abstract] *Physical Therapy,* Suppl. 671-R088.

PART TWO:
PATIENT ASSESSMENT

INITIAL INTERVIEW:
A CLIENT-CENTERED APPROACH

Judy R. Sotosky, MEd, PT, and Jeanne Melvin, MS, OTR, FAOTA

The single most important reason for obtaining a medical history and symptoms assessment from a patient is to gain an understanding of how the disease has affected and is affecting that person's life. This information provides guidance for the health professional's choice of intervention. The physical, psychological, and social responses of each individual to illness are unique. Incorporating these responses in treatment provides the challenge that forms the art and science of health care. Before taking a medical history, one must think about the purpose for which the information is to be used. Different parts of the interview may be more important than others for each health care professional. A thorough understanding of the rheumatic diseases, their clinical patterns, and medication regimes is essential for taking an effective and efficient medical history from a person with arthritis. This chapter reviews the initial assessment process relevant to occupational and physical therapists.

The National Arthritis Advisory Board (NAAB) and the Association of Rheumatology Health Professionals (ARHP) have identified essential competencies in the area of rheumatology needed by physical and occupational therapists new to this practice area. These include the skills to obtain a medical history, to assess the patient's expectations, pain status, disease activity level, difficulties in functional ability, and the impact of disease on all phases of the patient's life, and to set patient goals (Moncur, 1988; ARHP, 1991).

The impact of a rheumatic disease on a particular individual is defined in part by the characteristics of that individual. Using the World Health Organization model (Carr & Thompson, 1994), the information obtained in a patient interview can be organized into three categories: (1) **impairment** (organic changes or pathology) such as local joint inflammation and pain, (2) **disability** (changes in ability to perform activities of daily living), for example, inability to climb steps, and (3) **handicap** (changes in ability to fulfill normal role in society), for example, inability to hold down a job and provide income. Although there is not always a direct hierarchical relationship among these planes, a change in one may influence one or more of the others.

A good medical history and symptom assessment includes investigation of the disablement process. Nagi proposed a model of the disablement process that takes these concepts one step further (Guccione, 1994). It describes the progression of disablement as one of disease, impairment, functional limitation, and ultimately disability. This model has been expanded to include several human or social factors that may influence progression at various points (Figure 1). These parameters provide a comprehensive picture of the individual and the impact of the disease on his or her life, which is of paramount importance when considering treatment.

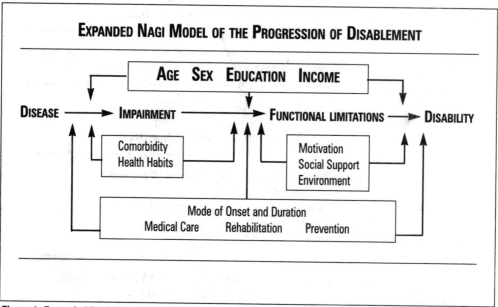

Figure 1: Expanded Nagi Model of the Progression of Disablement. Guccione, 1994, p. 410. Reprinted with permission.

HISTORY AND SYMPTOM INTERVIEW, A PATIENT-CENTERED APPROACH

A model for patient-centered medical history and symptom assessment in persons with rheumatic disease is outlined in Figure 2. The key components of this type of interview include the patient's perspective and goals, personal profile, prior and current treatments, rheumatic disease status, physical activity and functional ability, health habits, self-management, and psychosocial issues. Some of these topics are completely covered in the initial interview, and some are screened to determine if an in-depth assessment is needed.

This chapter is an overview of the initial interview, which ascertains the patient's medical history, the nature of the current illness, approach to self-management, and goals for treatment. It discusses several topics that have parameters unique to the rheumatic diseases. The actual physical assessment of the joints, which defines the nature of the impairment, is covered in chapter 6, musculoskeletal assessment, and chapter 7 on joint and soft tissue pain. The full assessment of disability and handicap is covered in chapter 8 on functional assessment, chapter 9 on locomotion, and chapter 3 on adherence.

HISTORY AND SYMPTOM INTERVIEW — A PATIENT-CENTERED APPROACH

CATEGORY	CONTENT
Patient's perspective and goals	What do they want from therapy? What are their goals? What are their treatment priorities?
Personal profile (demographics)	Age, sex, diagnosis, comorbidity, educational occupation, culture, living situation, language of choice.
Prior and current treatments	Medical (medications), surgical, rehabilitative, complementary medicine.
Rheumatic disease status ("impairment")	Onset, pattern, severity, variability, extraarticular and neurologic manifestations, fatigue, morning stiffness, swelling, gelling, pain, limited ROM, weakness.
Physical activity/ functional ability ("disability")	What activities have they given up because of the arthritis? What would they like to do? How has disease changed their functional ability? What functional activities are they able to do? What do they need to do?
Health habits	Diet, exercise, smoking, stress management, sleep pattern, relaxation skills, caffeine intake, alcohol and drug use.
Self-management	Knowledge of self-management skills. Specific lifestyle changes to improve health. Flare/pain management plan. Self-efficacy. Plan to improve health.
Pyschosocial	Response to illness: depression, anxiety, role changes.
Impact on life ("handicap")	Coping skills. Social support systems. Expectations/beliefs about illness and healing. Finances.

Figure 2: History and Symptom Interview—A Patient-Centered Approach

DIAGNOSIS AND COMORBID CONDITIONS

Does the patient know his or her diagnosis? Does he or she understand it? A person who does not know the diagnosis may be exhibiting denial, anxiety, or evidence of a breakdown in patient-physician communication. Any of these would influence treatment and patient education in different ways. It is best to determine the patient's understanding with an open question, for example, "What type of arthritis do you have?" Another question to ask is, "Are there other family members with this diagnosis?" This often reveals personal experiences and beliefs about the illness. Many patients are terrified of osteoarthritis (OA) because they have seen a relative crippled by rheumatoid arthritis (RA). Insight into the meaning of the disease to the patient is valuable in planning treatment (Carr & Thompson, 1994).

It is important to know if the person has other illnesses or conditions that can have an impact on treatment, for example, cardiac disorders, pulmonary disease, high blood pressure, or diabetes. Organ involvement associated with the rheumatic disease is referred to as "extraarticular manifestations." They are specific for each disease and are reviewed in the disease-specific chapters in Volume 2. For example, RA can affect the eyes, lungs, and heart.

AGE AND ONSET

Although age seems obvious, there are actually several different age questions. These include current age, age at first symptoms, and age at diagnosis. Frequently a lapse occurs between onset and diagnosis because of the delay in seeking medical attention for what are commonly referred to as "aches and pains." Lapses in time suggest that physical and/or functional difficulties in the present may have been developing over a long time. They also suggest that gradual adaptation has occurred in the patient's lifestyle. Looking at the age at which events occur helps the interviewer identify the developmental or maturational impact of the illness.

There can also be three distinct onsets: symptoms, diagnosis, and disability (Melvin, 1989). If you ask a patient, "When did you get rheumatoid arthritis?" or "How long have you had osteoarthritis?" he or she will most typically tell you the date the diagnosis was made. This can be years after symptoms began. The onset of symptoms gives a more accurate picture of how much joint damage or functional change has occurred.

The onset of disability may also differ significantly from the onset of arthritis. For example, if you ask a person disabled by arthritis in the knees, "How long have you had arthritis?" the person may say 10 years, possibly implying he or she has been disabled for 10 years, when in fact he or she may have been disabled for only 1 year (Melvin, 1989). Additional questions to ask are, "How long has the arthritis in your joints limited your ability to do things?" and "What does it keep you from doing?"

CURRENT AND PAST MEDICATIONS

Fast-acting medications (e.g., aspirin, nonsteroidal antiinflammatory drugs [NSAIDs], and analgesics) can alter patient performance on objective assessments, such as grip strength, range of motion, and so forth, in as little as 30 minutes. In fact, these are standard assessments in clinical trials of NSAIDs. Therefore, it is important to note the name, dosage, frequency, and regularity of the patient's current medications (Melvin, 1989). Unless carefully interviewed, patients who skip dosages or forego them altogether will not be detected. Most arthritis medications must be taken daily no matter how a person is feeling, because it is the constant level in the body that produces the result.

Assessing for medication side effects can facilitate therapy and treatment planning but requires knowledge of the side effects to look for, as patients may not be aware of symptoms or physical changes that can be related to medications. For example, NSAIDs can cause tiredness or lassitude and in the elderly decreased concentration, forgetfulness, light-headedness, and increased depression (Goodwin & Regan, 1982). Aspirin-containing medications can decrease hearing, which can cause significant impairment in the elderly with mild hearing loss. (The side effects of drugs used for arthritis are listed in Volume 2, chapter 3, Drug Management.)

Many NSAIDs lose their effectiveness over time. Some work for a few months and then stop being effective. Specific questions eliciting the patient's perception of efficacy can be invaluable in coordinating rehabilitation with medical management, for example, "Do you think your NSAID is helping?" The response might be, "Absolutely, if I am not able to take my afternoon dose, I hurt all over." Or it could be, "I don't know. I forgot to take it with me last weekend, and I couldn't tell the difference. It seemed to work well in the beginning." In the latter case the therapist should contact the physician with this finding. The patient will benefit far more from therapy if the inflammation is controlled by medication. Also, people should not take NSAIDs unless they are sure the medications are helping because there is a 25-30% risk of gastric ulcers with use of these medications. Not only can you die from a bleeding ulcer, but once you have one, you often cannot take NSAIDs in the future.

The proper use and understanding of medications can make or break a therapy program. Consider the following example. A patient with RA was instructed in an isometric strengthening program. The following week she reported that the exercises were making her joints worse, so she stopped doing them. But her joints remained painful. The fact that her joints did not get better after stopping the exercises was suspicious and indicated that the exercises might not be the aggravating factor. Inquiry regarding her medications revealed that she had been on a new NSAID for 2 months with minimal improvement. She also had other increases in systemic manifestations. She had not made the connection that the NSAID might not be working for her. It turns out that she was on the fourth NSAID prescribed in a short period of time, and she desperately wanted "this one to work." After some discussion, she contacted her physician, who changed her medication. This time the medication worked fairly effectively, and the patient was able to resume the exercises without any increase in symptoms.

Patients may omit reporting that they use narcotic pain medications on particularly bad days. Sporadic use of analgesics can skew objective assessments from one visit to the next, and persistent use without medical supervision may lead to additional health problems. Narcotic medications are generally not recommended for people with arthritis because they mask the pain without reducing the inflammation, and that results in increased stress on damaged joints.

In the medical treatment of the rheumatic diseases there are various classifications of medications used. An understanding of their mode of action, potential side effects and length of time of effect are important tools in treating these patients. Physical and occupational therapies work in conjunction with medical therapy; therefore the therapist should know the physical and neuropsychiatric impact of NSAIDs, slow-acting antirheumatic drugs (SAARDs), steroids, immunosupressive drugs, and analgesics (see Volume 2, chapter 3, Drug Therapy).

Finding out whether a person has had therapy or been previously treated for arthritis, of what that treatment consisted, and its effect can provide valuable information in treatment planning. This area of inquiry may also provide insight into the person's beliefs about arthritis and the potential for response to treatment (see chapter 3, Adherence, for an in-depth review of how a patient's beliefs in treatment affect treatment follow-through).

COMPLEMENTARY MEDICINE

It is now common to have patients who are actively participating in self-management of their health by seeking holistic or nondrug treatments. Previously called "alternative medicine," these treatments are not necessarily used in place of but to complement traditional medical care. Treatments that would be included in this category include acupuncture, Ayurvedic medicine, biofeedback training, chiropractic, craniosacral therapy, homeopathy, yoga, Qigong, Chinese medicine, herbal therapy, hypnotherapy, naturopathic medicine, certain nutritional or diet therapies, body-work therapies such as Feldenkrais and Alexander work, and others. Although in some circles these treatments are considered "unproven" and even irrational, all of these therapies are growing in popularity because of word-of-mouth referral by people these kinds of treatments have helped.

It is important to screen for these treatments, have a nonjudgmental approach, and solicit from the patient what the treatment consists of and how he or she has benefited from it. In all of the above treatments that involve active participation, patients generally learn many effective self-management methods. Additional information on the above methods is in *Alternative Medicine: The Definitive Guide* (The Burton Goldberg Group, 1995).

JOINT SYMPTOMS

Using the *pattern of joint involvement* as a guide, systematically ask the patient to describe the problems related to the joint. Doing this before the physical evaluation allows the health care provider to get a sense of current and past involvement in each joint and helps determine the scope of treatment needed. It also prevents overlooking problem sites that may have an impact on treatment outcome. Be a careful listener when soliciting subjective information about the intensity, volatility, and nature of the patient's condition. Such information will assist you in deciding what can be done during the examination, that is, how vigorous you can be, and it will help you tailor your evaluation to the individual.

Since knowing the pattern of joint involvement helps guide the initial assessment, a summary of the joints commonly affected by OA and ankylosing spondylitis are listed in Tables 1 and 2. For additional information refer to disease-specific chapters and Volume 2, chapter 4, Radiology, which has joint pattern diagrams for each disease. The details of doing a physical evaluation of the joints and differentiating joint and soft-tissue pain are discussed in detail in chapters 6 and 7 in this volume.

Pain is the most common symptom that causes a person with a musculoskeletal disorder to seek medical treatment. Two key pain questions applicable to rheumatic disease patients include, "Where does it hurt?" (Severity of pain can be assessed using a 0 to 10 scale or 10 cm visual analog scale; both scales are simple to use and have been shown to be valid and reliable in this population); and "What makes it feel better or worse?" (listen here for altered medication usage, over-the-counter medications, alcohol, or illegal drugs). Also investigate pain intensity related to activity.

Other questions may add to your understanding of the impact on the individual's life: "What are your best and worst times of day?" "Does your pain interfere with sleep?" (pain that interferes with sleep suggests more active disease). "Has your pain caused you to change your activities?" (the first activities to go are usually social and leisure activities, the loss of which can have a significant negative effect on a person's social role and psychological health).

MORNING STIFFNESS AND JOINT GELLING

Morning stiffness is a term used to describe the *generalized* stiffness associated with inflammatory polyarthritides that occurs throughout the body, not just in affected joints, upon awakening. The stiffness may last from a few minutes to several hours. The duration of the stiffness is an indicator of inflammatory disease activity: The longer the stiffness, the more active the disease. It is not uncommon for a person with active RA to report morning stiffness lasting several hours. Morning stiffness lasting fewer than 30 minutes indicates the disease is well controlled by medications.

To determine the duration of morning stiffness, ask "How long from the time you first wake up does it take for this excessive stiffness to wear off and leave you with only your regular stiffness? Does the morning stiffness limit your ability to do things?"

Persons with severe morning stiffness may be quite functionally limited during this period. The interview should take into account functional limitations from morning stiffness. For example, getting up during the night and in the morning, a person may not be able to use a standard-height toilet seat but is able to after the morning stiffness wears off. Self-management training should include ways to reduce morning stiffness (see chapter 12 on joint protection).

JOINTS COMMONLY AFFECTED BY OSTEOARTHRITIS

DISTAL INTERPHALANGEAL (DIP) JOINTS

PROXIMAL INTERPHALANGEAL (PIP) JOINTS

FIRST CARPOMETACARPAL (CMC) JOINTS

INTERCARPAL TRAPEZIAL JOINTS (PANTRAPEZIAL ARTHRITIS)

SPINE (CERVICAL, THORACIC, LUMBAR)

HIPS

KNEES

FIRST METATARSOPHALANGEAL (MTP) JOINTS

OA can affect the MCP and wrist joints, but these are not common sites.

Table 1: Joints Commonly Affected by Osteoarthritis (Moskowitz & Goldberg, 1988).

Persons with OA also have excessive joint stiffness in the morning, but it is localized to the affected joints rather than generalized and is commonly called "gelling." It is the same phenomenon that occurs following periods of inactivity. This usually abates with gentle movement. People with ankylosing spondylitis and psoriatic arthritis also tend to have localized stiffness in the morning unless they are having a flare of the disease.

People with fibromyalgia syndrome report excessive stiffness in the morning, but it is in the muscles and tendons rather than the joints, a distinction that is often hard for patients to discern. Some clinicians refer to this as "AM stiffness" to distinguish it from "morning stiffness," which is a specific term associated with inflammatory diseases.

FATIGUE

Fatigue has historically been considered a hallmark symptom of inflammatory disease, but experience with fibromyalgia has shown that fatigue can also result from a non-restorative sleep disorder. Fatigue is defined as an enduring, subjective sensation of debilitating, generalized tiredness or exhaustion (Belza, 1994). There is no single standard measure of fatigue, but several measures are available and are being investigated. The Fibromyalgia Impact Questionnaire (FIQ) uses visual analogue scales to assess "How tired have you been?" and "How have you felt when you got up in the morning?" (Burckhardt, Clark, & Bennett, 1991). Evaluation and treatment of fatigue is discussed in detail in chapter 8, Volume 2 on systemic lupus erythematosus.

Clinically useful areas of information to obtain about fatigue are (1) how fatigue interferes with function, (2) how the person copes with fatigue, and (3) what is the pat-

---

JOINTS COMMONLY AFFECTED BY ALKYLOSING SPONDYLITIS

SACROILIAC (SI) JOINTS

LUMBAR AND THORACIC SPINE

HIPS

SHOULDERS

KNEES

HEEL/FOOT PAIN (ACHILLES TENDON, PLANTAR FASCIA)

CERVICAL SPINE*

---

* Women are more likely to have cervical spine and peripheral joint involvement and less likely to have progressive spinal disease than men.

Table 2: Joints Commonly Affected by Alkylosing Spondylitis (Calin, 1988).

tern and severity of fatigue. Common patterns of fatigue in rheumatic disease patients are shown in Table 3.

SYMPTOM AND DISEASE VARIABILITY

Most forms of arthritis including OA are characterized by days when symptoms abate and other days when problems are worse. Different people experience different patterns of disease. It is helpful to get a general determination of the disability status of the person by finding out how often the patient is unable to function due to arthritis. For example, if a patient has 3-4 "bad" days a week, this is equivalent to being disabled 50% of the time. Even though the arthritis is not constant, this person would have difficulty maintaining a house or working full time.

ACTIVITY LEVEL

A review of functional assessment outcome tools frequently used with rheumatic disease patients (see chapters 4 and 8) may help to familiarize the health professional with functional activities commonly affected by arthritis.

General interview questions are useful in assessing global function: "What has changed in what you are able to do over the past 6 months, 1 year, 2 years?" "What can you not do that you want to do?" "What do you believe therapy will help you to do?" "What are your goals?" "What do you want to be able to do again?" "Has your pain caused you to change your activities?" (The first activities to go are usually social and leisure activities, the loss of which can have a significantly negative effect on the person's social role and psychological health.)

COMMON PATTERNS OF FATIGUE IN RHEUMATIC DISEASES

- **DECONDITIONING**—fatigue following minimal level of any physical activity

- **DEPRESSION**—fatigue all the time, no matter how much sleep, often excessive sleeping

- **FIBROMYALGIA SYNDROME (FMS)**—wake up feeling tired, exhausted, or unrefreshed

- **OSTEOARTHRITIS (OA)**—fatigue at end of day, early evening, or following physical activity

- **RHEUMATOID ARTHRITIS (RA)**—fatigue in early afternoon, refreshed by nap; systemic fatigue, resulting from disease flare, usually lasts all day and is not resolved with a nap

- **SYSTEMIC LUPUS ERYTHEMATOSUS (SLE)**—fatigue, exhaustion, not resolved with sleep, lessens with control of disease

Table 3. Common Patterns of Fatigue in Rheumatic Diseases

Consider an example of a 64-year-old commercial salesman with moderate OA of the knees. He has a history of knee injuries while in the armed forces about 40 years ago. He reports being "just about" able to make the end of his work day until the pain gets "real bad," but otherwise does what he wants. Further questioning revealed that over the past 10 years he has gradually given up most of his gardening and golf, now plans fewer social outings with his wife, and spends most of his leisure time in front of the TV because his knees hurt. When questioned, he stated, "I just thought it was part of getting old."

SOCIAL ROLES AND SOCIAL SUPPORTS

In broad terms this area includes the patient's life responsibilities and the support structure available from family, friends, neighbors, and others. Persons with rheumatic diseases who have stronger support networks tend to do better than those who do not. Keep this in mind when interviewing older persons with arthritis. They may be experiencing a decline of income, social isolation (as spouses and friends die and going out becomes more difficult), and a fear of losing their independence (Badley, 1995). The baby-boom generation is now in its 50s and finding itself sandwiched between caring for adolescents and sick or elderly parents. Volatile economic times have resulted in many adult children moving back into the family home. Many people in retirement are financially strained by helping unemployed children or caring for grandchildren. All of these situations can change the roles, responsibilities, and stresses that patients experience.

Recreation and social activities are generally the first to be sacrificed with reduced function or the development of pain. It is important to recognize the role of the above factors when getting an overall picture of the health and well-being of each individual (Guccione, 1994).

PATIENT GOALS AND EXPECTATIONS

A frank discussion of goals and expectations is helpful for therapist and patient in forming a positive working relationship. In addition this information can be used as a strong motivating force. People are more likely to work at a task if they know it is going to help them achieve their goals (see chapter 3 for an in-depth discussion of using goals for increasing patient motivation).

Consider also what the patient is willing and able to do to assist in self-management (Moncur, 1996). A patient with OA of the knee who can afford to purchase a cane may refuse to use one for reasons of vanity. If appearance is this important, avoiding a cane may be a strong motivator for participation in an aquatics exercise program or using joint-protection principles.

SELF-EFFICACY

Assessment of self-efficacy or a person's belief in his or her capacity to manage the illness is now becoming a part of the initial assessment of people with arthritis. The Self-Efficacy Scale developed by Lorig and colleagues (1989) is a self-administered question-naire that can provide invaluable insights into the patient's perception of self-manage-ment skills and provide an objective basis for self-management training. This assessment can also be given at the end of treatment to document the outcome of self-management training.

Persons who feel that they cannot do anything to change the arthritis pain are less likely to manage their arthritis successfully than those who feel reasonably certain that they can take steps to control their pain. When is it is not practical to administer the entire scale, selected questions can be asked during the medical history interview. Ask a simple question like, "on a scale of 0 to 100, with 0 meaning completely uncertain and 100 meaning completely certain, how certain are you that you can do back exercises three times this week?" Or, "How certain are you that you can make a large reduction in your arthritis pain by using methods other than taking extra medication?" (Lorig et al., 1989). The answer may give valuable insight into a patient's feelings of self-efficacy regarding a specific aspect of treatment. Responses lower than 70 suggest a greater likelihood of the person not accomplishing the goal (Lorig et al.).

Chapter 10, Patient Education for Self-Management, discusses self-efficacy in more detail and assesses its influence on health-status outcome and ways to modify a person's self-efficacy through education. Chapter 3, Adherence, reviews ways to assess patients to enhance follow-through with treatment.

SUMMARY

In the rheumatic diseases, as in most other conditions, patient evaluation is an ongoing process that is repeated over time. It helps health professionals to modify and mold programming to suit the individual (Moncur, 1989).

The medical history and symptom interview can play a key role in this treatment planning process by providing a wealth of information on patient status, beliefs, and expectations. By gaining an understanding of the impairments, functional limitations, and disabilities (Guccione, 1994) caused by the disease as well as modifying factors, health care providers are better able to apply their skills to meet the individual needs of patients.

Without giving unrealistic promises, it behooves therapists to provide patients with optimism and hope for the future. Most rheumatic diseases are chronic, lifetime diagnoses. Quality medical care and effective self-management can accomplish much, but they need to be reinforced by positive, active education and encouragement.

REFERENCES

ARHP. (1991). *Standards of practice: Occupational therapy and physical therapy competancies in rheumatology.*

Badley, E. M. (1995). The effect of osteoarthritis on disability and health care use in Canada. *Journal of Rheumatology, Suppl 43, 22,* 19-22.

The Burton Goldberg Group. (1995). *Alternative medicine: The definitive guide.* Fife, WA: Future Medicine Publishing.

Belza, B. (1994). The impact of fatigue on exercise performance. *Arthritis Care, 7,* 176-180.

Burckhardt, C. S., Clark, S. R., & Bennett, R. M. (1991). The Fibromyalgia Impact Questionnaire: Development and validation. *Journal of Rheumatology, 18,* 728-733.

Calin, A. (1988). Ankylosing spondylitis. In R. Schumacher (Ed.), *Primer on the rheumatic diseases* (9th ed.). Atlanta, GA: Arthritis Foundation.

Carr, A. J., & Thompson, P. W. (1994). Towards a measure of patient-perceived handicap in rheumatoid arthritis. *British Journal of Rheumatology, 33,* 378-382.

Goodwin, J. S., & Regan, M. (1982). Cognitive dysfunction associated with Naproxen and Ibuprofen in the elderly. *Arthritis and Rheumatism, 25,* 1013-1015.

Guccione, A. A. (1994). Arthritis and the process of disablement. *Physical Therapy, 74,* 408-414.

Lorig, K., Chastain, R. L., & Ung, E. (1989). Development and evaluation of a scale to measure perceived self-efficacy in people with arthritis. *Arthritis and Rheumatism, 32,* 37-44.

Melvin, J. (1989). *Rheumatic disease in the adult and child: Occupational therapy and rehabilitation* (3rd ed.). Philadelphia, PA: F. A. Davis.

Moncur, C. (1996). Physical therapy management of the patient with osteoarthritis. In J. M. Walker & A. Helewa (Eds.), *Physical therapy in arthritis.* Philadelphia, PA: W. B. Saunders.

Moncur, C. (1989). Adult with rheumatoid arthritis. In R. M. Scully & M. R. Barnes (Eds.), *Physical therapy.* Philadelphia, PA: J. B. Lippincott.

Moncur, C. (1988). Physical therapy competencies. In B. F. Banwell & V. Gall (Eds.), *Physical therapy management of arthritis.* New York: Churchill Livingstone.

Moskowitz, R., & Goldberg, V. (1988). Osteoarthritis. In R. Schumacher (Ed.), *Primer on the rheumatic diseases* (9th ed.), Atlanta, GA: Arthritis Foundation.

6 MUSCULOSKELETAL ASSESSMENT

A. Joseph Threlkeld, PhD, PT

At its core, the musculoskeletal evaluation is a means of gathering data to make or clarify a diagnosis, to plan treatment, to document change, or to assess the outcome of treatment. When conducted by a skilled therapist, the musculoskeletal evaluation assumes a much broader role. Not only are the necessary data gathered, but the process also communicates the therapist's competence and caring, and firmly establishes the essential interpersonal basis for the therapeutic relationship. This is particularly critical for patients with arthritis who are fearful of being hurt by the examination. Viewed in this broader context, this evaluation is a critical event in a complex, two-way communication process between therapist and patient, and for both physical and interpersonal reasons it may determine the eventual success or failure of the therapeutic intervention. The technical characteristics of the examination are certainly important, but the rehabilitation professional must take advantage of this unique opportunity to establish the patient rapport and trust necessary for successful treatment.

SUBJECTIVE EXAMINATION, PROVISIONAL DIAGNOSES, AND IRRITABILITY ESTIMATE

A thorough subjective history should precede the physical exam (see chapter 5 on the initial interview). The history must solicit the patient's chief complaint, detail the present symptoms or illness, explore precipitating events, carefully investigate the variation of the symptoms with respect to time of day and specific activity level, document prior treatment and results, chronicle concurrent local and systemic disease states or pathologies, and uncover relevant familial or social connections. Determining the number and pattern of joint involvement is relevant to both diagnosis and treatment planning for the rheumatologic diseases. The arthritides often present with typical and selective patterns of joint involvement, which helps to narrow the diagnostic possibilities and cues the examiner to more carefully assess commonly involved joints for clinical or subclinical changes. Systemic arthritides may also produce extraarticular changes (e.g., fever, fatigue, weakness) or can affect health and function of other organs (lungs, kidneys). From the information in the history, the therapist should make a mental list of the possible diagnoses, which will serve to guide the subsequent physical exam. The primary suspects on this list are usually medical diagnoses (e.g., osteoarthritis [OA], rheumatoid arthritis [RA], fracture). The therapist also needs to investigate secondary medical diagnoses such as joint instability, peripheral neuropathy, bursitis, and tenosynovitis. Secondary diagnoses may also be function related, for example, gait impairment, ineffective grasp, or insufficient sitting endurance to permit gainful employment. The primary diagnoses provide a prognostic framework and guidelines for precautions; but the secondary diagnoses, sometimes called the problems list, will more clearly guide the course of treatment, including self-management.

In addition to the provisional medical and functional diagnoses, the subjective examination must be used to determine the irritability of the patient's condition (Maitland, 1986). A patient with low irritability may report few or no painful symptoms at rest, but after performing an activity that exacerbates the condition will experience symptoms that diminish to negligible levels immediately or within an hour. A patient with low irritability can usually be thoroughly examined and considered for more aggressive forms of treatment. Conversely, a patient with high irritability often reports pain and symptoms at rest and may require many hours or even days of convalescence to return to tolerable symptomatic levels after performing activities that exacerbate the symptoms. High irritability often occurs during acute or subacute episodes of the systemic arthritides such as RA. Patients with high irritability must be examined with caution, and the therapist should selectively administer only those examination procedures that will yield the most crucial information to guide treatment selection. The therapist may have to accommodate joint irritability by collecting data over the course of several sessions while concurrently delivering treatment, and may also need to modify procedures to minimize musculoskeletal stress. By skillfully gathering valid information to clarify or establish the diagnosis and guide treatment while demonstrating compassionate respect for the patient's symptoms and discomfort, the clinician establishes the rapport and earns the trust that underpin a successful therapeutic relationship.

OBJECTIVE EXAMINATION
EXAMINATION PLANNING

The musculoskeletal evaluation should be conducted in a logical and somewhat stereotypic manner to assure consistent baseline data and maximize reevaluation and intertherapist reliability. Certain core tests and observations should always be undertaken, and additional clarifying tests included based on the history and the site of pathology, and to verify suspected primary and secondary diagnoses. The experienced examiner uses several tests, preferably ones that rely on different diagnostic approaches, to corroborate suspicions and reach a conclusion.

SCREENING EXAMINATION

A general screening examination of regions that are anatomically or kinetically linked to the area of complaint should always precede a differential musculoskeletal evaluation in order to assess the role of referred pain and identify contributing mechanical factors.

Kinetic linkage refers to a functional association of body parts such that a positional change in one region forces or encourages a compensatory positional change in one or more kinetically linked but potentially nonadjacent areas.

The screening exam is not intended to be comprehensive but is meant rather to scan for pathology outside of the specific region of complaint. For example, when a patient reports symptoms in the region of the tibiofemoral joint, the actual site of the pathology producing the symptoms might be the lumbosacral spine or the hip. In addition, biomechanical imbalances of the foot-ankle complex can generate abnormal lower-extremity forces that in turn can produce or exacerbate pathology in the knee. In the upper extremity, a person with limited supination of the forearms due to RA will often alter the posture of the cervicothoracic spine and shoulder girdles in order to accomplish hand tasks. The resulting abnormal stresses and overuse of the shoulders and upper back may produce concomitant functional problems (secondary diagnoses) that could be overlooked by a therapist focusing only on the hand dysfunction. More generally stated, symptoms localized to an extremity or axial region require a screening examination of the associated body quadrant. Suggested screening examinations for the upper and lower quarters are outlined in Tables 1 and 2.

Aside from its contribution to the diagnostic process, the screening examination is particularly important for identifying precautions and contraindications peculiar to an individual. For example, if a patient with osteoarthritic lumbar symptoms also has a significant but unrelated unilateral restriction of knee motion due to a prior fracture, the evaluative and treatment process for the lumbar dysfunction will have to be modified to accommodate and protect the restricted knee. The screening exam provides critical data for making safe and effective professional judgments.

As with all examination procedures, the screening examination should be conducted in a way that minimizes discomfort to the patient and avoids unnecessary exacerbation of irritable, inflammatory conditions. Recall that the purpose of the general screening examination is to determine if an unrecognized concomitant pathology or functional limitation exists, or if there is a need for detailed regional evaluation outside the area of chief complaint. Faced with an irritable, generalized inflammatory disease, the evaluator should cautiously conduct only the most essential and illuminating examination procedures and may need to gather data over the course of several visits.

DIFFERENTIAL MUSCULOSKELETAL EVALUATION

The key components of a specific, differential musculoskeletal evaluation that is focused on patients with rheumatologic symptoms can be outlined using variations of the scheme proposed by Kaltenborn (1989; Table 3). The sequence of the tests may vary with the preference of the therapist and should be arranged to minimize the discomfort and position changes necessary for the patient.

1. INSPECTION

Observation begins as the patient enters the clinic and continues throughout the exam. Note the patient's willingness to move, habitual postures, pain behaviors, gait pat-

UPPER-QUARTER SCREENING EXAMINATION

PURPOSE: To screen regions outside of the specific area of the patient's complaint.

GENERAL GUIDELINES:
Positive test results include significant malalignment, markedly asymmetric or reduced range of motion, reports of localized pain and/or reproduction of patient's primary symptoms. Positive results indicate that the region should be investigated in more detail to assess its possible contribution to the presenting pathology or if an unrelated pathology may be present in the region. If the patient can attain full active motion without pain or symptom reproduction, the examiner should apply gentle overpressure at the end of the patient's active motions to ensure that full available range is being used and to place additional stress on the joints and soft tissues.

CERVICAL SPINE
(1) Cervical Range of Motion: Rotation, lateral bending, flexion and extension. Use caution when assessing cervical extension in patients with a history of vascular disease, dizziness, altered consciousness, or blurred vision associated with head positioning.
(2) Cervical Quadrant Test: Maximal cervical rotation combined with cervical extension and contralateral cervical side-bending. Repeat to the other side. Cautions associated with the cervical range of motion exam should be observed.
(3) Spring Test: Patient prone and examiner applies gentle manual oscillatory posterior-to-anterior pressure to the dorsal tip of each accessible cervical spinous process (C2-C7) and upper thoracic region (T1-T4).

SHOULDER GIRDLE
(1) Shoulder abduction and rotation.
(2) Functional Tests: Hands behind head, then abduct and externally rotate shoulders. Hands behind the back on the lumbar spine, then slide the hands upward toward the scapulae (Apley's scratch test).

ELBOW
(1) Elbow flexion and extension.

FOREARM, WRIST, AND HAND
(1) Forearm pronation and supination.
(2) Wrist extension, flexion, radial and ulnar deviation.
(3) Hand function: Full fisting, full opening, digital abduction/adduction, and thumb opposition/deopposition (retropulsion).

UPPER-QUARTER NEUROLOGICAL SCREENING
Key neuromuscular function. Isometric manual muscle testing.
(1) Glenohumeral abduction: C5 nerve root; axillary nerve.
(2) Ulnohumeral flexion = C5, C6 nerve roots; musculocutaneous nerve.
(3) Ulnohumeral extension = C7 nerve root; radial nerve.
(4) Tip-to-tip pinch of the thumb and index finger = C8, T1 nerve roots; median nerve.
(5) Abduction of the small finger = C8, T1 nerve roots; ulnar nerve.
(6) Grip strength = not specific, includes C6-T1 nerve roots; radial, median, and ulnar nerves. Provides overall indicator of forearm, wrist and hand function.

UPPER-QUARTER NEUROLOGICAL SCREENING

Key dermatome and peripheral cutaneous sensation—light touch.

(1) Lateral deltoid muscle near deltoid tuberosity = C5 dermatome; axillary nerve.

(2) Lateral forearm over belly of brachioradialis muscle = C6 dermatome; radial nerve.

(3) Dorsum of hand in the web space of the thumb = not specific for dermatome (junction of C6 and C7); isolated region of sensation for radial nerve in the hand.

(4) Palmar tip of index finger = not specific for dermatome (junction of C6 and C7); isolated region of sensation for median nerve in the hand.

(5) Palmar tip of long finger = C7 dermatome; not always specific for peripheral cutaneous nerve (commonly median nerve but may be ulnar nerve).

(6) Palmar tip of small finger = not specific for dermatome (junction of C7 and C8); isolated region of sensation for ulnar nerve in the hand.

(7) Proximal third of the forearm on the ventral-medial aspect over the flexor muscle mass = C8 dermatome; ulnar nerve.

UPPER-QUARTER NEUROLOGICAL SCREENING

Deep tendon reflexes for nerve root and peripheral nerve.

(1) Biceps = C6; musculocutaneous nerve.

(2) Triceps = C7; radial nerve.

(3) Brachioradialis = C7; radial nerve.

LOWER-QUARTER SCREENING EXAMINATION

PURPOSE: To screen regions outside of the specific area of the patient's complaint.

GENERAL GUIDELINES:

Positive test results include significant malalignment, markedly asymmetric or reduced range of motion, reports of localized pain and/or reproduction of patient's primary symptoms. Positive results indicate that the region should be investigated in more detail to assess its possible contribution to the presenting patholo-gy or if an unrelated pathology may be present in the region. If the patient can attain full active motion with-out pain or symptom reproduction, the examiner should apply gentle overpressure at the end of the patient's active mo-tions to assure that full available range is being used and to place additional stress on the joints and soft tissues.

GENERAL LOWER-QUARTER AND TRUNK ALIGNMENT AND FUNCTION

Thoracic kyphosis, lumbar lordosis, knee valgus or varus, hindfoot pronation, hallux valgus. Observation of gait (velocity, symmetry, range of motion utilized, use of trunk rotation, arm swing, lateral trunk bending) including pain avoidance behavior.

THORACIC AND LUMBAR SPINE

(1) Thoracolumbar Range of Motion: Active trunk flexion and return from flexion (quality of motion, smoothness, halting, etc.), relative motion of the involved segments (shoulder girdle protraction, thoracic, lumbar, and hip flexion) and lateral deviations during flexion. Trunk side bending, rotation, and extension.

(2) Thoracolumbar Quadrant Test: Trunk extension with ipsilateral side bending and examiner overpressure at the shoulder stresses the ipsilateral lumbar facets while narrowing the lumbar intervertebral foramen (Magee, 1992).

(3) Spring Testing of the Thoracolumbar Spine. A patient prone on a treatment table then sequentially placing oscillatory posterior-anterior pressure on the individual spinous processes of the lumbar and thoracic spine. Moderate pressure applied through the hypothenar border of the examiner's hand and provide 4 or 5 oscilla-tions (1 to 2 Hz frequency) before moving to the adjacent spinous process. Complaints of specific stiffness and discomfort at one or a few adjacent spinal levels may indicate localized degenerative changes, while tenderness spanning larger regions may indicate a systemic inflammatory processes. It is unusual even in systemic arthritides for spring testing to elicit complaints of marked discomfort throughout the entire thora-columbar spine, and patient somatization of anxiety should be considered when it is present.

HIP AND KNEE

(1) Hip and Knee Range of Motion. Active hip flexion, abduction, adduction and extension, internal and external rotation. Knee flexion and full extension. A bilateral deep knee bend will further challenge functional range and strength in the lower extremities.

FOOT AND ANKLE

(1) Active talocrural dorsiflexion or plantarflexion; foot inversion supination and eversion/pronation.

LOWER-QUARTER NEUROLOGICAL SCREENING

Key neuromuscular function. Isometric manual muscle testing.

(1) Hip flexion = L2, 3 nerve roots; lumbar plexus.
(2) Knee extension = L3, 4 nerve roots; femoral nerve.
(3) Knee flexion = L4, 5, S1 nerve roots; sciatic nerve.
(4) Great toe extension = L5 nerve root; peroneal nerve.

LOWER-QUARTER NEUROLOGICAL SCREENING

Key neuromuscular function. Functional muscle testing.

(1) Ankle dorsiflexors (primarily tibialis anterior): Patient walks several steps on his or her calcanei maintaining full dorsiflexion demonstrating periods of single limb support during stance phase = L4, 5 nerve roots; peroneal nerve.
(2) Ankle plantar flexors (primarily gastrocsoleus muscle group): Patient walks several steps on the balls of his or her feet maintaining full plantarflexion demonstrating periods of single limb support during stance phase = S1, 2 nerve roots; tibial nerve.

LOWER-QUARTER NEUROLOGICAL SCREENING

Key cutaneous sensation. Light touch sensation.

(1) Lateral proximal thigh = L2 dermatome; Lateral femoral cutaneous nerve.
(2) Anteromedial thigh over vastus medialis oblique = L3 dermatome; saphenous nerve.
(3) Lateral calf at fibular neck = L4 dermatome; common peroneal nerve.
(4) Dorsum of foot = Not specific for dermatome (junction of L4 and L5); superficial peroneal nerve.
(5) Dorsal web space between 1st and 2nd toe = Not specific for dermatome (junction of L4 and L5); deep peroneal nerve.
(6) Posterolateral calcaneus = S1 dermatome; tibial nerve.
(7) Plantar surface of foot over 1st metatarsal head = L5 dermatome; medial plantar nerve.
(8) Plantar surface of foot over 5th metatarsal head = S1 dermatome; lateral plantar nerve.

LOWER-QUARTER NEUROLOGICAL SCREENING

Deep Tendon Reflexes.

(1) Quadriceps tendon = L4; femoral nerve.
(2) Achilles tendon = S1; tibial nerve.

Table 2: Lower-Quarter Screening Examination (continued)

terns, and other gross, static, and dynamic behaviors. An antalgic gait pattern with shuf-
fling of the feet, bilateral reduction of hip and knee angular excursion, lack of trunk rotation, and minimal arm swing tell the examiner that a widespread condition can be expected and a limited, cautious exam may be necessary. Observing simple maneuvers such as
the ability to place the hands symmetrically behind the head to pull the hair back or squat
to pick up a small object from the floor will guide the therapist in planning an effective
evaluation that is sensitive to the patient's condition and inflammatory status. This also
provides key data necessary to prescribe appropriate intervention and determine the
effectiveness of treatment. The patient must be clothed or draped so that the body segments under inspection are easily visible and permit dynamic evaluative motions without
restriction or undue embarrassment. Assorted sizes of elastic-waist shorts and tee-shirts
are excellent additions to the usual clinic linen.

Inspection of activities includes the patient's ability to perform activities of daily living. Performance of these activities represents a composite of the patient's range of
motion, strength, postural adaptation, and cognitive problem-solving ability. The patient's
use of aids (supports, braces, straps, or assistive devices) should be noted and their purpose, source, length of use, fit, and success investigated.

The postural alignment of body segments should be assessed when the patient is
standing and sitting. Habitual or compensatory postural malalignments may contribute
to musculoskeletal syndromes and often give significant insight into antalgic behaviors
or functional substitutions.

OBJECTIVE EVALUATION SCHEME

1. INSPECTION
   a. Activities of daily living
   b. Assistive devices
   c. Posture
   d. Shape
   e. Skin

2. PALPATION
   a. Skin and subcutaneous tissues
   b. Tendon sheaths and bursae
   c. Muscle and tendons
   d. Joints
   e. Nerves and blood vessels

3. NEUROLOGICAL
   a. Key muscles and reflexes
   b. Nerve trunks, peripheral nerves (& cranial nerves)
   c. Sensation
   d. General motor function and coordination

4. FUNCTION
   a. Active osteokinematic movement
   b. Passive osteokinematic movement
   c. Resisted movement
   d. Traction and compression
   e. Gliding and joint stability

5. SPECIAL ADDITIONAL TESTS
   a. Diagnostic imaging
   b. Laboratory tests
   c. Electrophysiologic testing
   d. Punctures—biopsies, fluid collection

Table 3: Objective Evaluation Scheme (modified from Kaltenborn, 1989)

The patient will naturally and unconsciously alter the postural platform to minimize discomfort and effort related to functional activities. The changes in both the static and dynamic alignment of the scapula and cervical spine in response to chronic arthritic change in a glenohumeral joint are excellent cases in point. The gross shapes of limbs and back and particularly of the joints are important in rheumatologic evaluation because of the linkage of the specific pathologies with predictable deformities such as the association of genu varum and tibiofemoral osteophytosis with OA of the knee.

The condition of the skin, changes in sweating patterns, and presence of scarring, discoloration, or abnormal hair growth may spur the therapist to additional inquiry about as yet overlooked trauma, previous procedures, and associated conditions. Dryness on the palmar surface of the hand often signals the early stages of carpal tunnel syndrome, a common complication of several rheumatic diseases.

2. PALPATION

This portion of the musculoskeletal evaluation relies on the examiner's knowledge of the relationship of surface landmarks to underlying anatomical details in order to correctly locate and isolate specific structures. Palpation of the joints for physical signs of heat, swelling, bogginess, and hypertrophy is central to any rheumatologic exam. The correlation of synovial inflammation and swelling with a patient's subjective report of pain upon palpation is far less than the examiner might expect. The patient's subjective reports of pain associated with the arthritides is dependent on a wide spectrum of physical, chemical, and psychological factors and have shown low correlations with joint inflammation and articular destruction (Amiado, 1988; Anderson et al., 1987; Kellgren, 1983). In this respect, the subjective intensity of tenderness upon palpation must be combined with the aforementioned physical manifestations to estimate the presence and intensity of synovitis.

Particularly in the limbs, palpable changes in synovial tissue and the adjacent connective tissue are apparent in regions of synovial outpouching and where bursae or tendon sheaths are superficial (see Table 4 and Box 1).

The search for tender points within muscles is also an important goal of palpation. A tender point is a predicable area in the muscle that is excessively tender to palpation. It should not be confused with a "trigger point," in which compression produces both pain at the site and referred pain in a predictable fashion outside of the area of compression, as classically associated with myofascial pain syndrome (Travell & Simons, 1983). A regional search for tenderness should include the skin, muscles, tendons, bursae, and joints. The discovery of tenderness hints that a pathologic process is present and warrants further examination. In this respect, tenderness is used as a flag for further examination. For example, the discovery of multiple or diffuse tender sites within the hip and shoulder girdle musculature raises the examiner's suspicion of fibromyalgia, but specific, unilateral tenderness immediately below the acromial arch may imply subdeltoid bursitis or supraspinatus tendinitis. Tenderness alone is not diagnostic but signals the need for additional testing to identify the pathology. Both examples (fibromyalgia and supraspinatus tendinitis) must meet specific criteria to warrant their diagnosis (Magee, 1992; Schumacher, Klippel, & Koopman, 1993). For additional information on fibromyalgia, see Box 2. When searching for tender points, the examiner must use a reasonable and reproducible amount of force. M. Certo recommends pressing hard enough to blanch the examiner's thumbnail bed (approximately 74 psi) while the American College of Rheumatology recommends using 4 kg of force (McCarthy, 1993; Schumacher et al., 1993). These are suggested maximums; less force may be necessary.

SYNOVITIS, BURSITIS, AND TENOSYNOVITIS: ASSESSMENT OF SWELLING

JOINT AND STRUCTURE

LOCATION

SHOULDER
1. Subacromial bursa
   Lateral aspect of deltoid immediately distal to acromion process.
2. Bicipital tenosynovitis (biceps tendon sheath of long head)
   Anterior aspect of deltoid within the intertubercular groove.

ELBOW
1. Ulnohumeral joint synovitis
   Posteromedial elbow immediately distal to the medial epicondyle of the humerus at the edge of the trochlear groove of the ulna. Partially covered by the ulnar nerve. Same synovial space as ulnohumeral joint.
2. Radiohumeral joint synovitis
   Posterolateral elbow immediately to the lateral epicondyle of the humerus at the articular circumference of the radial head. Surrounded by the annular ligament. Same synovial space as ulnohumeral joint.
3. Olecranon bursa
   Proximal posterior subcutaneous aspect of ulna overlying the olecranon process.

WRIST AND HAND
1. Radiocarpal synovitis (pouch of the radiocarpal joint)
   Dorsal surface of the radiocarpal joint immediately distal to the radius. Must be differentiated from overlying extensor tenosynovitis.
2. Dorsal wrist tenosynovitis (tendon sheaths of the wrist extensors, digital extensors and extensors/abductors of the thumb).
   Dorsal surface of the wrist, and extend approximately 1 inch, distal to the radiocarpal joint. Swelling is easily visible and outlines the length of the sheaths. It may be compressed by the dorsal retinaculum and be more apparent at the borders of the retinaculum.
3. Thumb carpometacarpal joint synovitis
   Swelling apparent over the lateral-volar aspect of the trapezial-metacarpal joint.
4. Metacarpophalangeal joint synovitis
   Dorsum of the MCP joints, full flexion reveals fullness in the valleys between the metacarpal heads.
5. Interphalangeal joint synovitis
   Symmetric swelling around the joint line.

KNEE

1. Suprapatellar pouch of the tibiofemoral joint
   Anterior aspect of the distal thigh, proximal to the patella. An extension of the tibiofemoral synovium positioned proximally beneath the distal quadriceps muscle. For minimal effusions, with the knee in extension, stroke and compress fluid from the medial side of the knee, tap the lateral side; a "bulge sign" or wave of fluid on the medial side indicates an effusion.

2. Anteromedial and anterolateral pouches of the tibiofemoral joint
   Anteromedial and anterolateral aspect of the knee just to either side of the patellar ligament and immediately proximal to the tibial plateau. Best palpated with the knee in slight flexion.

3. Pes Anserine bursitis
   Anteromedial aspect of the proximal tibial condyle approximately 2 cm distal to the tibiofemoral joint line. Beneath the combined tendons of the sartorius, gracilis, and semimembranosus muscles.

ANKLE AND FOOT

1. Talocrural joint synovitis
   Anterior aspect of the distal extent of the tibia. Most easily palpated with the foot in plantarflexion. Must be differentiated from the overlying extensor tendon sheaths.

2. Tenosynovitis of the tibialis anterior and the extensor digitorum longus tendons
   Dorsum of the foot passing across the talocrural joint and extending distally over the tarsals. Pass beneath the retinaculum at the talocrural joint.

3. Achilles tendonitis or tenosynovitis (Achilles peritenon)
   Posterior aspect of the distal calf surrounding the gastrocsoleus tendon and extending to the calcaneus.

4. Tenosynovitis of the tibialis posterior, flexor digitorum communis, and flexor halluces longus tendons
   Posterior aspect of the medial (tibial) malleolus. Associated with the neurovascular bundle passing into the foot.

5. Tenosynovitis of the peroneal tendons
   Posterior aspect of the lateral (fibular) malleolus (peroneus longus and brevis) and the anterior aspect of the lateral malleolus (peroneus tertius).

DETECTION OF SYNOVIAL AND BURSAL INFLAMMATION

ACUTE STAGE
- Skin erythema and elevated temperature.
- Palpation produces localized tenderness. Synovium or bursa may be enlarged and extend outside of its usual boundries into the adjacent soft tissue.
- Surface contour of the skin will be distorted over the structure with a visible increase in tissue volume; fluid motion may be detected on compression.
- Muscles that compress the inflamed bursa or pass through the involved synovial sheath have reduced strength due to pain.
- Patient selects a resting position for a joint with synovitis that maximizes joint volume.
- Crepitation may occur with joint motion. The probability of crepitation increases with each recurrence of inflammation.

CHRONIC STAGE
- Skin color and temperature often normal.
- Palpation produces localized tenderness and adjacent tissues may also be tender.
- Synovium or bursa may be enlarged and extend outside of its usual boundries into the adjacent soft tissue. The synovial and bursal tissues feel thick, dense, and boggy.
- Surface contour of the skin will be normal or minimally distorted over the structure unless the underlying bone shape has been remodeled. Fluid volume increases are often minimal and hard to detect.
- Generalized (nonspecific) decrease in muscle strength around the joint.
- Patient selects a resting position for a joint with chronic inflammation that minimizes periarticular soft tissue stress.
- Crepitation frequently present with joint motion.

Box 1: Detection of Synovial and Bursal Inflammation

DIAGNOSTIC CRITERIA FOR FIBROMYALGIA SYNDROME

- Widespread pain in muscles of the trunk and all four extremities, present for at least 3 months.

- Patient reports pain (not just tenderness) upon digital palpation of 11 out of 18 specific muscular sites using 4 kg of force.

Box 2: Diagnostic Criteria for Fibromyalgia Syndrome. Source: Wolfe, Smythe, Ynus, et al. (1990).

The solicitation of subjective reports of tenderness is only one aspect of palpation. The therapist must be able to vary the orientation of the palpating finger(s) and the amount of pressure applied to glean the available information from the specific tissues of interest. When examining for information other than tenderness, the most common palpation fault is to apply too much pressure, which in turn limits the therapist's sensory feedback to the relatively indiscriminant deep pressure sensors. A gentle palpating touch using an uncalloused region of the distal finger pulp will allow the sensitive light touch receptors to participate. Temperature differences are best detected by using the dorsal surface of the fingers (McCarty, 1993).

The skin and subcutaneous tissues are palpated for rheumatoid nodules and to detect displacement of fat pads on the plantar surfaces of the metatarsophalangeal joints, signs often associated with chronic inflammatory diseases such as RA. Increased localized skin temperature is indicative of an acute inflammatory process, whereas thinning of subcutaneous fat and changes in sweating patterns suggest chronic changes. Patients with RA may have warm, moist hands with palmar erythema indicative of vascular changes associated with the disease.

Tendon sheaths are palpated for warmth, volume (fullness), crepitation, catching, and nodular change. Inflammation may produce crepitus within a tendon sheath or connective tissue plane. This is best palpated during motion. In addition to static assessments, tendon sheaths and joints should be palpated during movement. Assessment of "lag" between active and passive ROM is a key assessment in determining impaired tendon gliding from tendinous stenosis.

Palpation related to nerves is primarily limited to percussion or tapping over the subcutaneous courses of peripheral nerves at sites of potential compression. Evoked paraethesias indicate pathologic irritability potentially caused by mechanical entrapment or metabolic compromise.

Upper-quarter pulses for routine palpation include those of the brachial, radial, and ulnar arteries. In the lower quarter, pulses include the femoral, popliteal, posterior tibial, and dorsalis pedis.

3. NEUROLOGICAL ASSESSMENT

Much of the neurological testing is included in the screening examination, specifically testing the neuromuscular function of key muscles, deep tendon reflexes, and sensory assessment. The neurological elements contained within the screening exam should be included in every complete musculoskeletal evaluation.

Patients with RA and OA of the cervical spine are at high risk of developing nerve-root compression, which is often painless and may be unnoticed until muscle atrophy or sensory loss occurs. The high incidence of peripheral entrapment neuropathies seen in rheumatic disease (RD) patients is attributed to the "double-crush" phenomenon, in which proximal compression in the cervical spine alters the physiology of the peripheral nerves and makes them susceptible to compression at a distal level. The cervical involvement may be clinical (symptomatic) or subclinical (asymptomatic). Once a peripheral entrapment neuropathy is determined, it is critical to assess potential cervical compression carefully. When a double-crush phenomenon exists, the distal entrapment will not respond to treatment unless the proximal entrapment is treated (Nakano, 1993).

In RD patients the most common peripheral entrapment neuropathies seen in the upper extremity are median neuropathy at the carpal tunnel, ulnar neuropathy at Guyon's canal and cubital tunnel, and brachial plexus at the thoracic outlet. In the lower extremity they are sciatic nerve at the piriformis muscle, posterior tibial nerve in the tarsal tunnel, and interdigital nerves between the third and fourth interspaces of the foot (Morton's neuroma) (Nakano, 1993).

General motor function and coordination of the upper quarter may be assessed by having the seated patient touch his or her nose with his or her index finger, then reach to touch the examiner's fingers, which are positioned at the limit of the patient's reach. The examiner's fingers are moved each time to gauge the patient's ability to accurately reach above and below shoulder level as well as ipsilaterally and contralaterally with respect to the patient's midline. Proprioceptive ability can be assessed by having the blindfolded patient actively move one upper extremity to match the examiner's passive placement of the contralateral upper extremity. Lower-quarter coordination and proprioception can be assessed through observational gait analysis and by standing with single limb support — eyes open and eyes closed (Rhomberg test).

4. FUNCTION

In addition to the gross motions evaluated during the screening examination, the active and passive osteokinematic range of motion of the suspect joints should be objectively assessed and recorded. When possible, deficits should be compared to uninvolved contralateral joints. If range of motion is less than normal, mild overpressure (gentle force applied by the examiner to move the joint in the direction of the active or passive motion) applied at the limit of the patient's available active and passive ranges of motion may be performed to discover any changes in the patient's subjective symptoms, as well as to assess the amount and type of resistance to further motion (endfeel).

The endfeel gives some insight about the cause of the restricted motion (Gould, 1990). A sudden, rigid stoppage of motion like that occurring during normal elbow extension (hard endfeel) implies a bony limitation, and a stiffly elastic stoppage like that occurring during normal glenohumeral external rotation (leathery endfeel) implies that tight connective tissue is limiting the motion. A hard endfeel often results from osteophytosis as in the loss of terminal extension of the osteoarthritic knee, while scleroderma provides many examples of motion losses with a leathery endfeel. The sensation of muscular spasm at the end of available range indicates that motion is limited by pain or spasticity, and a springy endfeel implies that a loose body or fibrocartilage is blocking joint motion and actually causing a slight rebound of motion in the other direction. An "empty" endfeel means that the examiner senses no mechanical resistance at the shortened pathological limit of motion but that the patient reports marked discomfort at any attempt to move the joint further.

An empty endfeel associated with significant pain is a cautionary flag to the examiner. A severe inflammatory state may exist, a serious medical condition (e.g. tumor, fracture) may be present, or the joint may have a marked subluxation or instability. When a joint provides no resistance to movement (lack of an endfeel) and the patient does not report pain, there may be significant joint disruption such as the complete loss of ligamentous integrity or marked bone-end resorption may be present, as with the mutilans deformity of the fingers, toes or ulnar styloid in RA, or psoriatic arthritis. When passive mobility differs from active mobility, extensor lag is present. The source of the lag should always be determined. In the presence of tenosynovitis the most common cause of lag is impaired distal or proximal gliding of the associated tendons. But it can also result from muscle weakness, tendon rupture, or a tendon nodule preventing excursion of the tendon.

Assessment of muscle strength (force-generating ability) is commonly performed by manual muscle testing (MMT) procedures (Kendall, McCreary, & Provance, 1993). These procedures are widely documented and are most useful for detecting and discriminating marked muscle weakness (rankings of 3 or less on a scale of 5) or for gross bilateral comparisons. For people with painful joints, resistance may need to be applied when the joint is positioned within the pain-free range because this avoids pain inhibition of muscle strength.

Aside from disuse or hypoactivity, a number of factors can reduce the force generating capacity of muscles: pain, inflammation (local or associated with systemic diseases such as RA), medications (particularly steroids), and denervation. This latter group of causes for muscle weakness does not respond to exercise intervention in the same way as simple weakness from hypoactivity, a fact that must be considered when designing intervention for weakness. The accuracy and reproducibility of strength measurements can be markedly improved over manual muscle testing through the use of objective dynamometers (hand-held or free-standing) (Deones, Wiley, & Worrell, 1994; Hayes & Falconer, 1992; Wadsworth, Krishnan, Sear, Harrold, & Neilsen, 1987). Objective dynamometry is particularly desirable for accurate documentation of incremental changes in strength over time and although widely used in the hand and the knee is just becoming the norm for other joints.

The response of a joint to decreased loading (traction) and increased loading (compression) should correlate with, respectively, the patient's subjective statements about symptom behavior in response to weight bearing and to rest in a supported position. The response to traction or compression will also prove valuable in selecting therapeutic interventions. Patients who have increased pain with compression and improve with traction may benefit greatly from the buoyant environment of a therapeutic pool.

Detectable losses of osteokinematic range of motion, patient complaints of symptom reproduction during motion, or an abnormal endfeel dictate the assessment of gliding motions at the involved joints. Gliding is often referred to as arthrokinematic motion or joint-play motion and may be defined as the subtle motions of joint surfaces with respect to one another that occur as part of the larger osteokinematic motions. Mechanically, these motions are referred to as slide, spin, and roll (Soames, 1995). An example is the arthrokinematic caudal glide of the humeral head within the glenoid fossa that must occur to allow full, pain-free osteokinematic abduction of the humerus. Due to the much larger surface length of the humerus with respect to that of the glenoid surface, pure osteokinematic abduction without concurrent downward gliding of the humeral head would result in a marked cranial translocation of the humeral head with respect to the glenoid cavity. Practically, a restriction of caudal glide causes the humerus to press into the coracoacromial arch during abduction and impinge on the supraspinatus tendon. Assessment of joint arthrokinematics and the useful application of the test results require the examiner to possess a detailed working knowledge of joint kinematics (Norkin & Levangi, 1992).

Joint stability, subluxation, and ligamentous and soft-tissue integrity should be assessed as part of the functional examination. Assessment can be done concurrent with an arthrokinematic assessment (Magee, 1992).

5. SPECIAL ADDITIONAL TESTS

A wide array of diagnostic imaging techniques is now available to depict both hard and soft tissues. Laboratory testing, particularly serological tests, are critical to the diagnosis of systemic arthritides. Electrophysiological testing (nerve conduction velocities and electromyography) can confirm and localize peripheral neuropathies and separate certain neuropathies from myopathies. Taps of synovial fluid and biopsies of the periarticular soft tissues are quite useful in delineating specific primary medical diagnoses and separating the arthritides from other categories of medical diagnoses. Finally, the examiner must always consider the diagnostic and treatment advantages provided by the wide array of practitioners within the health care team. The diagnostic challenges and complex sets of patient problem presented by the rheumatologic diseases are best met by a collaborative group working for the good of the patient.

SUMMARY

Based on the information gleaned from subjective and objective examinations and provided by outside sources or practitioners, the examiner must rule out unlikely diagnosis, choose a likely diagnosis, determine secondary and functional diagnoses, and decide whether additional information is necessary before proceeding with treatment. This is rarely an absolute decision. Rather many, but not all, of the diagnostic indicators will point toward one or a few likely possibilities. The initial selection of treatment must be based on this informed choice, with the caveat that treatment results must be closely monitored. Positive responses to treatment provide additional evidence that the diagnostic selection was correct, and further choices can be made. Equivocal or negative treatment responses send the examiner back to repeat key tests that may have given indefinite results or to start the examination process again in the hope of being more accurate and complete the second time. The probability of "getting it right the first time" increases with the experience and skill of the examiner, but willingness to reject a favored hypothesis and try again is the hallmark of a master clinician.

REFERENCES

Anderson K. O., Bradley L. A., McDaniel L. K., et al. (1987). The assessment of pain in rheumatoid arthritis. Validity of a behavioral observational method. *Arthritis and Rheumatism, 30*(1), 36-43.

Amiado, P. C. (1988). Pain dysfunction syndromes. *Journal of Bone and Joint Surgery, 70-A,* 944-949.

Deones, V. L., Wiley, S. C., & Worrell, T. (1994). Assessments of quadriceps muscle performance by a hand-held dynamometer and isokinetic dynamometer. *Journal of Orthopaedic and Sports Physical Therapy, 20,* 296-301.

Gould, J. A. (1990). *Orthopaedic and sports physical therapy* (2nd ed.). Philadelphia, PA: Mosby.

Hayes, L. W., & Falconer, J. (1992). Reliability of hand-held dynamometry and its relationship with manual muscle testing in patients with osteoarthritis of the knee. *Journal of Orthopaedic and Sports Physical Therapy 16,* 145-149.

Kaltenborn, F. M. (1989). *Manual mobilization of the extremity joints: Basic examination and treatment techniques* (4th ed.). Oslo, Norway: Olaf Norlis Bokhandel.

Kellgren, J. H. (1983). Pain in osteoarthritis. *Journal of Rheumatology* (supp 9) *10,* 108-109.

Kendall, F. P., McCreary, E. K., & Provance, P. G. (1993). *Muscles: Testing and function* (4th ed.). Baltimore, MD: Williams and Wilkins.

Magee, D. J. (1992). *Orthopedic physical assessment* (2nd ed.). Philadelphia, PA: W. B. Saunders.

Maitland, G. D. (1986). *Vertebral manipulation* (5th ed.). Boston: Butterworth.

McCarty, D. J. (1993). Differential diagnosis of arthritis: Analysis of signs and symptoms. In D. J. McCarty & W. J. Koopman (Eds.), *Arthritis and allied conditions: A textbook of rheumatology* (12th ed.). Philadelphia, PA: Lea & Febiger.

Nakano, K. K. (1993). Entrapment neuropathies and related disorders. In W. N. Kelly, E. D. Harris, S. Ruddy, & C. B. Sledge (Eds.), *Textbook of rheumatology.* Philadelphia, PA: W. B. Saunders.

Norkin, C. C., & Levangi, P. L. (1992). *Joint structure and function: A comprehensive analysis* (2nd ed). Philadelphia, PA: F. A. Davis.

Travell, J. G., & Simons, D. G. (1983). *Myofascial pain and dysfunction: The trigger point manual.* Baltimore, MD: Williams and Wilkins.

Schumacher H. R., Klippel J. H., & Koopman, W. J. (Eds.). (1993). *Primer on the rheumatic diseases* (10th ed.). Atlanta, GA: Arthritis Foundation.

Soames, R. W. (1995). Skeletal system. In P. L. Williams, M. M. Berry, P. Collins, M. Dyson, J. E. Dussek, & M. W. J. Ferguson (Eds.), *Gray's anatomy.* New York, NY: Churchill Livingstone.

Wadsworth, C. T., Krishnan, R., Sear, M., Harrold, J., & Neilsen, D. H. (1987). Intrarater reliability of manual muscle testing and hand-held dynametric muscle testing. *Physical Therapy, 67,* 1342-1347.

Wolf F., Smythe H. A., Ynus M. B., et al. (1990). The American College of Rheumatology 1990 criteria for the classification of fibromyalgia. Report of the multicenter criteria committee. *Arthritis and Rheumatism, 33,* 160-172.

JOINT AND SOFT TISSUE PAIN

Karen W. Hayes, PhD, PT, and Cheryl M. Petersen, MS, PT

Many conditions can manifest pain in or surrounding a joint, and conditions of soft tissues near the joint may be mistaken for some form of joint disease. The purpose of this chapter is to discuss clinical diagnostic techniques that formulate the basic evaluation framework to distinguish between painful conditions of the joint and those of the periarticular soft tissues such as muscle, tendon, ligament, joint capsule, bursa, or fascia.

SOFT-TISSUE DISORDERS

Soft-tissue disorders result from trauma, repetitive overload, faulty biomechanics, or disuse, or they occur as part of disease. Soft tissues react to these unusual stresses based on their structure, location, and the mechanical properties that determine their function. Unusual stresses cause structural and functional failure of the tissue components, acute inflammation, repair or remodeling, and structural and functional adaptation. Structural adaptation can affect the function of the tissue; for example, scarring can produce decreased tissue mobility. If overuse, disuse, disease, or faulty biomechanics are not corrected, further stress aggravates the condition and produces a chronic problem (Figure 1).

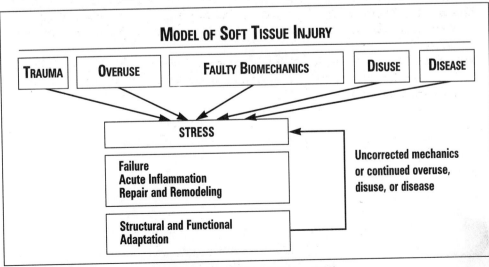

Figure 1. Model of Soft Tissue Injury (adapted from Klaiman & Gerber, 1996)

Many soft-tissue conditions are independent entities, but they may also occur in conjunction with rheumatic diseases such as rheumatoid arthritis and osteoarthritis. Inflammatory tendinitis, for example, can occur in conjunction with inflammatory arthritis or in response to altered function from repeated contact with an osteophyte. Soft-tissue conditions may be difficult to manage because some tissues such as tendon, ligament, and fibrocartilage have little or no vascular supply and are slow to heal. Some ligament injuries require up to 18 months for functional recovery and rarely achieve full structural recovery. Decreased vascularity may be aggravated by the concurrent presence of connective tissue disease or corticosteroid use (Klaiman & Gerber, 1996).

CLINICAL EXAMINATION

The clinical examination is the major approach to diagnosing painful soft-tissue conditions because laboratory and radiographic methods are often of little benefit. The clinical examination collects signs and symptoms from the patient through an interview and physical examination. The clinical examination is guided by the patient's chief complaint, which in joint and soft-tissue conditions is usually pain or limited function.

THE MEANING OF PAIN

Pain can provide valuable information about the patient's condition, but it may also be misleading in the diagnostic process because there is often a discrepancy between the location of the pain and the site of the lesion. Pain arising from a structure may be felt at the site of the structure, or it may be referred to a distant site. Distortion of the pain location may occur with irritation or compression of a spinal nerve root, which produces radiating pain. Distortion may also occur as a result of referred pain. Each periarticular structure has a segmental embryological derivation (Wadsworth, 1988). For example, the supraspinatus muscle and the glenohumeral joint capsule are derived embryologically from the fifth cervical segment (Magee, 1992). If a periarticular structure is involved, it refers pain to its segmental derivation; that is, a supraspinatus strain will refer pain to the C5 dermatome. Thus pain referring to a joint area may not arise from a joint structure. Pain that is referred to a joint area rarely is reproduced when the joint is moved. The practitioner must be careful to have the patient locate the pain and must always consider that the location may be an area of referred or radicular pain coming from a distant site.

THE INTERVIEW

Possible diagnoses are generated early in the patient interaction from the answers to the questions in the interview (Elstein, Shulman, & Sprafka, 1978; Payton, 1985). Each question provides a single data point and cannot, by itself, lead to an accurate diagnosis. Throughout the interview, however, the practitioner synthesizes the individual data points to create a profile of the problem and establish a working hypothesis. The responses to the questions in the interview guide the remainder of the clinical examination in an attempt to rule in or rule out possible diagnoses.

Interview questions should focus on current symptoms and their behavior, the history of the condition, and pertinent medical and family history. It is also important to determine the functional impact of the problem, that is, the extent to which the pain limits function, the amount of activity needed to initiate the pain, and the length of time the pain lasts once initiated (Maitland, 1970). This information can suggest how irritable the condition is. For example, if a patient has a supraspinatus tendon problem and experiences pain that lasts for 30 to 60 minutes after trying to brush her hair, the problem is considered irritable. Practitioners must plan their examination to avoid irritating the problem and preventing the patient from tolerating the entire examination. Tests that would aggravate the structure should be postponed until late in the examination. To clarify the condition, the examiner needs specific information about the onset of the condition, behavior, nature of the precipitating incident, if any, location of the symptoms, activities, positions, or behaviors that make the symptoms better or worse, progression of the symptoms, present treatment, and past management.

Information about the onset of the pain can suggest the type of the condition. For example, pain of recent onset and short duration suggests a traumatic or inflammatory origin. Pain of a more chronic and progressive nature often indicates joint incongruity (Sculco, 1981).

Information about the behavior of the pain can also suggest the nature of the condition. For example, if the pain is sharp, sudden, movable, and associated with giving way of the limb, a loose body (an isolated piece of cartilage or bone) could be in the joint. Nocturnal pain usually indicates inflammation or a serious problem.

The nature of the condition may also be suggested by the type of precipitating incident, if any. For example, a patient's report of pain related to repetitive motion suggests an overuse injury such as tendinitis or bursitis. A report of pain subsequent to a stretching activity indicates a muscular or ligamentous injury.

The location of pain may indicate the specific structure involved. For example, pain anterior to the acromion suggests a lesion in the supraspinatus tendon. The practitioner should be alert, however, that continued irritation or overuse of the tendon could cause the pain to refer throughout the entire C5 dermatome. Pain at the same location could also indicate a problem in the cervical spine involving the C5 nerve root with pain referred to the C5 dermatome.

Asking patients about positions and activities that make the condition better or worse provides the practitioner with clues regarding its structure as well as its irritability. For example, if the patient reports that activities involving shoulder abduction or any overhead activities cause the symptoms to increase, the practitioner could surmise that these activities are aggravating the supraspinatus muscle or tendon. Likewise, a patient may report that back pain is relieved when he or she is lying down and worsens when he or she sits. A recumbent position decreases compression on a protruded disc, and sitting increases the compression. The practitioner may logically begin to think that the patient has a disc protrusion.

The progression of the symptoms provides information about the direction of progression of the condition. Symptoms can start locally in the back and progress into the lower extremities, just as pain in the shoulder with the supraspinatus muscle or tendon problem could begin locally and develop referral pain throughout the related dermatome. These reports suggest that the condition is worsening.

Clues to the type of problem and ideas for management can be derived from the patient's reports of present treatment and past management. If the condition is recurrent, repeating previous successful treatments with subsequent relief helps confirm the diagnosis. For example, if deep-friction massage to the supraspinatus tendon has been successful in a previous episode and is successful again, the practitioner can feel confident that the previous supraspinatus tendinitis has returned. Relief with the use of antiinflammatory medications suggests that the condition is acute.

PHYSICAL EXAMINATION

The next step in determining the specific structures affected is a systematic physical examination. Physical examination of the joint and soft-tissue lesions is based on the function of the tissues and how they behave when subjected to various stresses (Cyriax, 1982; Ombregt, Bisschop, der Veer, & Van de Velde, 1995). During the physical examination, different stresses are applied in an attempt to reproduce the patient's symptoms, especially pain, and show dysfunction. It is important that the practitioner remind the patient to report the behavior of the particular pain or symptom that brought the patient to the office. Careful examination can serve to identify specific soft-tissue structure(s) and define their inflammatory status.

Four components of a typical physical examination include active motion, passive motion, resisted testing, and palpation. The responses of the patient's tissues to active, passive, and resistive stresses allow the practitioner to discriminate lesions in contractile tissues (muscle, tendon, enthesis) from those in inert tissues (capsule, ligament, bursa, fascia, nerve root, dura mater). It is often necessary to perform neurological tests such as sensory and deep-tendon reflex tests to clarify whether the problem arises from the soft-tissue structure or has a neurological origin.

Diagnosis of soft-tissue lesions by the functional behavior of the tissues is a popular and useful model for the clinical examination and provides a structure for the collection of patient data and a basis for clinical reasoning. The sensitivity, specificity, diagnostic accuracy, and reliability of the system, however, have been little studied. Individual components of the system appear to have low to moderate reliability (Hayes, Petersen, & Falconer, 1994; Patla & Paris, 1993) and questionable diagnostic accuracy (Franklin et al., 1996), but the entire system including the patient interview appears to have high inter-rater reliability of diagnostic classification (Pellecchia, Paolino, & Connell, 1996). Diagnostic accuracy of the entire system has not been studied. Regardless of the potential limitations of the system, diagnosis by behavior of tissues and structures during function is currently the only clinical means available. Done carefully, it provides reasonable accuracy and can be confirmed by more expensive and invasive methods.

ACTIVE MOTION

Active motion is used to identify the area of the problem, the patient's willingness to move, and his or her functional range of motion and strength. The patient is asked to move the various joints, and the examiner observes the patient's responses and complaints of pain. Various diagnoses may already be suggested during this initial phase, but definitive diagnoses should not be made at this time.

PASSIVE MOTION

Passive motion assesses the amount and direction of any limitations of motion, the palpable sensation at the end of passive motion (endfeel), the sequence of pain reported by the patient and endfeel noted by the practitioner during endfeel testing (pain/resistance sequence), and the presence or absence of a painful arc of motion.

PATTERN OF RESTRICTION

The amount and direction of limitation of motion are examined to determine the presence or absence of a capsular pattern of restriction. Cyriax (1982) proposed that each joint has a specific, proportional pattern of motion restriction that indicates involvement of the entire joint capsule. For example, at the shoulder he defined the capsular pattern as some limitation of abduction, more limitation of external rotation, and less limitation of internal rotation (with specific proportions) based on normal ranges of about 90 degrees of each glenohumeral motion (Cyriax). While the concept of patterns of restrictions at various joints is generally upheld by clinical experience, the specific proportions Cyriax proposed are controversial (Hayes et al., 1994). When a clinical capsular pattern is detected, involvement of the entire joint capsule is suggested. A pattern of motion limitation that deviates from the capsular pattern (noncapsular pattern) can indicate ligamentous or partial capsular adhesions, extraarticular involvement or internal derangement (Cyriax).

ENDFEEL

Endfeel is interpreted to indicate the anatomical structures that limit passive motion. An endfeel that feels extremely hard is interpreted as bone contacting bone. For some motions such as elbow extension, this bony endfeel is normal, but a bony endfeel can also mean that pathology such as advanced osteoarthritis (OA) is present and that trying to regain motion will be futile. An endfeel that is firm but still gives indicates that ligaments or the joint capsule are stopping motion. For many joints this capsular endfeel is normal, but in OA, for example, the end of the range of motion, and thus the capsular endfeel, occur earlier than anticipated. Some passive motions end with a muscle-spasm endfeel, indicating that muscles have acted to stop the motion, presumably due to pain. Spasm endfeels are common in joints that are inflamed. Multiple joint muscles may also stop motion when they are lengthened across all joints; this muscular endfeel feels firm but with more give than a capsular endfeel. When loose bodies are present in the joint, the endfeel may feel springy; a springy block would be detected when a meniscus in the knee joint is torn or when a piece of articular cartilage has loosened from the articular surface. Some motions end when other parts of the body prohibit further motion. This tissue-approximation endfeel feels rather soft as one body part compresses another. Empty end-feels occur when patients are unwilling to complete the motion (Cyriax, 1982).

PAIN-RESISTANCE SEQUENCE

The sequence of pain reported by the patient and resistance felt by the examiner during passive endfeel testing guides the vigor of treatment (Cyriax, 1982) and is often interpreted as an indicator of relative chronicity. Pain occurring before resistance is felt by the examiner suggests a lesion with active inflammation for which stretching would be inappropriate. Pain occurring synchronously with resistance suggests a lesion with less active inflammation for which gentle stretching might be tolerable, while pain occurring after resistance suggests a lesion without inflammation for which vigorous stretching would be appropriate.

PAINFUL ARC

A painful arc of motion suggests that a structure is being pinched in the arc of motion and relieved earlier and later in the range (Cyriax, 1982). Such a pattern of motion would be seen in subacromial bursitis, when the inflamed bursa is not irritated during early abduction but is compressed during midrange abduction and is decompressed once again during end-range abduction. A painful arc may also be seen if loose bodies are positioned in the joint so that they are compressed during part of the range of motion.

RESISTED CONTRACTIONS

Resisted testing determines the reaction of the contractile unit (muscle, tendon, enthesis) to muscle contraction. This type of resisted testing is performed to optimize discrimination of contractile from inert problems. The joint is positioned in midrange so that the capsule, ligaments, and other inert tissues are slack. An isometric test specific to the muscle or muscle group is done with maximal stabilization to prevent joint movement and muscle substitution. Contractions that are strong and painless suggest no lesion. Those that are strong and painful suggest a minor lesion of muscle or tendon such as a first-degree strain. Weak and painful contractions usually indicate a major lesion of a muscle or tendon such as a second-degree strain, but could indicate a fracture. Weak and painless contractions indicate a complete rupture of a muscle or tendon (third-degree strain) or neurological involvement (Cyriax, 1982).

The relationship among the passive, active, and resisted components is used to discriminate inert from contractile-tissue lesions. When active and passive motions are painful and limited in the same direction, and resisted contractions are not painful, an inert structure is implicated. For example, if the anterior capsule of the shoulder were sprained, pain and limitation of motion would be elicited both actively and passively during external rotation, extension, horizontal abduction, and from 90 to 180 degrees of flexion when the anterior capsule is being stretched, but no pain or limitation would be present on active or passive internal rotation and horizontal adduction, or during isometric resisted testing of any muscles. When active and passive motions are both painful in one direction, active motions are painful in the opposite direction, and resisted isometric contractions are painful, a contractile structure is implicated. For example, if the brachialis muscle were strained, active and passive elbow extension would be painful (the muscle is stretched), and active and resisted elbow flexion would be painful due to the contraction of the muscle.

PALPATION

After possible diagnoses are generated based on the results of active, passive, and resistive testing, static and dynamic palpation are used to identify whether the structure or structures suggested by the previous portions of the test are tender and to determine the presence of swelling, heat, or crepitus.

SPECIAL TESTS

The physical examination may also include special tests of joint and soft-tissue function. These tests are needed when the basic examination has not led to reproduction of the symptoms or identification of the dysfunction. Special tests may also help make a more specific clinical diagnosis, that is, identify the particular part of the structure involved. Various tests are used to assess the mobility and integrity of specific portions of the joint capsule, capsular ligaments, extraarticular ligaments, joint surfaces, or the ability of nerve structures to move within the soft tissues.

IMAGING IN SOFT-TISSUE DIAGNOSIS

Once a working musculoskeletal diagnosis has been established, treatment may often begin without further testing. If the condition is not responsive to therapy or if the clinical examination is inconclusive, diagnostic imaging is useful. Only recently have there been imaging methods available that are effective for confirming lesions in soft tissues. Most imaging methods provide the most useful information if they are done bilaterally. Although radiographs are often requested before the clinical examination is performed, they can be misleading because radiographically detectable changes are often asymptomatic. They are more useful if examined after the clinical examination to clarify clinical impressions.

Plain radiographs can be used to detect fractures and bony involvement such as spondylolisthesis or osteophytes, or to screen for congenital abnormalities. They are helpful in detecting instability using flexion, extension, or stress views in which force is applied manually to the joint. Radiographs are used routinely to screen for chronic conditions such as osteoarthritis (Karl & Floberg, 1995). A radiograph is the study of choice to rule out bone infection, tumor, or fracture with avascular necrosis, although they may appear normal for several weeks. Although used to detect osteoporosis, bone must have lost up to 30% of its mineral before plain radiographs can detect the loss. Plain radiographs are not very helpful in examining soft-tissue structures, but they can help to identify areas of edema or effusion (White, 1993).

Magnetic resonance imaging (MRI) is much more specific for soft-tissue involvement (Deutsch & Mink, 1989; White, 1993). Thorough assessment of extraosseous structures (cartilage, tendons, ligament, muscles) and intraosseous marrow is possible with MRI due to its fine soft-tissue contrast. It is also the study of choice for soft-tissue tumors (Karl & Floberg, 1995). Magnetic resonance imaging has been useful in clarifying conditions such as spinal cord injuries, acute herniated discs, epidural hematoma, avascular necrosis of the femur and scaphoid bones, lateral epicondylitis, tenosynovitis, rotator-cuff injuries, and injuries to the knee menisci and joint ligaments.

Computed tomography (CT) provides excellent cross-sectional anatomic definition of both muscular and skeletal systems simultaneously. Computed tomography can distinguish density differences of about 1% and allows discrimination between contiguous soft-tissue structures (in contrast, plain radiography detects density differences of about 5%). Computed tomography is particularly valuable in detecting lateral disc herniation and skeletal abnormalities such as spinal stenosis, osteochondral fractures, or intraarticular loose bodies (Karl & Floberg, 1995).

Nuclear skeletal imaging (bone scans) can reveal the presence of disease before it can be detected clinically or on plain radiographs. Its role traditionally has been in the detection of metastatic disease, but with recent technological advances it is used to evaluate traumatic and sports-related injuries such as myositis ossificans and inflammatory lesions in the skeleton such as reflex sympathetic dystrophy. Because bone scanning represents metabolism and not anatomy, it has high sensitivity (detecting disease in symptomatic people) but lower specificity (ruling out disease in people without disease). Any increase in metabolic activity of bone, regardless of the reason, will appear abnormal on the scan (Karl & Floberg, 1995).

Diagnostic ultrasound is also helpful and less expensive than some other forms of imaging, but its usefulness is confined to extraarticular lesions because sound waves do not penetrate bone (White, 1993). Ultrasound is especially useful in characterizing certain soft-tissue masses such as differentiating a Baker's cyst from other causes of popliteal swelling, but it is not a major imaging tool for the musculoskeletal system (Karl & Floberg, 1995).

LABORATORY STUDIES AND INJECTIONS

Injections of local anesthetic agents are often used to corroborate a clinical diagnosis. Once the involved structure has been identified clinically, it may be injected with a local anesthetic. After 5 minutes, the movements that reproduced the symptoms are repeated. If the symptoms are relieved, the diagnosis is considered to be accurate (Ombregt et al., 1995).

Laboratory studies such as the erythrocyte sedimentation rate, white blood cell counts, uric-acid levels, genetic markers, and rheumatoid factor are essential for diagnosis of rheumatoid arthritis, gout, or others of the various rheumatic disorders (Sculco, 1981), but they are not useful in determining a specific soft-tissue lesion.

Finally, aspirations of joint or extraarticular fluid may be necessary to determine the nature of the fluid. Analysis of joint effusion is particularly useful in infectious and crystal-induced lesions (Sculco, 1981; Stern, 1981) and following joint trauma. Synovial biopsy aids in diagnosis of pigmented villonodular synovitis.

DIAGNOSIS

To illustrate the use of this systematic examination, the next section of this chapter presents types of findings common to various soft-tissue and joint disorders (Biundo, 1993; Corrigan & Maitland, 1983; Salter, 1983; Sheon, Moskowitz, & Goldberg, 1987)

LIGAMENT SPRAIN

Ligaments reinforce the joint capsule at points of stress, hold bone ends together, guide joint motion, and provide stability to the joint. A ligament can be torn or stretched as a result of trauma or habitual postures that produce a lengthened position such as when a genu valgus position elongates the medial collateral ligament at the knee. Patients typically complain of pain on movements that stress the ligament or of giving way if a ligament is completely torn.

Active and passive movements that stress the ligament are painful. During the acute phase, range of motion may be limited due to protective muscle spasm, but range of motion may be excessive if the condition is not acute. Passive movements, if limited, are limited in a noncapsular pattern. The joint demonstrates a spasm endfeel if the condition is acute, or a capsular endfeel if the condition is chronic. In the acute phase, the patient complains of pain before the examiner feels resistance to the passive movements. When the condition is more chronic, the examiner feels resistance before the patient complains of pain. Because muscles are not involved, resisted contractions will be strong and painless. During palpation, the examiner may produce tenderness, or feel swelling or a breach or rupture in the area of the ligament. Specific ligamentous stress testing can identify laxity of specific ligaments. With third-degree sprains, there may be associated capsular tearing with bony subluxation or dislocation detectable radiographically.

BURSITIS

A bursa is a flattened pouch of synovial membrane that is situated between two tissue layers to reduce friction by creating a discontinuity between those tissues (Williams & Warwick, 1980). Thus, a bursa allows two structures to glide over each other smoothly. On occasion, the bursa may become irritated, fill with synovial fluid, and become inflamed. The inflammation is often from infection but rarely from acute trauma (Kessler

& Hertling, 1983). Patients complain of pain with movements of the joint that compress the bursa. The most common sites for bursitis are beneath the acromion at the shoulder, at the greater trochanter of the hip, at the patella in the knee, and over the olecranon at the elbow, although it can occur at any bursa.

On testing, patients experience pain with active and passive movements that compress the bursa. A painful arc is often present either actively or passively, and movement is limited in a noncapsular pattern. The examiner detects a spasm or empty endfeel, especially if the condition is acute and the patient is avoiding compressing the bursa. In the acute phase, the patient complains of pain before the examiner feels resistance to the passive movements. When the condition is more chronic, the examiner feels resistance before the patient complains of pain. Resisted testing produces strong but painful contractions if the condition is acute and the contraction compresses the bursa, although resisted testing may also be negative (strong and painless). While bursae are normally not palpable, if the bursal area is accessible, the examiner can palpate swelling over the inflamed bursa.

TENDINITIS AND MUSCLE STRAINS

Tendons and muscles provide motion and stability to joints. Tendons may be contained within a sheath (paratenon) or may be unsheathed. Tendinitis is a lesion of a tendon; tenosynovitis is a lesion of a tendon sheath (paratenonitis). Both tendinitis and tenosynovitis involve inflammation and degeneration and usually result from overuse, tissue fatigue, or rheumatic disease (Kessler & Hertling, 1983). Muscle strains, on the other hand, involve muscle-tissue tears of various magnitudes (from fiber tears to complete rupture) and result from trauma (Kessler & Hertling).

During the interview patients report that they experience pain during certain movements. When questioned closely it becomes apparent that pain is produced when the involved structure is stretched actively or passively and when the muscle contracts actively or against resistance. On testing, active motion produces pain in the pattern described above, that is, painful stretching and painful contraction of the muscle. Active movements that stress the muscle or tendon may also be limited by pain. Passive movements of the joint that do not stretch the muscle produce no pain, and endfeels are normal for the joint. However, if the condition is acute, the patient may complain of pain before the examiner feels resistance to the passive movements. When the condition is chronic, the examiner may feel resistance before the patient complains of pain, but endfeel testing will usually be pain free.

The examiner will provoke pain on resisted testing. If the response is strong but painful, a first-degree strain is suggested. A weak and painful contraction suggests a second-degree strain, and a weak but painless contraction suggests a third-degree strain because the tendon or muscle is completely ruptured and is no longer able to generate force. On palpation, the examiner will produce pain and feel swelling, trigger points, or atrophy in the muscle. In second- and third-degree strains, the examiner may feel a breach in the muscle. In tenosynovitis, crepitus is common.

LOOSE BODIES

Loose bodies are diagnosed infrequently. They usually occur when a small fragment of articular cartilage or bone breaks away, either due to OA or as a result of trauma (Cyriax, 1982). They can occur in the knee, hip, ankle, shoulder, elbow, wrist, spine, and temporo-mandibular joints. Over time, loose bodies can enhance joint damage (Hettinga, 1985). On interview, patients complain of clicking on specific movements, locking, or giving way, if the loose body is caught between articular surfaces. They may also complain of pain on compression of the joint.

Active and passive motions are limited in a noncapsular pattern, and a painful arc may be present. The examiner detects a spasm endfeel if the condition is acute or a springy block if a cartilage fragment interferes with joint motion. In the acute phase, patients complain of pain before the examiner feels resistance to the passive movements. When the condition is more chronic, the examiner feels resistance before patients complain of pain. Resisted testing produces contractions that are strong and painless because muscles are not involved. Palpation is negative. If loose bodies are bony, they may be seen radiographically.

OSTEOARTHRITIS

Osteoarthritis is usually considered to be a progressive disease of joints characterized by joint destruction, often in response to abnormal stresses such as compression, immobility, or hypermobility. It is common in the weight-bearing joints of older men and women. Osteoarthritis is considered to be noninflammatory, although secondary synovitis may occur (Brandt & Slemenda, 1993; Magid, 1981) (see chapter 5, Volume 2).

On interview, the patient may complain of stiffness more than pain and may report creaking in the joint. Both active and passive motion are limited in the capsular pattern for the involved joint with a capsular endfeel at the early termination of motion. The examiner may also feel a spasm endfeel if the condition is acute. If acute, pain is reported by the patient before the examiner feels resistance to passive movements. In more chronic stages, the examiner feels resistance before the patient complains of pain. Resisted movements are painless and strong because muscles are not involved. On palpation, the examiner may feel osteophytes, bony hypertrophy, and occasionally swelling. Passive accessory tests show limitations in all directions of the joint capsule. Radiographs may show osteophytes and joint space narrowing.

INFLAMMATORY JOINT PAIN

In inflammatory joint disorders such as rheumatoid arthritis, patients usually complain of pain more than stiffness. As in osteoarthritis, both active and passive motion are limited in a capsular pattern, with spasm endfeels in the acute phase and capsular endfeels in the more chronic phase. If acute, pain is reported by the patient before the examiner feels resistance to passive movements. In more chronic stages, the examiner feels resistance before the patient complains of pain. Resisted testing of any muscle may be painful if the condition is very acute, but resisted testing usually produces strong, painless contractions. The synovium may be tender to palpation, and the examiner may detect joint effusion. Radiographs show effusion, osteoporosis, joint-space narrowing, and osteolytic areas. Later, subluxation and dislocation are common. In very late stages, ankylosis is seen. Laboratory tests show rheumatoid factor and elevated white blood cell counts and erythrocyte sedimentation rates.

COMMON CONDITIONS AT DIFFERENT JOINT REGIONS

In the next portion of this chapter, we show how selected conditions manifest in specific structures at specific joints. These conditions are only examples of common conditions practitioners encounter in the clinic; we make no attempt to provide exhaustive coverage of the wide variety of conditions that practitioners could encounter. We present the material in tabular form for quick reference (Tables 1-7) but caution the reader that conditions will often not present as described here. Presentation will differ depending on whether the condition is acute or chronic, minor or major. Many patients experience more than one condition simultaneously, and that confuses the interpretation of data. The practitioner must compile a list of possible diagnoses and, using all of the patient's data, develop a profile that explains the results. We present the material as it would be encountered in the clinic. The patient arrives with a complaint of pain in or around a particular joint area. Questioning elicits key symptoms, and examination uncovers key signs. The combination of signs and symptoms leads to a likely diagnosis.

It is obvious that many of these conditions present similar findings. It is only by examining how the structures function in conjunction with the information gathered from the patient and imaging techniques, laboratory tests, and local injection of anesthetic agents that the practitioner can detect a pattern of dysfunction that suggests what structure is at fault.

Once the correct musculoskeletal diagnosis has been made, it must be managed appropriately to prevent recurrence. The principles of rehabilitation that physical and occupational therapists use to manage soft-tissue lesions include resolving the current problem and, more importantly, preventing recurrence by identifying the cause of the problem and correcting it or helping the patient find ways to compensate without putting other tissues and structures at risk. While complete discussion of treatment is beyond the scope of this chapter, these principles translate into treatment goals of relieving pain and inflammation, promoting tissue healing, preventing or reducing fibrosis and scarring, restoring appropriate flexibility, strength, and endurance, correcting mechanical faults and alignment, and teaching the patient self-management skills.

SPINE PAIN: KEY CLINICAL FINDINGS OF SELECTED CONDITIONS

SPINE

INTERVIEW STATEMENTS	PHYSICAL FINDINGS	LIKELY CONDITION
Patient complains of pain that increases with activity and decreases with rest. Minimal decrease in pain from weight bearing to non–weight bearing.	**Active and Passive Motion:** Pain and limitation in a capsular pattern (limited extension and side bending and rotation to the right) **Resisted Testing:** Negative **Palpation:** Pain and swelling over facet joint, local muscle guarding in area **Special Tests:** Passive accessory intervertebral motion and passive physiological intervertebral motion testing painful and limited; distraction painful **Imaging:** Negative	**Right cervical facet joint dysfunction, typical of OA (unilateral or bilateral) or RA (usually bilateral)**
Patient complains of pain that increases in weight bearing and decreases in non–weight bearing; spinal and lower extremity pain.	**Active and Passive Motion:** Pain and limitation in a noncapsular pattern (limited flexion, right lateral flexion) **Resisted Testing:** Negative **Palpation:** Local and nonspecific muscle guarding **Special Tests:** Compression painful; distraction relieves pain; neurological testing and EMG will show positive neurological involvement **Imaging:** MRI shows disc herniation	**Left lumbar disc herniation**

Table 1: Spine Pain: Key Clinical Findings of Selected Conditions

SPINE

INTERVIEW STATEMENTS	PHYSICAL FINDINGS	LIKELY CONDITION
Patient complains of neck pain (dull aching) associated with stiffness. Pain is often constant and made worse by sudden movements or physical activity involving the neck. Pain radiates into the left arm due to nerve root pressure, following cervical extension or excessive use of the arm and occasionally following minor trauma or overuse.	**Active and Passive Motion:** Painful extension, left side bending and rotation **Resisted Testing:** Negative **Palpation:** Possible cervical, upper trapezius area, and scapular tenderness **Special Tests:** Positive neurological testing related to the nerve root level involved (sensory changes in dermatome, motor changes in myotome, segmentally related deep tendon reflex changes), positive upper limb tension tests **Imaging:** Degenerative changes (spurs, osteophytes) may be seen on X-ray	**Cervical spondylosis with left radiculopathy**

HIP PAIN: KEY CLINICAL FINDINGS OF SELECTED CONDITIONS

HIP

INTERVIEW STATEMENTS	PHYSICAL FINDINGS	LIKELY CONDITION
Patient complains of groin pain, especially on weight bearing or lying on the involved side, and stiffness after inactivity.	**Active and Passive Motion:** Pain and limitation in a capsular pattern (limited flexion, abduction, internal rotation, and slight extension) **Resisted Testing:** Negative **Special Tests:** Limited distraction, long axis traction, posterior glide; positive joint scouring and Fabere[a] tests **Imaging:** Radiography shows osteophytes, joint narrowing, bony sclerosis; bone scans show increased activity at joint margins **Other:** Negative ESR and synovial fluid	**Osteoarthritis**
Patient complains of pain in lateral aspect of proximal thigh; may report blow or overuse; aggravated by climbing stairs and lying on the involved side.	**Active and Passive Motion:** Limited especially in external rotation (noncapsular pattern) **Resisted Testing:** Painful resisted abduction **Palpation:** Tender and swollen lateral aspect of greater trochanter **Special Tests:** None **Imaging:** Positive sonogram but not often used **Other:** Relief with anesthetic injection into trochanteric bursa	**Trochanteric bursitis**

[a]The patient reports pain when the involved hip is flexed, abducted, and externally rotated with the heel resting on the opposite straight leg above the knee, and then passively moved into further abduction, external rotation, and extension.

Table 2: Hip Pain: Key Clinical Findings of Selected Conditions

HIP

INTERVIEW STATEMENTS	PHYSICAL FINDINGS	LIKELY CONDITION
Patient complains of pain in groin area; may report history of overuse or slipping and stretching the upper thigh.	**Active Motion:** Painful adduction; may be limited by pain **Passive Motion:** End range of abduction painful **Resisted Testing:** Painful resisted adduction **Palpation:** Tender over the musculotendinous junction or enthesis **Special Tests:** None **Imaging:** Positive sonogram but not often used **Other:** Relief with anesthetic injection into adductor tendons	**Adductor tendinitis**
Patient complains of abrupt onset of groin and thigh pain, at first only with weight bearing and later during non–weight bearing and even at rest. May report use of high doses of corticosteriods, trauma, or having a connective tissue disorder (SLE, RA).	**Active and Passive Motion:** Decreased range of all motions due to pain and later due to bony destruction **Resisted Testing:** Negative **Palpation:** Negative **Special Tests:** None **Imaging:** Positive MRI bone scan, radiographs, CAT scan	**Osteonecrosis of the femoral head**
Patient complains of intermittent sharp pain, sudden twinges, and giving way.	**Active and Passive Motion:** External rotation and flexion painful and limited (noncapsular pattern) **Resisted Testing:** Negative **Palpation:** Unremarkable **Special Tests:** None **Imaging:** CT scan, radiographs may show bony fragments	**Loose body**

KNEE PAIN: KEY CLINICAL FINDINGS OF SELECTED CONDITIONS

KNEE

INTERVIEW STATEMENTS	PHYSICAL FINDINGS	LIKELY CONDITION
Patient complains of pain with weight bearing; stiffness, especially in the morning and after prolonged sitting.	**Active and Passive Motion:** Pain and limitation in a capsular pattern (flexion more limited than extension) **Resisted Testing:** Negative **Palpation:** May be bony hypertrophy, creaking **Special Tests:** Compression may be painful **Imaging:** Radiographs show decreased joint space, osteophytes, bone scans show increased activity at joint margins	**Osteoarthritis**
Patient complains of pain with pressure on the kneecap following prolonged kneeling or direct trauma.	**Active and Passive Motion:** Flexion may be painful and limited **Resisted Testing:** Painful extension **Palpation:** Pain/swelling superficial to the kneecap **Special Tests:** Compression painful; distraction relieves pain **Imaging:** Positive sonogram but not usually done	**Prepatellar bursitis**

Table 3: Knee Pain: Key Clinical Findings of Selected Conditions

KNEE

INTERVIEW STATEMENTS	PHYSICAL FINDINGS	LIKELY CONDITION
Patient complains of pain with knee extension activities, such as sit/stand, stairs, walking/running; may report occasional sensation of weakness or giving way.	**Active Motion:** Pain in extension and may be limited by pain **Passive Motion:** End of range of knee flexion painful **Resisted Testing:** Extension painful **Palpation:** Tenderness/swelling in tendon; crepitus with passive movements of the tendon **Special Tests:** Negative **Imaging:** Negative	**Patellar tendinitis**
Patient complains of diffuse swelling of the calf, pain, and sometimes erythema and edema of the ankle. May report having a knee condition with synovial effusion.	**Active and Passive Motion:** End range limitation of flexion and extension with discomfort **Resisted Testing:** Negative **Palpation:** Swelling in the popliteal region **Special Tests:** None **Imaging:** Positive sonogram or arthrogram	**Baker's cyst (common secondary to RA, OA, or internal derangement of the knee)**
Patient complains of pain and a sensation of weakness while weight bearing in knee extension, and lateral tibial rotation; reports being hit on the outside of the leg with the foot planted.	**Active and Passive Motion:** Pain in knee extension and lateral tibial rotation **Resisted Testing:** Negative **Palpation:** Pain, breach, or swelling over the medial collateral ligament **Special Tests:** Positive valgus stress test[a] and Apley's distraction[b] **Imaging:** MRI shows tear (but not often done)	**Medial collateral ligament sprain**

[a] The supine patient demonstrates laxity and may complain of pain when a valgus force is imparted to the extended or slightly flexed knee.
[b] The prone patient complains of pain when a distraction force with internal and external tibial rotation is applied to the flexed (90 degrees) knee through the tibia.

KNEE

INTERVIEW STATEMENTS	PHYSICAL FINDINGS	LIKELY CONDITION
Patient complains of intense pain when the leg was planted with the knee in a flexed and laterally rotated position.	**Active and Passive Motion:** Pain and limitations in a non-capsular pattern **Resisted Testing:** Negative **Palpation:** Medial tibial plateau tender **Special Tests:** Positive McMurray's[c] and Apley's compression[d] tests **Imaging:** Positive MRI	Medial meniscus tear (sometimes associated with RA)

[c] The supine patient complains of pain and a click is heard or felt when a valgus force with external tibial rotation is applied to the fully flexed knee while the knee is moved into extension.
[d] A click is heard or felt at the joint line or the patient complains of pain when the examiner applies a compression force through the tibia and internally and externally rotates the tibia of the prone patient whose knee is flexed 90 degrees.

Table 3: Knee Pain: Key Clinical Findings of Selected Conditions (continued)

ANKLE PAIN: KEY CLINICAL FINDINGS OF SELECTED CONDITIONS

ANKLE

INTERVIEW STATEMENTS	PHYSICAL FINDINGS	LIKELY CONDITION
Patient complains of pain and swelling over the Achilles tendon related to overuse or inadequate footwear.	**Active Motion:** Pain and possible limitation in plantar flexion **Passive Motion:** Pain at end of range in dorsiflexion **Resisted Testing:** Plantar flexion painful **Palpation:** Pain and swelling over the Achilles tendon; crepitus on plantar/dorsiflexion **Special Tests:** Negative **Imaging:** Positive sonogram but not usually done	**Achilles tendinitis**
Patient complains of pain when standing; located over the metatarsal head area with callusing over the area; may report abnormal mechanical stress or joint disease such as RA.	**Active and Passive Motion:** Hypermobility into pronation **Resisted Testing:** Negative, but there may be associated intrinsic foot weakness **Palpation:** Pain/tenderness over the metatarsal head area **Special Tests:** Negative **Imaging:** Negative	**Metatarsalagia**

ANKLE

INTERVIEW STATEMENTS	PHYSICAL FINDINGS	LIKELY CONDITION
Patient reports sensory and motor changes in the distribution of the posterior tibial nerve distal to the tarsal tunnel; burning pain on the plantar surface of the foot; may report direct trauma or chronic irritation, pain worse on weight bearing.	**Active and Passive Motion:** May be associated with hypermobility into pronation **Resisted Testing:** Muscles innervated by the posterior tibial nerve distal to the tarsal tunnel weak **Palpation:** Unremarkable **Special Tests:** Positive neurological examination; positive percussion test **Imaging:** Negative **Other:** Slowed or blocked conduction on nerve conduction studies; relief with injection of corticosteroid	**Tarsal tunnel syndrome**
Patient complains of heel pain, especially with initial weight bearing after rest; may report trauma from athletic activity, prolonged walking, etc.	**Active and Passive Motion:** May be associated with increased pronation or supination **Resisted Testing:** Negative **Palpation:** Tenderness over the medial calcaneal plantar tuberosity **Special Tests:** Negative **Imaging:** Radiographs may show calcaneal spur **Other:** Relief with injection of corticosteroid	**Plantar fasciitis**

Table 4: Ankle Pain: Key Clinical Findings of Selected Conditions (continued)

ANKLE

INTERVIEW STATEMENTS	PHYSICAL FINDINGS	LIKELY CONDITION
Patient reports pain, swelling, and restricted ankle movement; may report trauma, overuse, or a rheumatic disease such as RA or spondyloarthropathy.	**Active Motion:** Pain during ankle plantar flexion and inversion and may be limited by pain **Passive Motion:** Ends of range of ankle dorsiflexion and eversion are painful **Resisted Testing:** Ankle plantar flexion and inversion are painful **Palpation:** Tender and swollen posteriar tibialis tendon above, behind, or just below the medial malleolus; crepitus during motion **Special tests:** None **Imaging:** Positive sonogram but not usually done **Other:** Injection of corticosteroid produces relief	**Posterior tibial tenosynovitis**

SHOULDER PAIN: KEY CLINICAL FINDINGS OF SELECTED CONDITIONS

SHOULDER

INTERVIEW STATEMENTS	PHYSICAL FINDINGS	LIKELY CONDITION
Patient reports gradual onset of generalized shoulder pain with severe loss of shoulder mobility; may complain that lying on the affected shoulder is painful.	**Active and Passive Motion:** Pain and limitation in a capsular pattern (external rotation more limited than abduction which is more limited than internal rotation) **Resisted Testing:** Negative **Palpation:** Unremarkable **Special Tests:** Accessory movements (limited lateral distraction, anterior glide, inferior glide, posterior glide) **Imaging:** Arthrography shows decreased volume of capsule **Other:** Relief with corticosteroid injection into the glenohumeral joint and subacromial bursa	**Adhesive capsulitis**
Patient complains of pain usually over the outer aspect of the shoulder which can radiate down the arm; pain occurs following overuse or trauma to the shoulder. May be recurrent.	**Active Motion:** Painful and possibly limited abduction; possible painful arc **Passive Motion:** Painful arc **Resisted Testing:** Painful abduction **Palpation:** Tender/swollen over tendon **Special Tests:** Negative **Imaging:** Negative **Other:** Relief with anesthetic injection and use of corticosteroids	**Supraspinatus tendinitis**

Table 5: Shoulder Pain: Key Clinical Findings of Selected Conditions

SHOULDER

INTERVIEW STATEMENTS	PHYSICAL FINDINGS	LIKELY CONDITION
Patient feels or hears a sudden painful "snap" in the shoulder following a history of recurrent tendinitis; reports a loss of strength and mobility in the shoulder.	**Active Motion:** Loss of abduction to about 20 degrees **Passive Motion:** Full abduction **Resisted Testing:** Abduction weak and painless **Palpation:** Breach, swelling in tendon **Special Tests:** Positive drop arm test[a] **Imaging:** Arthrography of the shoulder shows communication between joint and subacromial bursa.	**Supraspinatus rupture**
Patient, more frequently female, complains of progressive muscle weakness in shoulders and other proximal muscles, joint and muscle pain, difficulty in climbing stairs, getting in and out of a chair, fatigue, and possible difficulty breathing and swallowing.	**Active Motion:** Pain and weakness in all shoulder, trunk, and hip muscles **Passive Motion:** In early stages, full range; in later stages may be limited by muscle weakness **Resisted Testing:** Proximal limb and neck muscles weak and painful **Palpation:** Proximal muscles are typically tender and atrophied **Special Tests:** None **Imaging:** MRI shows inflammation **Other:** Elevated serum levels of CPK, aldolase, lactic dehydrogenase, and the transaminases; EMG shows myopathic motor unit potentials and fibrillation potentials; muscle biopsy shows inflammation; may have decreased tidal volume on pulmonary function tests and arrythmias on ECG	**Polymyositis**

[a]The patient is unable to support the arm in shoulder abduction when the examiner raises it passively to 90 degrees.

Table 5: Shoulder Pain: Key Clinical Findings of Selected Conditions (continued)

SHOULDER

INTERVIEW STATEMENTS	PHYSICAL FINDINGS	LIKELY CONDITION
The patient is likely to be over 50 years old and female; complains of symmetrical stiffness and discomfort in the shoulders (it can also affect the neck, upper arms, lower back, and hips); onset is often sudden.	**Active Motion:** All shoulder movement limited and painful **Passive Motion:** Limited shoulder movement **Resisted Testing:** Strength unimpaired but may be painful **Palpation:** Tenderness around shoulders **Special Tests:** None **Imaging:** X-rays negative; MRI shows nonspecific inflammation in shoulder synovial tissue **Other:** Elevated ESR, positive response to low-dose prednisone	**Polymyalgia rheumatica**
Patient is likely to be middle aged; reports ache or pain in the shoulder with movement. Reports no pain at rest. After a month or two, reports pain with movement becoming more severe with constant aching. May state that pain is worse at night and especially if he/she lies on that side. May also report reoccurrence at the other shoulder.	**Active and Passive Motion:** Pain and limitation in a capsular pattern (external rotation more limited than abduction which is more limited than internal rotation) **Resisted Testing:** Negative **Palpation:** Negative **Special Tests:** None **Imaging:** Radiographs show soft-tissue swelling **Other:** Intraarticular steriod injection provides relief, elevated ESR	**Monoarticular RA (synovitis)**

Table 5: Shoulder Pain: Key Clinical Findings of Selected Conditions (continued)

ELBOW PAIN: KEY CLINICAL FINDINGS OF SELECTED CONDITIONS

ELBOW

INTERVIEW STATEMENTS	PHYSICAL FINDINGS	LIKELY CONDITION
Patient complains of localized tenderness over the lateral epicondyle with wrist extension combined with forearm supination/pronation activities; related to overuse of the wrist extensors.	**Active Motion:** Pain and possible limitation with wrist extension **Passive Motion:** Painful at end of wrist flexion with elbow extension **Resisted Testing:** Painful wrist extension **Palpation:** Tender over the lateral epicondyle, swelling possible **Special Tests:** Negative **Imaging:** Negative **Other:** Relief with local steroid injection	**Lateral epicondylitis**
Patient reports sensory and motor changes in the ulnar nerve distribution distal to the elbow; may describe nocturnal paresthesias and numbness; may report repeated pressure on nerve.	**Active Motion:** Limitation of wrist flexion, ulnar deviation and intrinsic hand and finger motions due to weakness **Passive Motion:** Negative **Resisted Testing:** Ulnar nerve muscles distal to elbow (hand intrinsics and flexor carpi ulnaris) are weak **Palpation:** With ulnar nerve pressure, pain or paresthesia in the ulnar nerve distribution; atrophy of hypothenar area **Special Tests:** Positive neurological examination (decreased or absent sensation in ulnar distribution); positive percussion test **Imaging:** Negative **Other:** Slowed or blocked nerve conduction; postural clawing of ring and little fingers	**Ulnar nerve entrapment**

ELBOW

INTERVIEW STATEMENTS	PHYSICAL FINDINGS	LIKELY CONDITION
Patient reports tenderness to pressure over tip of elbow; onset may be insidious or secondary to trauma.	**Active and Passive Motion:** Pressure/pain at end of flexion **Resisted Testing:** Negative **Palpation:** Swollen and tender to pressure over the olecranon area **Special Tests:** Negative **Imaging:** Positive sonogram but not usually done **Other:** Aspiration shows clear or blood-tinged fluid; relief with corticosteroid injection	**Olecranon bursitis**
Patient complains of pain and stiffness: may report having arthritis, trauma, or a period of immobilization.	**Active and Passive Motion:** Pain and limitation in a capsular pattern (flexion more limited than extension) **Resisted Testing:** Negative **Palpation:** Unremarkable **Special Tests:** Accessory movements (limited humeroulnar distraction and caudal glide: limited humeroradial distraction and palmar glide) **Imaging:** Radiographs may show joint space narrowing and osteophytes, bone scans show increased activity at joint margins	**Osteoarthritis**

Table 6: Elbow Pain: Key Clinical Findings of Selected Conditions (continued)

WRIST PAIN: KEY CLINICAL FINDINGS OF SELECTED CONDITIONS

WRIST

INTERVIEW STATEMENTS	PHYSICAL FINDINGS	LIKELY CONDITION
Patient complains of pain around the base of the thumb, increased with pinch grip; may report trauma, or have generalized osteoarthritis.	**Active and Passive Motion:** Pain and limitation in a capsular pattern (limitation of extension and abduction) **Resisted Testing:** Negative **Palpation:** Possible bony changes ("squaring") or dorsal subluxation; crepitus with CMC movements **Special Tests:** Positive joint compression **Imaging:** Radiographs (performing a pinch grip) including an oblique view show joint space narrowing and osteophytes	**Osteoarthritis of the first CMC joint**
Patient shows discreet swelling on the dorsum of the wrist; may state that wrist extension produces discomfort.	**Active and Passive Motion:** Discomfort at end range of extension or flexion **Resisted Testing:** Negative **Palpation:** Cystic, tender swelling on the dorsum of the wrist; may only be evident on full wrist flexion **Special Tests:** Negative **Imaging:** Negative **Other:** Aspiration shows thick, jelly-like fluid; injection of corticosteroid provides relief	**Ganglion**

WRIST

INTERVIEW STATEMENTS	PHYSICAL FINDINGS	LIKELY CONDITION
Patient complains of pain on radial side of the wrist, radiating into forearm or thumb; made worse by movements of the thumb or wrist; may report repetitive lateral pinch activities.	**Active Motion:** Painful and possibly limited thumb abduction and extension and wrist extension and radial deviation **Passive Motion:** Painful thumb flexion **Resisted Testing:** Thumb abduction and extension and wrist extension and radial deviation painful **Palpation:** Tender swelling on radial side of the wrist **Special Tests:** Finkelstein's[a] test positive **Imaging:** Negative **Other:** Relief with local injection of corticosteroid	**Tenosynovitis of first compartment tendons (abductor pollicis longus and extensor pollicis brevis (de Quervain's tenosynovitis)**
Patient reports sensory (pain or paresthesia) and motor changes in the hand; may report repetitive wrist motion; nocturnal paresthesia or pain; associated with flexor tenosynovitis in patients with RA or with osteophytes in patients with OA.	**Active Motion:** Limitation of some finger and thumb movements due to weakness of muscles supplied by median nerve distal to the carpal tunnel **Passive Motion:** Negative **Resisted Testing:** Muscles supplied by the median nerve distal to the carpal tunnel may be weak **Palpation:** May be tender over the tunnel **Special Tests:** Positive neurological examination (sensory changes in median nerve distribution); positive percussion test and Phalen test[b] **Imaging:** Negative **Other:** Slowed or blocked conduction on nerve conduction studies	**Carpal tunnel syndrome**

[a]Patient complains of pain in the first compartment with full thumb flexion, adduction, and wrist ulnar deviation.
[b]Patient reports reproduction of sensory symptoms when the dorsums of the hands are placed together and the wrists are flexed maximally and held for up to 60 seconds.

Table 7: Wrist Pain: Key Clinical Findings of Selected Conditions (continued)

REFERENCES

Biundo, J. J. (1993). Regional rheumatic pain syndromes. In H. R. Schumacher (Ed.), *Primer on the rheumatic diseases* (10th ed., pp. 277-287). Atlanta, GA: Arthritis Foundation.

Brandt, K. D., & Slemenda, C. W. (1993). Osteoarthritis: A. Epidemiology, pathology and pathogenesis. In H. R. Schumacher (Ed.), *Primer on the rheumatic diseases* (10th ed., pp. 184-188). Atlanta, GA: Arthritis Foundation.

Corrigan, B., & Maitland, G. D. (1983). *Practical orthopaedic medicine.* London: Butterworth.

Cyriax, J. (1982). *Textbook of orthopaedic medicine: Volume I: Diagnosis of soft tissue lesions* (8th ed.). London: Balliére Tindall.

Deutsch, A. L., & Mink, J. H. (1989). Magnetic resonance imaging of musculoskeletal injuries. *Radiologic Clinics of North America, 27,* 983-1001.

Elstein, A. S., Shulman, L. S., & Sprafka, S. A. (1978). *Medical problem solving: An analysis of clinical reasoning.* Cambridge, MA: Harvard University Press.

Franklin, M. E., Conner-Kerr, T., Chamness, M., Chenier, T. C., Kelly, R. R., & Hodge, T. (1996). Assessment of exercise-induced minor muscle lesions: The accuracy of Cyriax's diagnosis by selective tension paradigm. *Journal of Orthopaedic and Sports Physical Therapy, 24,* 122-129.

Hayes, K. W., Petersen, C., & Falconer, J. (1994). An examination of Cyriax's passive motion tests with patients having osteoarthritis of the knee. *Physical Therapy, 74,* 697-707.

Hettinga, D. L. (1985). Inflammatory response of synovial joint structures. In J. A. Gould & G. J. Davies (Eds.), *Orthopaedic and sports physical therapy: Volume two* (pp. 87-117). St. Louis, MO: Mosby.

Karl, R. D., & Floberg, J. A. (1995). Radiologic assessment of the musculoskeletal system. In W. G. Boissonault (Ed.), *Examination in physical therapy practice: Screening for medical disease* (2nd. ed., pp. 365-397). New York: Churchill Livingstone.

Kessler, R. M. & Hertling, D. (1983). *Management of common musculoskeletal disorders: Physical therapy principles and methods.* Philadelphia: Harper & Row.

Klaiman, M. D., & Gerber, L. H. (1996). General considerations for managing tendon injuries. *Bulletin on the Rheumatic Diseases, 45,* 1-6.

Magee, D. J. (1992). *Orthopedic physical assessment* (2nd. ed.). Philadelphia: W. B. Saunders.

Magid, S. K. (1981). Osteoarthrosis (osteoarthritis, degenerative joint disease). In J. R. Beary, C. L. Christian, & T. P. Sculco (Eds.), *Manual of rheumatology and outpatient orthopedic disorders: Diagnosis and therapy* (pp. 183-196). Boston: Little, Brown.

Maitland, G. D. (1970). *Peripheral manipulation* (2nd ed.). Worcester, MA: Butterworth.

Ombregt, L., Bisschop, P., der Veer, H. J., & Van de Velde, T. (1995). General principles. In L. Ombregt, P. Bisschop, H. J. der Veer, & T. Van de Velde, *A system of orthopaedic medicine* (pp. 1-100). London: W. B. Saunders.

Patla, C. E., & Paris, S. V. (1993). Reliability of interpretation of the Paris classification of normal end feel for elbow flexion and extension. *Journal of Manual & Manipulative Therapy, 1,* 60-66.

Payton, O. D. (1985). Clinical reasoning process in physical therapy. *Physical Therapy, 65,* 924-928.

Pellecchia, G. L., Paolino, J., & Connell, J. (1996). Intertester reliability of the Cyriax evaluation in assessing patients with shoulder pain. *Journal of Orthopaedic and Sports Physical Therapy, 23,* 34-38.

Salter, R. B. (1983). *Textbook of disorders and injuries of the musculoskeletal system* (2nd. ed.). Baltimore, MD: Williams & Wilkins.

Sculco, T. P. (1981). Hip pain. In J. R. Beary, C. L. Christian, & T. P. Sculco (Eds.), *Manual of rheumatology and outpatient orthopedic disorders: Diagnosis and therapy* (pp. 101-105). Boston: Little, Brown.

Sculco, T. P. (1981). Hip pain. In J. R. Beary, C. L. Christian, & T. P. Sculco (Eds.), *Manual of rheumatology and outpatient orthopedic disorders: Diagnosis and therapy* (pp. 101-105). Boston: Little, Brown.

Sheon, R. P., Moskowitz, R. W., & Goldberg, V. M. (1987). *Soft tissue rheumatic pain: Recognition, management, prevention* (2nd. ed.). Philadelphia: Lea and Febiger.

Stern, R. (1981). Arthrocentesis and intraarticular injection. In J. R. Beary, C. L. Christian, & T. P. Sculco (Eds.), *Manual of rheumatology and outpatient orthopedic disorders: Diagnosis and therapy* (pp. 23-28). Boston: Little, Brown.

Wadsworth, C. T, (1988). *Manual examination and treatment of the spine and extremities.* Baltimore, MD: Williams & Wilkins.

White, D. M. (1993). Diagnostic imaging. *PT Magazine, 1*(6), 66-72.

Williams, P. L., & Warwick, R. (1980). *Gray's anatomy* (36th British ed.). Philadelphia: W. B. Saunders.

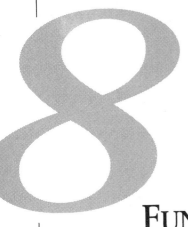

FUNCTIONAL ASSESSMENT

Catherine Backman, MS, OT(C)

Arthritis can have a substantial effect on a person's functional performance. Studies have established both an immediate and long-term relationship between arthritis and limitations in function (Guccione, 1994). Furthermore, the type of arthritis and severity of symptoms also contribute to the individual's ability to perform everyday activities. For example, in one study individuals with rheumatoid arthritis (RA) experienced functional limitations in a wide variety of activities in comparison with matched control subjects, while individuals with osteoarthritis (OA) experienced difficulties in a more limited range of household chores, shopping, and leisure pursuits (Yelin, Lubeck, Holman, & Epstein, 1987). Assessment of functional performance is an important part of establishing rehabilitation goals. In addition, research on the functional abilities and limitations of persons with chronic conditions helps rehabilitation practitioners and others understand the process of disablement, and our understanding may in turn lead to more effective treatment.[1]

This chapter begins with a definition of terms, identifies some special considerations when assessing the person with arthritis, outlines a traditional approach to assessing function for the purpose of treatment planning, introduces new approaches to assessing function, illustrates one of the new approaches with a case study, and concludes with a brief note about the role of standardized testing and the relationship between functional assessment and outcome measures.

DEFINITION OF TERMS

Two conceptual frameworks guide the content of this chapter: the World Health Organization (WHO) classification of impairment, disability and handicap (WHO, 1980), and the Occupational Performance Model (Canadian Association of Occupational Therapists [CAOT], 1991; Pedretti, 1996). These frameworks, listed in Table 1, include the following definitions of terms used throughout the chapter:

[1]For a review of arthritis and the process of disablement, see Guccione, A. A. (1994). Arthritis and the process of disablement. *Physical Therapy, 74,* 408-414.

Impairment refers to physiological deficits or limitations such as decreased range of motion (ROM). *Disability* is a restriction or lack of ability to perform everyday activities resulting from the impairment, such as inability to dress oneself as a result of limited ROM. *Handicap* refers to the social disadvantage of impairment or disability that prevents or limits the individual in fulfilling a usual role or occupation. For example, the lack of accessibility in the workplace may limit people's ability to work when arthritis causes disabilities or impairments. The assessment approaches discussed in this chapter deal predominantly with disability and handicap issues and the assessment of impairment is addressed in other chapters (e.g., musculoskeletal evaluation in chapter 6).

The occupational performance model is discussed fully in other sources (CAOT, 1991; Pedretti, 1996) and only key terms will be introduced here. *Occupational performance* refers to the ability to perform tasks that are necessary to fulfilling the individual's social roles in a manner appropriate to his or her developmental stage and physical, social, and cultural environments. The occupational performance model is defined by three performance areas: self-care, work and productivity, and leisure. *Self-care* includes self-maintaining tasks (eating, dressing, bathing, functional mobility); *work and productivity* include home management, school, and paid and unpaid work; and *leisure* refers to quiet and active recreational activities, play, and socialization. This chapter encompasses assessment of all three areas of occupational performance. It will not address the assessment of *performance components*, that is, the physical (sensorimotor), psychosocial, and cognitive components that are part of the occupational-performance model, because they are indicative of the level of impairment rather than disability and handicap. Finally, the occupational performance model emphasizes that function occurs within a specific *temporal and environmental context* (Pedretti), so the importance of assessing function will be discussed in a way that is specific to how, why, and where the individual fulfills his or her typical daily activities. Thus, "occupational performance" is almost synonymous with "function"; it provides a specific vocabulary to help define the many aspects of how and where people function.

Using occupational performance as a framework ensures that all tasks related to self-care, productivity, and leisure will be considered when evaluating the client. Although the term activities of daily living (ADL) seems to imply all tasks involved in everyday living, the trend in rehabilitation is to define ADL as the activities limited to self-maintenance, to use instrumental activities of daily living (IADL) to refer to household and community living tasks; and to define school, work, and leisure activities separately from ADL and IADL. Therefore, the all-encompassing framework of occupational performance seems better suited to discussion of functional assessment.

FUNCTIONAL ASSESSMENT—DEFINITION AND PURPOSE

Functional assessment has been defined as "the measurement of purposeful behavior in interaction with the environment, which is interpreted according to the assessment's intended uses" (Halpern & Fuhrer, 1984, p. 3). This is a good definition for rehabilitation practitioners, because it highlights the importance of meaningful occupations or activities (purposeful behavior), the context in which the client functions (interaction with the environment), and the reason for assessment (intended uses).

THE RELATIONSHIP BETWEEN TERMS USED IN THE WHO CLASSIFICATION SYSTEM AND THE OCCUPATIONAL PERFORMANCE MODEL (OPM)

WHO TERM	EXAMPLES	OPM TERMS

pathology	arthritis
	    joint inflammation
	    tenosynovitis
	    cartilage erosion	

impairment	joint motion/restriction muscle strength/weakness endurance/fatigue	performance components

disability	ability/inability to
	    dress
	    bathe
	    prepare meals
	    clean home
	    use work tools (computer, hammer)
	    play
	    pursue hobbies
		occupational performance areas
		    self-care
		
		    productivity/work
		
		    leisure

handicap	ability to fulfill roles relevant to age, gender, family expectations, societal/cultural/physical environment e.g., worker mother	developmental, sociocultural, and physical environments occupational roles

Shaded portion of table refers to the topic of functional assessment as addressed in this chapter.

Table 1: Terms Used in the World Health Organization (WHO) Classification System and the Occupational Performance Model (OPM)

There are at least four purposes of functional assessment: (a) to describe functional status in preparation for treatment planning or consultation, (b) to measure change and monitor progress, (c) to facilitate communication and decision making, and (d) to evaluate programs and conduct research (Backman, 1994). The method or measurement tools selected should match the purpose of the assessment. For example, if the purpose is to describe functional status in the area of self-care at a given time, possibly to determine if intervention is required, then a descriptive measure such as the Physical Self-Maintenance Scale (Lawton & Brody, 1996) might be appropriate for quickly screening basic self-care abilities (Law, 1993). If the purpose is to describe function for the purpose of treatment planning, and to recommend assistive devices, a more detailed assessment may be necessary, such as an ADL checklist (see appendix 2) or a more standardized approach such as the Klein-Bell Activities of Daily Living Scale (Klein & Bell, 1982). If the purpose is to facilitate decision making jointly with the client and family regarding the client's functional ability at home, then perhaps measurement is less important than developing an understanding of the client in context, and an ethnographic approach (described by Spencer, Krefting, & Mattingly, 1993) to interview and observe performance might be more appropriate. This approach is discussed in more detail in the section on contemporary approaches to assessment.

Many factors influence the assessment of self-care, work, and leisure. The importance of functionally relevant goals and outcomes to help identify health care priorities in an environment of escalating costs, societal demands for accountability, and managed care systems suggests the need for quick, reliable, and quantifiable measures. "Evidence of successful and efficient functional outcomes is expected to be the major mechanism by which organizations will convince third-party payers to cover services" (Velozo, 1994, p. 946). The trend toward client-centered or consumer-driven health services, an approach that respects the client's goals and priorities, suggests an individualized assessment process that is contextual and, by definition, unlikely to consist of measurement of standardized items of performance. Yet in order to develop a comprehensive treatment plan, some practitioners find itemized checklists useful for the identification of specific problems that require intervention. Because these and other external factors are often contradictory, it is not surprising to experience frustration or confusion when they surface in the clinical setting. By the end of this chapter the reader will have some strategies for responding to these issues.

Special Considerations When Assessing People with Arthritis

Functional assessment is only one part of the evaluation of the person with arthritis. Several factors that are associated with inflammatory arthritis such as morning stiffness, fatigue, and joint inflammation should be considered during the assessment of occupational performance, and these were addressed in more detail in the previous chapters. Variation in functional performance is to be expected when people have arthritis. For example, an assessment of ADL conducted before morning stiffness has eased may yield results that differ from the same assessment conducted in the afternoon. Fatigue may fluctuate and change performance, as will the number of active joints. Acutely inflamed joints also mean painful joints, so the client may be able to demonstrate some, but not all, activities in a single session. It is therefore important to enquire about the client's typical daily function in addition to what is observed at the moment, to ask about the duration of morning stiffness, the onset of fatigue, and the pain experienced during daily activities in order to obtain a reasonable estimate of day-to-day performance.

Psychosocial factors such as emotional stress may also have an impact on performance. Sometimes it may be difficult to differentiate psychosocial factors influencing function versus functional limitations influencing psychological well-being. From a practical perspective, it is necessary to be sensitive to each person's unique situation as well as the possibility that assessing function and dysfunction may be discouraging to some people. In most cases, this sensitivity is demonstrated by creating an atmosphere of mutual respect where the goal is to work together to identify and resolve problems. Psychosocial issues are discussed more fully in chapter 3.

Many people with arthritis will have learned strategies or selected special equipment to enable them to perform necessary and important activities in their own environments. Observation of performance in the clinical setting may differ from that observed in the client's home, school, or workplace because even simple things like the heights of chairs and countertops and the size or shape of handles on tools and utensils may make the difference between the ability to complete a task or not. Interpretation of assessments conducted in the clinic should carefully consider these variations.

ASSESSMENT FOR THE PURPOSE OF TREATMENT PLANNING: TRADITIONAL APPROACH

SCREENING ASSESSMENT

Typically, the need for a full functional evaluation is determined by asking a few key questions in the form of a screening assessment. This may stand alone (see the screening form, appendix 1) or be part of a more thorough initial assessment. For example, therapists at The Arthritis Society, British Columbia and Yukon Division, include key questions about self-care, work, and leisure within their initial general assessment guidelines, which also include a history and musculoskeletal examination. Responses to screening questions will most likely produce one of three outcomes: They may (a) indicate the need for a more detailed assessment of self-care, work and leisure tasks; (b) identify a minor problem that can be easily resolved (e.g., provision of a jar opener to assist with the task of opening containers); or (c) indicate that there are no functional problems requiring investigation or intervention.

DETAILED OBSERVATIONS AND CHECKLISTS

When the client and therapist agree that self-care, work, or leisure tasks are problematic, an observational assessment is indicated so that the therapist can observe first-hand how the client performs. In addition to describing occupational performance at a given time, observational assessments provide cues that the therapist can use when planning intervention and education strategies. For example, the methods used to dress, prepare a meal, or complete a work task may demonstrate inefficient or potentially harmful postures and may suggest the need for instruction on principles of joint protection and energy conservation. When observational assessments are impractical, an itemized checklist or detailed interview may be the only reasonable substitute. The ADL checklist provided by Melvin (1989) is frequently used with arthritis patients in the United States. The checklist section pertaining to occupational performance has been reprinted in appendix 2. Similarly, Melvin's interview questions regarding work assessment may also elicit useful information about the client's work day that helps the therapist to formulate practical recommendations to enhance performance. These, too, are appended as a resource (see appendix 3).

Perceived advantages to the itemized-checklist approach include its comprehensiveness and the opportunity to identify specific tasks that may be accomplished more easily with the provision of an assistive device or alternative method. The systematic review of a number of tasks representative of everyday living may serve to identify problems from a functional, rather than impairment-specific, perspective. This is important when funding sources want documentation of functional limitations and goals for treatment rather than descriptions of discrete physical limitations (i.e., restricted joint ROM or reduced muscle strength). Disadvantages include the lack of standardization in administration and interpretation, lack of quantification or scoring mechanisms to indicate changes when the assessment is repeated, and the fact that no one checklist can possibly contain the unique constellation of activities that is applicable to the person being assessed. Nevertheless, checklists may be the preferred approach in some settings.

CONTEMPORARY APPROACHES TO ASSESSING FUNCTION

Health reform takes on different forms in different regions of the world. In Canada, the management of health funds through regional (instead of central government) health boards and the need to demonstrate measurable functional outcomes to ensure ongoing funding mean that the assessment approach used with all clients needs to be integrated with outcome measures and empirical evidence that the approaches used have demonstrated reliability, validity, and clinical utility even when the primary purpose is treatment planning. In other words, assessment for the purpose of treatment planning is also expected to provide data that can be used for assessing functional outcomes and measuring the effects of the services provided. In response to this type of demand, several contemporary approaches to assessing function are emerging in both practice and research arenas.

CLIENT-CENTERED ASSESSMENT OF OCCUPATIONAL PERFORMANCE

Client-centered practice refers to the client leading the process of problem identification, priority setting, and treatment planning. Since clients seek health care based on their own priorities and identification of problems, it makes sense to develop assessments based on their perceptions rather than asking them to feed into a system that requires the practitioner to set problems and treatment plans. "If the person is no longer the problem definer, it is unlikely that he or she will be the problem solver either. This disparity can "reduce the client's self-determination and sense of control over health, often leading to what may appear as noncompliance" (Pollack, 1993, pp. 298-299). The MACTAR[2] Patient Preference Disability Questionnaire (Tugwell et al., 1987) and the Canadian Occupational Performance Measure (COPM) (Law et al., 1994) are two examples of client-centered approaches to assessing function.

The MACTAR was designed for clinical trials with people who have arthritis, with the belief that there is increased potential for demonstrating changes in disability if the focus of the measure is "on those activities directly affected by inflammation and judged to be important by the patient" (Tugwell et al., 1987, p. 446). The interviewer asks clients to "Please tell me which activities are affected by your arthritis?" and presents a menu of examples, including mobility, self-care, work and leisure activities to ensure that patients understand that all activities are of interest if affected by their arthritis. Up to 10 specific activities are identified and prioritized by asking "Which of these activities would you most like to be able to do without the pain or discomfort of your arthritis?" and "Which of these activities would you next most like to be able to do without the pain or discomfort of your arthritis?" To measure change at subsequent visits, patients are asked if there is improvement in their ability to do the 10 priority activities identified at baseline. When compared to traditional functional questionnaires, the MACTAR demonstrated a greater magnitude of change in functional status, probably because the items were selected by the patients (Tugwell et al.).

Somewhat similar to the MACTAR, but designed to be used with any client regardless of medical diagnosis, the COPM is a semistructured interview that asks clients if they need to, want to, or are expected to perform tasks in each of the three areas of occupational performance (self-care, productivity, and leisure). Then the client is asked if he or she is having difficulty performing any of the identified tasks. Up to five tasks or activities are prioritized and labeled as problems and subsequently rated by the client on a 1 to 10 scale indicating the client's ability to perform the task and the client's satisfaction with task performance (1 = low ability and satisfaction; 10 = high ability and satisfaction). Ratings are summed and divided by the number of problems to yield performance and satisfaction scores that can be used as an outcome measure when the rating process is repeated after intervention. (Because a 10-point scale is used and the summed ratings are divided by the number of problems rated, the highest possible score for each of performance and satisfaction is 10). "Through this process the true priorities of the clients become evident; these priorities often differed from the therapists' initial ideas" (Pollack, 1993, p. 300).

Both the MACTAR and COPM are excellent tools for an initial evaluation that helps rehabilitation practitioners to focus on problems from the clients' perspective, and both have been used in outpatient and inpatient settings with people who have arthritis. Neither tool is proposed to replace reliable and valid functional- or physical-status measures, although both the MACTAR and COPM may be more effective in identifying client priorities in occupational performance than the traditional ADL checklist. After using the MACTAR or COPM for problem identification and validation with the client, additional assessment tools may be necessary to determine the factors contributing to

---

[2] MACTAR is an acronym composed of letters from McMaster, Toronto, and arthritis, and it indicates the locations of the arthritis research and treatment programs of the test's authors.

each problem. For example, it may be necessary to conduct a detailed self-care evaluation, ROM and muscle-strength evaluation, hand assessment, or evaluation of home or work-site. However, since the priority occupational performance difficulties have been clearly identified, there is less chance that valuable time will be wasted on unnecessary evaluations or that the client will wonder about the purpose or relevance of the evaluation and intervention plans. All three occupational-performance areas of self-care, work, and leisure can be addressed in an initial assessment with the MACTAR or the COPM, which can be especially useful when assessment tools specific to each domain are either not available or are inappropriate for a client. Therefore, either the MACTAR or the COPM is highly recommended as an initial assessment for all clients with arthritis. To illustrate this approach, the COPM is used in the case example later in this chapter.

Trombly (1995) calls the identification of occupational-performance problems as the first step in assessment the "top-down" approach (as opposed to the "bottom-up" approach of assessing performance components such as joint ROM or hand strength first). There is a greater likelihood of understanding the context (i.e., the social, cultural, and physical environment) within which the individual functions when one takes the top-down approach. The problems identified and prioritized from the client's perspective will indicate the relative importance of observing function in the home, school, workplace, or community recreation site, where the subtle but important contributions of sociocultural roles and expectations, and environmental helps and barriers, can be observed.

Lessons from Ethnographic Approaches: The Importance of Context

Jette (1994) emphasizes that in order to understand why a person is more or less able to do the activities he or she needs or wants to do, it is important to consider both the person's physical capacities and the person's ability to perform in relevant situations and environments. He also defines three perspectives on situational need or context:

1. *How the individual defines the disablement situation and reacts to it (e.g., denial, depression).*

2. *How others (e.g., spouse, children, friends) define the disablement situation and set expectations for the individual (e.g., sick-role expectations).*

3. *Characteristics of the physical environment itself (e.g., environmental barriers) (p. 383).*

Understanding the context in which the person functions helps to explain why two people with very similar pathologies (e.g., acute episode of rheumatoid arthritis) and similar impairments (e.g., limitations in grip strength, finger dexterity, shoulder and elbow ROM) have quite different abilities to function at home and work: One person lives alone in an apartment, is independent in self-care and household management, and is self-employed as an organizational change consultant, while the other person is having difficulty managing a household with school-aged children and finds it necessary to leave her job as a secretary due to loss of finger dexterity for word processing. In this example, it is the environment and productivity requirements that cause disability in the latter case.

Spencer, Krefting, and Mattingly (1993) offer suggestions for incorporating ethnographic methods into assessment of function. This is especially important when the culture, environment, and socioeconomic experience of the client differ from that of the occupational or physical therapy practitioner, and these methods provide useful suggestions for understanding the client's perspective. Typically, document review in health care settings consists of reading the health record or medical reports; incorporation of ethnographic methods suggest that document review include personal items such as photographs, mementos, essays, or other work that is representative of the client and family's life experiences. Instead of a standard home assessment that utilizes a checklist of the physical environment, an ethnographic approach would be to assume the role of a participant-observer, with the client and family in their own home, workplace, or community recreational facilities doing the activities that have meaning to the client.

This type of evaluation helps the practitioner to understand the client as a whole person in a world of his or her own, rather than as someone with a chronic illness. In clinical practice settings clients are often seen at their most vulnerable, when they are having an acute flare of their symptoms, recovering from surgery, or other similar circumstance that presents them as people with chronic illness. The author can recall several situations in which seeing a former client outside of the health care environment presented an entirely different picture than when that person was a patient. For example, the social role was the predominant feature when a chance meeting enabled me to observe a young mother with her family at the county fair, instead of the active joint count that precipitated her last outpatient visit. Priority problems in the former view related to managing two young children and all their paraphernalia when planning a picnic lunch and day on the fairgrounds, while the focus in the latter view became the number of inflamed joints and whether or not ice and splints should be prescribed. Contextual assessment approaches help to identify the clients' strengths and assets as well as problems, instead of focusing on problems in isolation. In this way, intervention plans can be developed that take advantage of client strengths and opportunities, set reasonable treatment goals to enhance adherence, and create a partnership between client and therapist to resolve relevant problems instead of relying on standard protocols for problems typical of clients with similar diagnoses.

Ethnographic approaches adapt techniques used in qualitative research to the assessment process. At first glance, this may seem impractical for the typical outpatient rheumatology clinic, especially if home or worksite visits are not permitted. However, the intent of this approach is to better understand people's experience with their arthritis, instead of making assumptions based on medical diagnosis and impairment-based measures such as joint counts, range of motion, and muscle strength. If the practitioner understands the meaning of important roles to the client and understands something of the cultural and physical environment, then the practitioner is more likely to propose interventions that will be effective. Even though it may not be practical to apply some of the methods describe above, reading reports of ethnographic approaches may provide useful explanations to help therapists reflect upon their practices.

For example, Llorens, Umphred, Burton, and Glogoski-Williams (1993) propose a communication system to assist practitioners in learning more about their client's perspective. Coined "LEARN," for listen, explain, acknowledge, recommend, and negotiate, this system can be used to guide interviews with the client or client's family, without the requirement of time-consuming community-observation methods. The process of applying the LEARN methodology to assessment of function in a person with arthritis can be outlined as follows:

1. Listen to the person's explanation of functional abilities and limitations. This occurs naturally if using the MACTAR or COPM approach or a similar interview.

2. Explain the approach to arthritis management and resolution of functional problems that guides the therapist's practice. Beliefs about managing inflammation, principles of joint protection, educational strategies, etc., are shared at this step.

3. Acknowledge differences. Some "tried and true" treatments will be unacceptable to some people because they do not seem to make sense within their personal explanatory model. This provides a hint underlying situations that are often labeled as non-adherence to treatment recommendations.

4. Recommend interventions, techniques, or strategies that will address the problems identified by the client.

5. Negotiate acceptable or reasonable ways of implementing the recommendations, given the client's unique situation and beliefs.

A reasonable way of obtaining more information about values and beliefs in the outpatient setting is to invite family members to accompany the person with arthritis to a treatment session. Topics to discuss could be related to roles such as household management, meal preparation, and caregiving, as well as the meaning or value associated with each role by the members of the household. By way of illustration, Spencer and colleagues point out that meal preparation and family dining can hold great meaning for some people and serve as a "ritual function in anchoring relationships" (Spencer et al., 1993, p. 307) or are seen as a gift or sign of caring that require attention and effort. In these cases, an "energy conservation program that suggests the use of a microwave oven to prepare food would not be acceptable to someone who spends 2 days preparing lunch for guests" (p. 307). The LEARN strategy, especially the negotiation step, may be useful to reach a reasonable compromise between the therapist and client in order to achieve a realistic intervention plan that addresses the client's valued role as well as the therapist's recommendations related to joint protection and energy conservation.

TOOLS THAT ASSESS OCCUPATIONAL PERFORMANCE AND PERFORMANCE COMPONENTS

To assess function fully, it is not enough to ask what activities can and cannot be done, but also why they cannot be done (Fisher, 1992). In effect, this statement asks about the relationship of impairment, disability, and handicap, or the relationship between occupational performance and performance components. In rheumatologic rehabilitation this could be phrased as the relationship between functions and symptoms such as pain and fatigue, or as the relationship between function and physical components such as ROM, joint laxity, or muscle strength.

Gerber and Furst (1992) noted that while symptoms such as pain and fatigue are important to measure, they seldom provide direction for intervention strategies. The researchers developed the National Institutes of Health (NIH) Activity Record (ACTRE) in order to assess symptoms with respect to daily activities. Essentially the ACTRE is a daily log in which the client identifies the activity, how long it was done, how strenuous it was, its association with pain, fatigue, enjoyment, meaningfulness, difficulty, and whether it was well done. This presents a profile of function that is "conducive to developing quantifiable treatment goals and can be used to determine treatment efficacy" (Gerber & Furst, p. 86). One of the unique contributions of the ACTRE is that it can identify patterns of daily activity that are associated with the client's perceptions of competence and satisfaction. It may also highlight particularly troublesome times of day or activities that create difficulties. The ACTRE and an information packet and computer scoring program are available from NIH (see address in the list of references).

Little seems to be known about the relationship between occupational performance and performance components. A few studies have correlated the scores of occupational performance (for example, preparing a meal) with the scores of a performance component assessment (for example, cognitive function). Such studies demonstrate that there is some relationship, but much of the variance remains unexplained (Trombly, 1995). Guccione (1994) reviewed several studies that examined the relationship between selected physical components and functions, citing (a) a study of older adults with musculoskeletal impairment, which explained about 15% of the variance in scores on functional abilities; and (b) a predictive study that noted the relationship between musculoskeletal impairment and future functional decline in the elderly. This same study "noted that the impact of musculoskeletal impairment of the hand was chiefly on basic ADL, whereas lower extremity impairment affected instrumental ADL such as housekeeping, meal preparation, and shopping more" (p. 412). Hewlett, Young, and Kirwan (1995) in a study of dissatisfaction with function in 50 adults with RA found moderate and significant correlations among functional status, pain, and psychological status. This implies that addressing these variables through interventions such as education programs about pain relief or relaxation may reduce dissatisfaction with function (Hewlett et al.).

As Guccione (1994) pointed out, an impairment does not always result in a functional limitation, and few studies have attempted to correlate functional status with the magnitude of impairment. An assumption seems to exist that when people with arthritis have difficulty with functional activities it is due to joint pain, restricted motion, fatigue, or residual weakness. Aside from the fact that each of these reasons would suggest different interventions at the discrete level of physical components instead of the potentially more meaningful level of occupational performance, it also seems reasonable to propose that there is more to function than the physical limitations imposed by joint pathology. Most practitioners can recall clients with marked physical limitations who found a way to pursue work and social roles despite their arthritis, and other clients who experienced dramatic role limitations in the presence of only mild joint disease. To better understand why this happens requires the concurrent evaluation of occupational performance areas and performance components. A contemporary approach to the simultaneous evaluation of IADL and discrete skills that comprise performance components is the Assessment of Motor and Process Skills (AMPS; Fisher & Kielhofner, 1995).

The AMPS is an IADL evaluation that begins by taking into account motivational aspects of performance. It is comprised of familiar tasks that the client needs, wants, or is expected to do. The client chooses a familiar task from a list of IADL tasks provided by the therapist. The client performs the tasks and the therapist scores the performance on 16 motor and 20 process skill items (see Table 2). Motor skills include *transports, grips, calibrates, moves, and stabilizes*; process skills include those planning skills necessary to perform such as *chooses, uses, handles, restores, accommodates, and benefits*. For example, when opening a bread bag and removing two slices of bread to make a sandwich, the motor skills *grip* and *manipulate* are observed when the client opens the twist tie and grasps the bread slices; simultaneously, the process skill *handle* is observed and represents the client's knowledge of how a twist-tie works and that the bread bag must be supported when reaching inside for the slices. Skill items are assigned an ordinal score by the rater, but one of the unique aspects of the AMPS is that the raw data are subjected to many-faceted Rasch analysis, which takes into account the severity of the therapist rating the test and the difficulty of the IADL tasks observed. This feature requires raters to be trained and their rating pattern calibrated before they can administer the AMPS (the test center address is at the end of the chapter). However, it also results in the rank-ordering of more than 50 IADL tasks so that once a subject's AMPS performance has been analyzed on two or three tasks it is possible to predict which IADL tasks the subject can complete successfully, and which the subject will be likely to find difficult.

Several studies have contributed to the development of the AMPS as a reliable and valid measure of IADL (Fisher & Kielhofner, 1995). Furthermore, use of the AMPS in research projects is beginning to contribute to a greater understanding of function. For example, Park, Fisher, and Velozo (1994) investigated the effect of the environment on IADL performance of a group of 20 adults over 60 years of age residing in retirement complexes. The subjects included several with various forms of arthritis. Subjects were evaluated in their homes and in the occupational therapy clinic. Results suggested there was no difference between the two settings for the motor skill items, but there was a statistically significant difference in performance of the process skill items between the two settings. For 10 of the 20 participants, performance in the home was consistently better than in the clinic. This study lends support to the idea that environment and familiarity of tools and supplies used in a task influence performance for some people.

I've used the AMPS to evaluate IADL performance in a variety of outpatients with arthritis during home visits. It takes only about 10 minutes to observe a client complete a task, although an additional 20-30 minutes are required for scoring the assessment. However, this is offset by the usefulness of the information obtained by following the AMPS structured observation guidelines. It becomes possible to pinpoint some of the difficulties underlying functional problems. One might assume that the major source of functional limitations in people with arthritis is in the domain of motor skills, but in many cases a process-skills deficit can be identified, implying that a different treatment

ASSESSMENT OF MOTOR AND PROCESS SKILLS ITEMS

MOTOR SCALE		PROCESS SCALE	
stabilizes	flows	paces	terminates
aligns	moves	attends	searches/locates
positions	transports	chooses	gathers
walks	lifts	uses	organizes
reaches	calibrates	handles	restores
bends	grips	heeds	navigates
coordinates	endures	inquires	notices/responds
manipulates	paces	initiates	accommodates
		continues	adjusts
		sequences	benefits

Table 2: Items in the Assessment of Motor and Process Skills. Source: Fisher, A., & Kielhofner, G. (1995).

approach may be more effective. People who demonstrate process-skill deficits may require more intervention along the lines of planning and adapting activities, whereas those who demonstrate effective process skills turn out to be "natural problem solvers."

PERSON-ENVIRONMENT ASSESSMENTS

THE WORKPLACE

The multidisciplinary field of ergonomics contains several suggestions for the evaluation of worksites and the "fit" between worker and workstation, including ergonomic checklists or job analysis. Such tools can be useful guides for an initial visit to the client's place of work, but every workplace is unique. Some of the items will be irrelevant, and there may be additional workplace issues missing from the checklist or situational analysis. Space does not permit the reprinting of an ergonomic checklist here, but samples can be found in Grandjean (1985) and Jacobs (1991). It is important to ask the worker to identify sources of difficulty or potential difficulty, and investigate accordingly. There is no substitute for common sense.

To make recommendations for accommodating the symptoms of joint disease at work, it may be useful to interview the person about the whole work day, from start to finish. That is, begin by asking the person to describe the process of preparing for work in the morning: time of rising from bed; effects of morning stiffness, if any; the need to care for others in the household and the availability of others to offer assistance; and how long the process takes from rising to leaving the home. Also consider transportation to work such as the method and length of commute, and the opportunity to structure the work day with frequent rest breaks (which may range from 30 seconds at the end of a 10-minute task to 15-30 minutes for laying down and relaxing following lunch). Melvin (1989) proposed several questions for structuring an interview (see appendix 3).

Assessments of worker skills may have a place in evaluating persons with arthritis, especially if a client is investigating new job options and wants to determine his or her physical capacity for essential job tasks. Work samples and work simulators may help estimate the client's capacity to do the job, identify job tasks that could stress vulnerable joints, and provide sufficient data to suggest appropriate modifications to traditional work methods to help the worker accommodate the sequelae of joint disease such as pain, reduced motion, and fatigue. As an example, Cathey, Wolfe, and Kleinheksel (1988) used the BTE work simulator in a study of adults with either fibromyalgia or rheumatoid arthritis. They were able to document a relationship between work capacity and functional status as measured by the Health Assessment Questionnaire (HAQ). This study presents one example of the utility of a work simulator to estimate work capacity and learn more about the work abilities of people with arthritis.

THE HOME

Typically, home assessments review the physical accessibility of the home and the individual's ability to function using his or her own equipment. They therefore include a review of the individual's ability to enter and move about the home, and gain access to essential home furnishings and equipment in the kitchen, bedroom, bathroom, living room, and any other areas of importance. An assessment can consist of a logical progression through the client's home, starting at the entry and moving through each room in sequence. The client demonstrates how he or she opens doors, turns on lights, moves about, sits, rises, and uses appliances and equipment such as stove, television, and telephone. Cooper, Rigby, and Letts (1995) offer a review of available assessment tools for evaluating access to the home and community.

One commercially available tool for assessing clients' interaction with their home environment is the Safety Assessment of Function and the Environment for Rehabilitation (SAFER; Community Occupational Therapists & Associates, 1991). The SAFER is a checklist of 97 items intended to be completed in consultation with the client in his or her home. Each item is checked in one of three columns, indicating that the item was addressed, is not applicable to that situation, or there is a problem with that item. There is space for comments to describe the problem, barriers, or potential solutions.

FUNCTIONAL ASSESSMENTS AND OUTCOME MEASURES

Functional assessment is receiving increased attention in rehabilitation literature due to the emphasis on "outcomes that matter," and it is generally assumed that people's abilities to engage in their daily activities are important indicators of the success of rehabilitation programs. While some functional assessments can be used as outcome measures, not all outcome measures provide a comprehensive assessment of function. Program evaluation and outcome research rely on measures that are quantifiable, reliable, and valid measures of specific outcomes such as mortality, cost of treatment, pain, function, and health-related quality of life.

Van der Heide and colleagues reviewed 32 reports of clinical trials assessing drug efficacy in people with RA and noted that 14 of the trials used functional status as an outcome (Van der Heide et al., 1994). They cited the HAQ and the Arthritis Impact Measurement Scales (AIMS), both self-report instruments, as the most frequently used functional-outcome measures in these trials.

Many instruments designed as functional outcome measures, like the HAQ and AIMS, may help classify or distinguish among people of varying abilities but do not help the clinician identify the reasons for functional limitations or provide enough information for problem identification to guide intervention plans. On the other hand, they may more or less duplicate the function of a screening assessment and identify whether or not a more detailed functional assessment is required. It is therefore necessary to put outcome measures in the appropriate perspective: A quick, easy-to-use, self-administered functional outcome measure can add to database information and be of subsequent value in describing the level of disability of a group of clients upon admission and discharge from a program. Even if it does not aid in the assessment and identification of problems relevant to specific clients, it does not detract from the process either, and just might contribute to the pool of evidence that indicates that an arthritis treatment program is an important service deserving of funding.

FUNCTIONAL STATUS INDEX

Recently the Functional Status Index (FSI; Jette, 1987) has been used to evaluate self-reported functional abilities of people with arthritis. Many other assessments focus on basic ADL, but this instrument takes a broader view of functional status and adds IADL and social roles. Unlike many functional-assessment instruments, the FSI also asks the client to report the level of difficulty and pain experienced when performing the functional activities. The FSI asks respondents to rank the degree of assistance they required in a list of 18 activities during the 7 days prior to assessment, on a scale of 0 (independent) to 4 (unable to do). Pain and difficulty are scored on a scale of 1 (no pain or no difficulty) to 4 (severe pain or difficulty). FSI items are categorized into five indices: gross mobility, home chores, personal care, hand activities, and social or role activities. ICCs for interrater reliability for 149 people with RA ranged from 0.64 for the hand-activities index to 0.89 for the social-roles index for the ability-dependence rating scale; from 0.71 for the gross-mobility index to 0.82 for the social-role index for the pain rating scale and the difficulty rating scale. Test-retest reliability ICCs ranged from 0.40

for the social roles index to 0.87 for the home-chores index on the ability-dependence rating scale; 0.69 for the personal care index to 0.88 for the gross-mobility index for the pain and difficulty rating scales. Validity was assessed by comparing observed performance of tasks by a physical therapist with the patients' self-report and resulted in correlations ranging from 0.71 to 0.95. All of these data lend support to the use of the FSI as a reliable and valid self-report measure of functional status. Because the FSI was developed specifically for people with arthritis, it highlights typical functional problems experienced by people with arthritis such as buttoning clothes and turning faucets that may not be included in other generic functional assessments.

When selecting instruments such as those previously mentioned, consider several characteristics. These include the breadth of content, the instrument's sensitivity to changes in status, the reliability of the test procedures, the validity of the test, the resulting data, and the overall feasibility of the instrument for the setting(s) and individual(s) to which it will be applied (Backman, 1994). The content should match the anticipated range of activities that are part of the client's everyday activities. If the intent is to measure the effects of intervention or changes in disease status, then the instrument should be responsive to meaningful changes in functional capacity. Estimates of the instrument's reliability and validity should be based on clients similar to those who will be tested. Furthermore, test administrators should do their own evaluation of test reliability prior to collecting data to ensure consistent application and interpretation of test procedures. The resulting data should be in a form that is conducive to the purpose of the evaluation: For example, if it is to communicate with the client and team members, it needs to be in a format that will make sense to this group.

In contrast to outcome measures that address function, other standardized functional assessments tend to address occupational performance in more detail. This makes them unwieldy for outcome-measures databases but potentially useful for noting specific performance problems. As long as function remains an important outcome, functional assessments and outcome measures are not mutually exclusive. Further discussion of outcome measures is in chapter 17.

APPLICATION OF THE COPM — CASE EXAMPLE

Caroline was a 36-year-old single woman employed as a ticket agent for a major airline. She was referred to outpatient OT for conservative management of carpal tunnel syndrome secondary to rheumatoid arthritis. Her work performance was inconsistent due to numbness and tingling in her hands and fingers: Her keyboard skills were slower than usual, and she made more mistakes than before. She also reported waking up during the night with severe pain in one or both wrists and hands.

Caroline's RA was diagnosed about 6 years ago. Although she had had episodes of painful, swollen joints in the past, she reported that her medications had controlled her arthritis pretty well. Only rarely had she needed to take days off from work. Until the past month her arthritis had been only a minor and occasional barrier to fulfilling her life roles.

The Canadian Occupational Performance Measure (COPM; Law et al., 1994) identified issues of importance to Caroline that were affecting her occupational performance. A semistructured interview conducted by the therapist elicited Caroline's report of the self-care, work, and leisure tasks she needs to do in a typical day and the tasks that present difficulty. Caroline selected the most important problems, named them, and rated them in terms of her performance and satisfaction with her performance. Results of the COPM indicated that Caroline has three important issues to address: inability to sleep through the night, declining speed, ease, and accuracy with her computer keyboard skills at work, and trouble with gardening as a leisure pursuit.

Caroline's COPM scores for this initial assessment and a follow-up assessment are shown in Figure 1. As a result of the initial assessment, Caroline's OT identified the need to evaluate Caroline's computer workstation and to do a physical assessment of her hands and wrists, but it was not necessary to conduct a detailed self-care or home evaluation because Caroline indicated no problems in these areas. Intervention included adjusting the heights of Caroline's office chair and work surface, trading keyboards with a colleague who had a split keyboard that was easier for Caroline to use, adding a wrist support mat proximal to the keyboard, and implementing a 1-minute ROM break for her upper limbs every half hour or so at work. Intervention for the sleeping problem included night-resting splints and education regarding sleeping positions and mattress and pillow selection. Although the OT also suggested day splints, Caroline preferred a trial period with night splints and workplace modifications before considering the daytime wrist splints. Intervention for the third problem, gardening, consisted of a review of gardening tools and methods and ideas for container gardens. Caroline expressed an interest in fitness, and the OT also referred Caroline to a physical therapist for specific recommendations that could be incorporated into a community exercise group.

Reassessment of these three problems indicated that Caroline's performance score improved from 5.7 to 8.3, and her satisfaction with her performance improved from 3 to 6.7 (the highest possible score on the COPM is 10). At the follow-up visit, the OT suggested that Caroline consider other ways of managing her arthritis to maintain her engagement in work and other valued activities at the best possible level. Caroline agreed that she probably was not as knowledgeable as she could be and that the education program the OT proposed might be worthwhile. They could identify this as a potential problem (e.g., potential for decline in work and self-care activities due to limited knowledge of self-management principles) and rate it in the same way the initial problems were scored.

This case study highlights several issues. First, it is not necessary to conduct multiple or time-consuming assessments of function if the client clearly identifies priority problems to guide intervention. Caroline's OT was tempted to follow a protocol of functional wrist splints for daytime use, workstation modification, night splints (full-length, given the diagnosis of RA), and to embark on a program of joint-protection and energy-conservation techniques without considering Caroline's priorities or readiness to learn. The therapist in this example would have omitted leisure, since her outpatient practice rarely presents time to get beyond basic functional tasks. Yet, with the use of the COPM, Caroline's priorities were addressed first, and the OT was able to offer interventions that

CAROLINE'S COPM RESULTS

	INITIAL ASSESSMENT		REASSESSMENT	
OCCUPATIONAL PERFORMANCE PROBLEMS:	PERFORMANCE	SATISFACTION	PERFORMANCE	SATISFACTION
1. computer keyboard use	6	2	8	6
2. sleeping through the night	4	2	9	8
3. gardening	7	5	8	6
SCORING: (sum of performance or satisfaction number of problems) ÷number of problems)	17/3 = 5.7	9/3 = 3.0	25/3 = 8.3	20/3 = 6.7

Figure 1. Caroline's COPM Results

made a difference. Joint-protection and energy-conservation were introduced through the gardening interventions, which encouraged Caroline receptivity to additional recommendations in self-management principles. The assessment process was efficient and effective, and it encouraged negotiation between therapist and client that respected the client's decisions and right to choose without compromising the therapist's responsibility to provide an informed opinion.

In contrast, another client with the same diagnosis identified different problems. Sarah was a 36-year-old mother of two preschool-aged children with a similar diagnosis to Caroline: Sarah was diagnosed with RA 4 years ago. It was reasonably well controlled with her medications, but she noticed increased pain and swelling in her hands and wrists. When the therapist used the COPM as Sarah's initial assessment, Sarah identified meal preparation, dressing her 2-year-old (especially tiny buttons and snap fasteners), lifting and carrying groceries, and vacuuming as priority problems. When discussing the results of the COPM with Sarah, the therapist suggested a physical assessment of Sarah's upper limbs (similar to Caroline) as well as an IADL assessment to evaluate household management activities (unlike Caroline's results, which didn't identify this occupational performance area as an issue). Caroline and Sarah function in different environments with different roles, so although they had similar impairments, they had quite different disabilities.

Part of the reason the COPM and similar approaches to assessing occupational performance are effective is that they consider the context in which the client functions. Others have found context to be a very important factor that also helps to address the issue of decreasing lengths of stay on treatment programs (Haley, Coster, & Binda-Sundberg, 1994). The "contextual emphasis has helped the physical therapy staff to focus intervention on the most relevant functional competencies in order for the patient to return to his or her environment and maintain as much independence in mobility (across all relevant contexts) as possible" (Haley et al., p. 449).

CONCLUSION

The focus of this chapter has been the evaluation of the occupational performance areas of self-care, work, and leisure. Both traditional measures of functional status and contemporary approaches have been discussed, and both have a place in assessing function. Some of the issues to consider when making choices about how to assess function include the purpose of the assessment, the importance of direct observation of performance, and conducting assessments in the context of the client's daily living situation. Contemporary approaches that consider the client's priorities include the MACTAR and COPM, and the incorporation of ethnographic methods into assessment protocols offers some suggestions for assessing the client in context. "A contextual approach does not preclude assessment of other aspects of performance; rather, it creates a frame of reference for the other data that might be collected. . . . Real-life tasks provide cues and reinforcers for ongoing performance that are removed when we break a task down or simulate task performance" (Dunn, 1993, pp. 357, 358). The discrepancy between capacity and performance is documented in the outcome literature (Spencer et al., 1993) and one way to overcome this is to assess individuals in their own environments. To miss this opportunity may result in a distorted picture of the person's functional ability as well as the chance to observe the person's strengths and analyze the nature of the circumstances under which he or she routinely function (Spencer et al.).

Some of the assessment methods proposed may appear to be too time-consuming to consider within the context of the therapist's practice. Christiansen (1993) challenges therapists to "accept assessment approaches with greater costs in exchange for information of greater value that will lead to increased efficacies in intervention" (p. 259). In order to assist people with rheumatologic conditions to cope with the disabilities and handicaps that often result from the disease, it is necessary to conduct an assessment that provides accurate data to fulfill this goal and promote optimal occupational performance.

- To obtain a copy of the NIH Activity Record (ACTRE) write to:

   Gloria Furst, MPH, OTR
   National Institutes of Health
   Building 10, Room 6S235
   9000 Rockville Pike
   Bethesda, MD 20892

- For more information on the Assessment of Motor and Process Skills (AMPS) contact the

    AMPS Project
    Department of Occupational Therapy
    Colorado State University
    Fort Collins, CO 80523

- To obtain a copy of the Canadian Occupational Performance Measure (COPM) write to the

    Canadian Association of Occupational Therapists
    Carleton Training & Technology Centre
    1125 Colonel By Drive, Suite 3400
    Ottawa, ON, Canada K1S 5R1

- To obtain a copy of the Safety Assessment of Function and the Environment for Rehabilitation (SAFER) contact the

    Community Occupational Therapists & Associates
    3103 Bathurst Street, Suite 200
    Toronto, ON, Canada M6A 2A6

REFERENCES

Backman, C. (1994). Assessment of self-care. In C. Christiansen (Ed.), *Ways of living: Self-care strategies for special needs* (pp. 51-76). Bethesda, MD: American Occupational Therapy Association.

Canadian Association of Occupational Therapists. (1991). *Occupational therapy guidelines for client-centered practice.* Toronto, ON: CAOT Publications.

Cathey, M. A., Wolfe, F., & Kleinheksel, S. M. (1988). Functional ability and work status in patients with fibromyalgia. *Arthritis Care & Research, 1,* 85-98.

Christiansen, C. (1993). Continuing challenges of functional assesments in rehabilitation: Recommended changes. *American Journal of Occupational Therapy, 47,* 258-259.

Community Occupational Therapists & Associates. (1991). *Safety assessment of function and the environment for rehabilitation (SAFER).* Available from COTA, 3103 Bathurst St., Suite 200, Toronto, ON, Canada M6A 2A6.

Cooper, B., Rigby, P., & Letts, L. (1995). Evaluation of access to home, community and workplace. In C.A. Trombly, (Ed.), *Occupational therapy for physical dysfunction* (4th ed., pp. 55-72). Baltimore, MD: Williams & Wilkins.

Dunn, W. (1993). The issue is . . . Measurement of function: Actions for the future. *American Journal of Occupational Therapy, 47,* 357-359.

Fisher, A. G. (1992). Functional measures, part 2: Selecting the right test, minimizing the limitations. *American Journal of Occupational Therapy, 46,* 278-281.

Fisher, A., & Kielhofner, G. (1995). Skill in occupational performance. In G. Kielhofner, (Ed.), *A model of human occupation: Theory and application,* (2nd ed., pp. 113-138). Baltimore, MD: Williams & Wilkins.

Gerber, L., & Furst, G. P. (1992). Validation of the NIH activity record: A quantitative measure of life activities. *Arthritis Care and Research, 5,* 81-86.

Grandjean, E. (1985). *Fitting the task to the man: An ergonomic approach.* London: Taylor & Francis.

Guccione, A. A. (1994). Arthritis and the process of disablement. *Physical Therapy, 74,* 408-414.

Haley, S. M., Coster, W. J., & Binda-Sundberg, K. (1994). Measuring physical disablement: The contextual challenge. *Physical Therapy, 74,* 443-451.

Halpern, A. S., & Fuhrer, M. J. (Eds.). (1984). *Functional assessment in rehabilitation.* Baltimore, MD: Paul H. Brooks.

Hewlett, S., Young, P., & Kirwan, J. (1995). Dissatisfaction, disability and rheumatoid arthritis. *Arthritis Care & Research, 8,* 4-9.

Jacobs, K. (1991). *Occupational therapy: Work-related programs and assessments* (2nd ed.). Boston: Little, Brown & Co.

Jette, A. M. (1987). The functional status index: Reliability and validity of a self-report functional disability measure. *Journal of Rheumatology, 14* (suppl. 15), 15-19.

Jette, A. M. (1994). Physical disablement concepts for physical therapy research and practice. *Physical Therapy, 74,* 380-386.

Klein, R. M., & Bell, B. (1992). Self-care skills: Behavioral measurement with Klein-Bell ADL Scale. *Archives of Physical Medicine and Rehabilitation, 63,* 335-338.

Law, M (1993). Evaluating activities of daily living: Directions for the future. *American Journal of Occupational Therapy, 47,* 233-237.

Law, M., Baptiste, S., Carswell, A., McColl, M. A., Polatajko, H., & Pollock, N. (1994). *Canadian occupational performance measure* (2nd ed.). Toronto, ON: CAOT Publications.

Law, M., & Letts, L. (1989). A critical review of scales of activities of daily living. *American Journal of Occupational Therapy, 43,* 522-528.

Law, M., & Usher, P. (1988). Validation of the Klein-Bell activities of daily living scale for children. *Canadian Journal of Occupational Therapy, 55,* 63-68.

Lawton, M. P., & Brody, E. M. (1996). Assessment of older people: Self-maintaining and instrumental activities of daily living. *Gerontologist, 4,* 179-186.

Llorens, L. A., Umphred, D. B., Burton, G. U., & Glogoski-Williams, C. (1993). Ethnogeriatrics: Implications for occupational therapy and physical therapy. *Physical and Occupational Therapy in Geriatrics, 11,* 59-69.

Melvin, J. L. (1989). *Rheumatic disease in the adult and child: Occupational therapy and rehabilitation* (3rd ed.). Philadelphia: F. A. Davis.

Park, S., Fisher, A. G., & Velozo, C. A. (1994). Using the assessment of motor and process skills to compare occupational performance between clinic and home settings. *American Journal of Occupational Therapy, 48,* 697-709.

Pedretti, L. W. (1996). Occupational performance: A model for practice in physical dysfunction. In L.W. Pedretti, (Ed.), *Occupational therapy: Practice skills for physical dysfunction* (4th ed., pp. 3-12). St. Louis, MO: Mosby.

Pollack, N. (1993). Client-centered assessment. *American Journal of Occupational Therapy, 47,* 298-301.

Spencer, J., Krefting, L., & Mattingly, C. (1993). Incorporation of ethnographic methods in occupational therapy assessment. *American Journal of Occupational Therapy, 47,* 303-309.

Trombly, C. A. (1995). Theoretical foundations for practice. In C.A. Trombly (Ed.), *Occupational therapy for physical dysfunction* (4th ed., pp. 15-27). Baltimore, MD: Williams & Wilkins.

Tugwell, P., Bombardier, C., Buchanan, W. W., Goldsmith, C. H., Grace, E., & Hanna, B. (1987). The MAC-TAR patient preference disability questionnaire: An individualized functional priority approach for assessing improvement in physical disability in clinical trials in rheumatoid arthritis. *Journal of Rheumatology, 14,* 446-415.

Van der Heide, A., Jacobs, J. W. G., Van Albada-Kuipers, G. A., Kraaimaat, F. W., Gleenen, R., & Bulsma, J. W. J. (1994). Physical disability and psychological well being in recent onset rheumatoid arthritis. *Journal of Rheumatology, 21,* 28-32.

Velozo, C. A. (1994). The issue is: Should occupational therapy choose a single functional outcome measure? *American Journal of Occupational Therapy, 48,* 946-947.

World Health Organization. (1980). *International classification of impairment, disability and handicap.* Geneva, Switzerland: Author.

Yelin, E., Lubeck, D., Holman, H., & Epstein, W. (1987). The impact of rheumatoid arthritis and osteoarthritis: The activities of patients with rheumatoid arthritis and osteoarthritis compared to controls. *Journal of Rheumatology, 14,* 710-717.

SCREENING ASSESSMENT

Name: _____ Age: _____

Diagnosis: _____ Disease Duration: _____ Date: _____

Presenting Problem: _____
_____

EATING	use knife & fork (cut food)	
	raising cup to mouth	
	lifting food to mouth (soups, solids)	
DRESSING	upper body (shirts, sweaters)	
	feet (socks, shoes, pantyhose)	
	lower body (pants, skirts)	
	fastenings (buttons, zippers, laces)	
GROOMING	comb hair	
	wash face	
	brush teeth	
	shave	
HYGIENE	manage toilet	
	bathe/shower	
TRANSFERS	chair	
	toilet	
	tub/shower	

Appendix 1. Screening Assessment Form

TRANSFERS	bed
	car
	public transit
AMBULATION	walking distance/tolerance (how far, how long can you walk?)
	walking aids
HOUSEHOLD	meal preparation
	cleaning chores
	house/yard maintenance
WORK	note major work tasks and ability to do them
LEISURE	note major hobbies and ability to pursue them

ACTIVITIES OF DAILY LIVING CHECKLIST

The purpose of this questionnaire is to discover any difficulties you might have in the stated area with which the therapist may be able to help you. Please complete the following questionnaire putting a check (√) in the appropriate column or drawing a line through the question if it is not applicable.

SELF-CARE SECTION	EASILY	WITH DIFFICULTY	NOT AT ALL	SOLUTION
BEDROOM: CAN YOU...?				
move from place to place in bed				
roll to right and then to left side				
turn and lie on abdomen				
sit up in bed				
get into bed				
get out of bed				
DRESSING: ARE YOU ABLE TO PUT ON AND TAKE OFF THE FOLLOWING ARTICLES?				
WOMEN				
brassiere				
girdle				
garter belt				
panties				
slip				
stockings				
socks				
shoes				
dress with front opening				
dress with side opening				
dress with back opening				
blouse				

SELF-CARE SECTION	EASILY	WITH DIFFICULTY	NOT AT ALL	SOLUTION
skirt				
sweater				
coat				
hat				
gloves				
slacks				
MEN				
vest or undershirt				
shorts				
trousers				
shirt				
sweater				
socks				
shoes				
suit jacket				
tie				
coat				
hat				
gloves				
MEN & WOMEN: CAN YOU MANAGE...?				
zippers				
buttons, large				
buttons, small				
hooks and eyes				
snap dome fasteners				
buckles				
safety pins				

SELF-CARE SECTION	EASILY	WITH DIFFICULTY	NOT AT ALL	SOLUTION
belts				
putting hand in: back pocket				
putting hand in: side pocket				
brushing clothes				
hanging up/putting away clothes				
putting on splints				
TOILET: CAN YOU MANAGE...?				
getting on and off toilet				
adjusting clothes for toilet needs				
using toilet paper				
flushing toilet				
maneuvering bedpan				
getting to toilet at night				
BATH: CAN YOU MANAGE...?				
getting into a bath				
out of a bath				
into a shower				
turning taps (tub & sink)				
washing: feet				
hands				
back				
chest				
neck				
face				
hair				
drying self				
drying between toes				

Appendix 2. ADL Checklist (Melvin, 1989) (continued)

SELF-CARE SECTION	EASILY	WITH DIFFICULTY	NOT AT ALL	SOLUTION
PERSONAL CARE: CAN YOU MANAGE...?				
brushing teeth				
using dental floss				
using electric razor				
safety razor				
trimming: fingernails				
toenails				
brushing and combing hair				
WOMEN				
applying makeup				
setting hair				
shaving legs				
shaving under arms				
using sanitary napkins/tampons				
douching				
grooming eyebrows				
application of contraceptives				
AMBULATION: CAN YOU...?				
walk unaided or with cane				
with crutches				
walk up steps (if applicable)				
walk down steps				
walk up a slope				
walk down a slope				
turn around				
walk on rough ground				
get up and down a curb				

SELF-CARE SECTION	EASILY	WITH DIFFICULTY	NOT AT ALL	SOLUTION
AMBULATION: CAN YOU...?				
cross a street in 30 seconds on a green light				
get down to the floor and up again				
stand for more than half hour				
get on and off living room chair				
get on and off kitchen chair				
EATING: CAN YOU...?				
use a fork				
use a spoon				
cut meat				
butter bread				
drink from a cup				
drink from a glass				
stir coffee, tea, etc.				
pour from a bottle				
pour a cup of tea or coffee				
HOUSEHOLD ACTIVITY SECTION	EASILY	WITH DIFFICULTY	NOT AT ALL	SOLUTION
FOOD PREPARATION: CAN YOU...?				
do grocery shopping				
open tin cans				
open jars				
open packaged goods				
reach shelves above countertop				
reach shelves below countertop				
prepare vegetables: peel				
slice				

Appendix 2. ADL Checklist (Melvin, 1989) (continued)

HOUSEHOLD ACTIVITY SECTION	EASILY	WITH DIFFICULTY	NOT AT ALL	SOLUTION
FOOD PREPARATION: CAN YOU...?				
bake a cake or cookies:				
measure dry ingredients				
measure liquids				
break an egg				
use an eggbeater				
stir batter				
knead dough				
pour batter into pan				
open oven door				
place pan in oven				
roll dough				
use a saucepan				
fill a saucepan				
carry pan to stove				
remove hot dish from oven				
drain vegetables				
pour hot water from kettle				
pour tea and/or coffee into cups				
DINING: CAN YOU...?				
set table				
carry to table: full glass				
full cup & saucer				
full plate				
hot casserole				
(other)				

HOUSEHOLD ACTIVITY SECTION	EASILY	WITH DIFFICULTY	NOT AT ALL	SOLUTION
CLEAN UP: CAN YOU...?				
scrape and stack dishes				
wash dishes				
scrub pots and pans				
pick up object from floor				
wipe up spills on floor				
sweep floor				
use dustpan				
mop floor				
shake mop				
wash floor				
clean refrigerator				
clean oven				
dispose of garbage				
(other)				
OTHER HOUSEHOLD ACTIVITIES: CAN YOU MANAGE...?				
laundry: hand-washing				
wringing				
machine washing				
hanging on line				
ironing blouse or shirt				
folding sheets				
hanging dress on hanger				
dust/clean—high & low surfaces				
vacuuming/carpet sweeper				
making beds				
changing beds				

Appendix 2. ADL Checklist (Melvin, 1989) (continued)

HOUSEHOLD ACTIVITY SECTION	EASILY	WITH DIFFICULTY	NOT AT ALL	SOLUTION
OTHER HOUSEHOLD ACTIVITIES: CAN YOU MANAGE...?				
cleaning bathtub				
picking up a pin				
threading a needle and sewing				
using scissors				
handling coins				
feeding pets				
(other)				
TRANSPORTATION: CAN YOU...?				
get onto a bus				
stand on bus holding				
overhead bar				
descend from bus				
get into a car (open car door)				
get out of a car				
drive a car				
MISCELLANEOUS: CAN YOU...?				
manage medicine bottles				
take own medicine				
use a telephone				
open an envelope				
write for 15 minutes				
hold a book				
turn the pages				
shuffle and hold a hand of cards				
strike a match (cigarette lighter)				
smoke a cigarette or pipe				

HOUSEHOLD ACTIVITY SECTION	EASILY	WITH DIFFICULTY	NOT AT ALL	SOLUTION
OTHER HOUSEHOLD ACTIVITIES: CAN YOU MANAGE...?				
wind a clock				
wind a watch				
type				
care for garden				
mow lawn				
sweep porch				
open and close: a door				
window				
drawer				
reach shelves at head level				
open milk cartons				
turn taps on and off				
MISCELLANEOUS: CAN YOU...?				
use pull-chain light				
use light switches				
manage wall-plugs				
push buzzer, doorbell				
use spray cans				
open doors with knobs				
open doors with keys				
pour milk from bottle to glass				
operate stove burners and oven				
operate sink taps				
open and close refrigerator				
use wall-plug				
(other)				

Appendix 2. ADL Checklist (Melvin, 1989) (continued)

HOUSEHOLD ACTIVITY SECTION	EASILY	WITH DIFFICULTY	NOT AT ALL	SOLUTION
CHILD CARE OR GRANDCHILD CARE: CAN YOU...?				
lift a small child (under age two)				
bathe a child				
fix child's hair				
dress small child				
change diapers				
do personal hygiene for small children				
ENDURANCE:				
does an average day's housework make you:				
extremely tired				
quite tired				
only slightly tired				

What activity during the week is the most strenuous for you?

ASSISTANCE:

Who will do heavy cleaning duties, e.g., waxing floor, washing windows?

How often is he/she available?

HOUSEHOLD
ACTIVITY SECTION

DAILY ROUTINE:

Briefly describe your average daily routine or schedule:

RECREATIONAL OR LEISURE INTERESTS:

Difficulties with these activities due to the arthritis? Please list:

Reprinted from: Melvin (1989).

WORK ASSESSMENT QUESTIONS

by Jeanne L. Melvin

PREPARING FOR WORK

1. What are the effects of morning stiffness when preparing for work and at the beginning of the work day?

2. How hectic or stressful is the morning preparation time? Is there anything that could make the morning time more manageable? For example, morning time can be hectic if a young child or more than one child must be readied for school.

3. What are the person's scheduled work hours?

TRANSPORTATION

4. How does the person get to work? Commuting will be made easier or more difficult depending on the level of stiffness at the beginning of the day and fatigue at the end of the day.

5. What is the person's commute time and distance?

WORK SETTING

6. What are the physical working conditions? If a desk or work station is used, what type are they? What type of seating is available?

7. Where is this work area in relation to other facilities, for example, the cafeteria, restrooms, meeting rooms, parking?

8. What are the walking, standing, and sitting requirements of the job? Does the person walk to other floors or buildings or sit in one place all day? Are there elevators or escalators?

9. What are the writing or hand-skill requirements?

10. What level of strength is needed to do the job? What is the weight of material that must be lifted, carried, lowered, pulled or pushed? Is this work done in a standing, sitting or walking posture? Levels of strength needed in work are described as sedentary, light, medium, heavy, and very heavy work.

11. What are the stooping, kneeling, crawling, and crouching requirements, in terms of frequency and duration?

12. What are the climbing and balancing requirements, in terms of frequency and type, e.g., are ladders, stairs, or scaffolds used?

13. If the person works in a confined space, does this create excessive strain on the joint?

14. What are the environmental risk factors of the workplace? Consider the exposure to toxic chemicals and fumes, heat or cold, sun, dangerous mechanical processes, radiation, air pollution, excessive noise, and inadequate lighting. These factors can create additional physical and psychological stress at work.

LUNCH AND REST BREAKS

15. What are the nature, quality, and length of breaks?

16. Does the person hurriedly eat junk food from a machine for lunch at his or her desk in a busy office while working? Or is there a pleasant, relaxed area in which to eat and take a 45- to 60-minute lunch break?

17. Is a pleasant, smoke-free rest area available? (Even smokers hate smoke-filled rooms).

18. Is there a quiet place where the person could practice a relaxation exercise?

19. If the person eats in a cafeteria, can he or she handle the tray, dishes, cups, and so forth?

20. Does the person take advantage of available rest breaks, and if so, how?

21. Nutrition and eating patterns can have a major influence on fatigue. For example, sugar and caffeine create a temporary energy high that a few hours later depletes energy and causes fatigue. Mild dehydration, associated with not drinking water or liquids for long periods of time, can also bring on fatigue. Eating foods high in fat can slow one's metabolism, which also increases the feeling of tiredness.

WORK ACTIVITIES

22. What activities at work aggravate joints or symptoms the most? How does the person handle these activities? What adaptive methods are used?

23. What power or control does the person have to alter the work to reduce joint stress or accommodate symptoms?

INTERPERSONAL RELATIONSHIPS

24. Are the person's supervisor and co-workers supportive and pleasant to work with, or is there interpersonal strife?

25. Do the person's supervisor and co-workers know that the person has arthritis or back pain? If yes, what is their reaction? If no, how does this affect the person at work?

26. What are the sources of psychological stress on the job? For example, what is the nature of the person's relationship with the boss and co-workers? What is the amount of work to be done? What is the schedule? Is the person bored at work?

27. Does the person avoid taking actions at work that would reduce his or her pain, such as stretching during breaks, using orthosis, using ice packs, or using a cane, because others would react negatively?

Reprinted from: Melvin (1989).

LOCOMOTOR DYSFUNCTION: EVALUATION AND TREATMENT

Carol A. Oatis, PhD, PT

Locomotor dysfunction is one of the most common complaints of patients with arthritis. These complaints arise from both joint and soft-tissue changes in the lower extremities and spine and are associated with all the major rheumatic diseases. In addition, individuals with rheumatic diseases are frequently deconditioned from limited activity and may have systemic involvement of the cardiovascular and pulmonary systems that contributes to a further decrease in locomotor capacity (Philbin, Groff, Ries, & Miller, 1995). Ambulation and mobility, in turn, are critical for maintaining physical fitness. The role of intervention, then, is to optimize the individual's locomotor ability while minimizing those factors that could further the destruction of the involved joints. The purposes of this chapter are to discuss the principles of optimal gait and their application to arthritis-related gait deviations, to review methods of clinical gait evaluations and discuss the interpretation of their results, to describe the common alterations in the gait patterns of individuals with arthritis, and to discuss which factors to consider in the treatment of gait dysfunctions.

OPTIMAL GAIT

A common treatment goal for people with arthritis is "to improve gait." Inherent in this goal is the assumption that there is a gait pattern that is "better." However, what is that "better" gait? Is an "improved" gait safer, more comfortable, more normal? What is "normal gait"? Is normal gait achievable for patients with arthritis?

A common concept of a normal locomotion pattern is one in which each limb segment exhibits normal kinematic behavior. Many studies have demonstrated altered joint excursions during locomotion in persons with arthritis (Gyory, Chao, & Stauffer, 1976; Marshall, Myers, & Palmar, 1980; Messier, 1994; Messier, Loeser, Hoover, Semble, & Wise, 1992; Murray, Gore, & Clarkson, 1971; Quinn & Mote, Jr., 1992; Shih, Wu, & Lo, 1993). Studies have also demonstrated a change toward normal joint movements following surgical intervention, yet complete normalization of joint excursions is rarely achieved (Brown,

Hislop, Waters, & Porell, 1980; Collopy, Murray, Gardner, DiUlio, & Gore, 1977; Stauffer, Smidt, & Wadsworth, 1974). Thus one must ask if normal kinematic behavior is achievable for some individuals with arthritis and, indeed, if it is even desirable. Holt (1993) has reported that during treadmill walking nondisabled persons chose stride frequencies that tended to minimize metabolic cost, maximize head stability, and minimize the variability of lower-extremity joint-action coordination. However, he suggested that persons with disabilities might choose other optimizing criteria such as pain relief or balance. Clinical experience suggests that pain is a frequent optimizing criterion for individuals with arthritis.

What, then, are the essentials of optimal gait? To answer this question, it is useful to put the function of locomotion in perspective. Locomotion is goal oriented: People walk to transport themselves somewhere. An individual walks to get to work, go to the kitchen, or answer the telephone. Thus one factor of successful locomotion is that it allows the goal to be accomplished. Lundgren-Lindquist, Aniansson, & Rundgren (1983) studied 205 men and women, all 79 years of age, and reported that none exhibited a self-selected comfortable walking speed fast enough to cross a street in the time allotted by a standard traffic light. Only 32% of women and 72% of men achieved the recommended pedestrian norm when walking at their maximum speed. Regardless of their kinematic patterns, many of the elders in this study exhibited unsuccessful gait patterns because they were unable to cross the street with the light. Similarly, a successful gait for some individuals might be measured by the individual's ability to cross a room and answer the telephone before it stops ringing. Thus one criterion for successful gait is that it allows the individual to **accomplish the desired task successfully.** In addition, the individual must cross the street without being struck by oncoming traffic or cross the room without falling. Thus another element of successful gait is safe **accomplishment.**

Because locomotion is goal oriented, another factor in a successful gait is the need for the individual to possess enough energy following the ambulation to complete the desired task. For example, after crossing the room to answer the telephone the individual must have enough energy remaining to speak into the telephone. Thus another criterion of successful gait is adequate residual energy to accomplish the task after the walk.

Safe accomplishment of the task with residual energy describes the overriding elements of a successful gait. During a clinical gait assessment, it is easy for the clinician to concentrate on the pattern of joint motions and lose sight of the more general aspects of the gait. A closer inspection of the discrete tasks within the gait will help the clinician to focus on the essential ingredients of a successful gait. Das and McCollum (1988) suggested that the primary task of ambulation is forward progression. These authors noted that the tasks of the stance phase are support and propulsion, and that the three tasks of the swing phase are foot clearance, appropriate foot placement, and the transfer of angular momentum to maximize efficiency. Similarly, Winter (1989) described three necessary but insufficient elements of safe ambulation: upward support of the body, upright posture and balance, and adequate motor control of the foot for appropriate clearance and placement (Table 1).

Optimal gait must be safe by using adequate support to avoid falls, exhibit sufficient foot clearance to avoid tripping, and must have sufficient propulsive force to provide

ELEMENTAL TASKS OF GAIT	
STANCE PHASE	SWING PHASE
Upright support	Foot clearance
Balance	Appropriate foot placement
Propulsion	Transfer of angular momentum

Table 1: Elemental Tasks of Gait (Das & McCollum, 1988; Winter, 1989)

forward progress. In addition, it must be efficient so that enough energy is conserved during ambulation to allow accomplishment of the real task at hand such as talking, working, or eating.

Examining the elemental components of a successful gait may be more useful to the clinician working with people who have arthritis than images of an "ideal" kinematic pattern of movement to identify the source of a patient's gait pathology. How this perspective can be used to interpret data derived during evaluation is discussed below.

CLINICAL GAIT ASSESSMENT AND ITS INTERPRETATION

OBSERVATIONAL GAIT ANALYSIS

By far the most common mode of clinical assessment is visual inspection of the pattern of movement. Visual inspection was systematized in Observational Gait Analysis (OGA) first developed at Rancho Los Amigos Medical Center, Downey, California (Malouin, 1995; Pathokinesiology Department and Physical Therapy Department, 1996). This approach relies heavily on an understanding of normal kinematic patterns. The evaluator observes the person's ambulation and then identifies and records the deviation from normal movement of each joint or limb segment during each phase of the gait cycle (Figure 1). The form encourages the examiner to follow a single joint or limb segment through the entire gait cycle to identify abnormal behavior. Although its reliability has been shown to be only moderately acceptable, OGA remains the most often used clinical assessment tool for gait (Eastlack, Arvidson, Snyder-Mackler, Danoff, & McGarvey, 1991; Krebs, Edelstein, & Fishman, 1985).

RELATIONSHIP BETWEEN OGA RESULTS AND IMPAIRMENTS

A list of typical gait deviations identified by OGA in individuals with arthritis is presented in Tables 2-4. These are a guide to common gait abnormalities rather than an

GAIT ANALYSIS: FULL BODY
RANCHO LOS AMIGOS MEDICAL CENTER
PHYSICAL THERAPY DEPARTMENT

Reference Limb: L ☐ R ☐

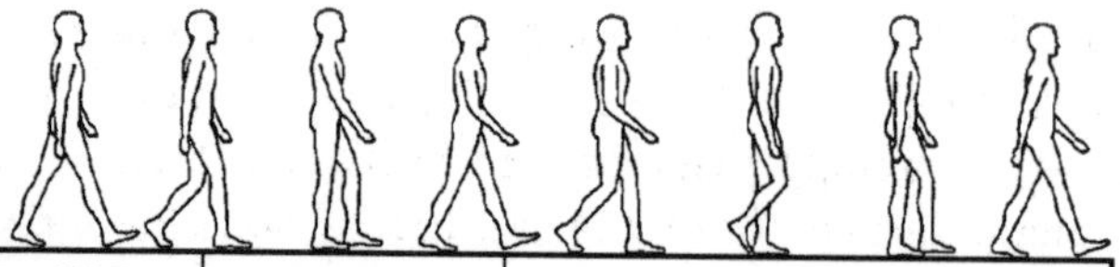

☐ Major Deviation
▨ Minor Deviation

		Weight Accept		Single Limb Support		Swing Limb Advancement			
		IC	LR	MSt	TSt	PSw	ISw	MSw	TSw
TRUNK	Lean: B/F								
	Lateral Lean: R/L								
	Rotates: B/F								
PELVIS	Hikes								
	Tilt: P/A								
	Lacks Forward Rotation								
	Lacks Backward Rotation								
	Excess Forward Rotation								
	Excess Forward Rotation								
	Ipsilateral Drop								
	Contralateral Drop								
HIP	Flexion: Limited								
	Excess								
	Inadequate Extension								
	Past Retract								
	Rotation: IR/ER								
	Ad/Abduction: Ad/Ab								
KNEE	Flexion: Limited								
	Excess								
	Inadequate Extension								
	Wobbles								
	Hyperextends								
	Extension Thrust								
	Varus/Allgus: Vr/Vl								
	Excess Contralateral Flex								
ANKLE	Forefoot Contact								
	Foot-Flat Contact								
	Foot Slap								
	Excess Plantar Flexion								
	Excess Dorsiflexion								
	Inversion/Eversion: Iv/Ev								
	Heel Off								
	No Heel Off								
	Drag								
	Contralateral Vaulting								
TOES	Up								
	Inadequate Extension								
	Clawed								

MAJOR PROBLEMS

WEIGHT ACCEPTANCE

SINGLE LIMB SUPPORT

SWING LIMB ADVANCEMENT

EXCESSIVE UE WEIGHT BEARING ☐

NAME _____

DIAGNOSIS _____

Figure 1. Gait Analysis: Full Body. © 1996 LAREI, Rancho Los Amigos Medical Center, Downey, CA 90242.

exhaustive list. Tables 2-4 also present some of the possible underlying pathologies that could be direct explanations of the deviations identified by OGA.

If patients appeared in the clinic exhibiting only one of the gait deviations listed in Tables 2-4, the clinician's task of identifying and treating that dysfunction would be quite straightforward. However, rarely does an individual with arthritis exhibit a single gait deviation. Most arthritides affect multiple joints and consequently many joints may be incapable of normal movement during the gait cycle. In the presence of multiple deviations, one of the challenges in drawing conclusions from data gathered during OGA is choosing the most important deficits toward which to direct treatment. In addition, motion at one joint influences the motion at adjacent joints. Particularly when the limb is in contact with the ground, the motion at distal joints is reflected to the more proximal joints. Therefore, separating the primary deviation from those compensatory deviations is another challenge to the clinician. For example, inadequate knee extension at push-off may be the direct result of a knee flexion contracture. However it may also be the result of insufficient plantar-flexion strength to stabilize the ankle as the body translates over the fixed limb or the result of a hip flexion contracture. Thus the impairments listed in Tables 2-4 may be the direct cause of the deviation. But the deviation could also be the result of movement abnormalities at adjacent joints. How, then, can a clinician use observations of gait to direct treatment?

The gait deviations exhibited by individuals with arthritis generally stem from one of several possible impairments: pain, joint stiffness, joint instability, joint deformity, or muscle weakness. Having identified gait deviations through OGA, the clinician must attempt to relate those abnormalities to other clinical measures of impairment. For example, identification of a knee flexion contracture may explain the inadequate knee extension used at ground contact and later during push-off. Of course, when clear links exist between impairments and gait pathology, the ideal solution is to eliminate the impairment: Reduce the flexion contracture, strengthen the muscle, or reduce the pain. Unfortunately, in chronic disorders such as arthritis, complete resolution of an impairment is unlikely. In addition, because the gait problems of individuals with arthritis are usually a complex intertwining of deviations, the effects of changing one deviation on the remaining gait pattern must be considered. The clinician may realize that improving one segment of the gait pattern will have negative repercussions on other factors of the gait. In other words, the clinician must focus on the issue of optimization.

Consideration of walking speed will help illustrate this dilemma. It is well known that there is a strong positive relationship between walking speed and joint excursion (Eberhart, Inman, Saunders et al., 1947; Murray, 1967). As an individual walks more slowly, the joint excursions decrease. The reverse is also true. The OGA revealed that the patient has decreased hip and knee flexion in early stance and inadequate extension later in stance. The clinician has also noted that the patient is walking abnormally slowly (approximately 0.5 m/sec compared to the normal 1.3 m/sec). The treatment goal is to normalize the gait pattern, which suggests trying to increase joint excursions. However, in order for joint excursions to be increased feasibly, walking speed must also be increased. Is increasing walking speed a reasonable goal? It may be for some persons such as those whose joint involvement is slight or whose impairments have been reduced.

FOOT AND ANKLE ARTHRITIS:
TYPICAL OGA FINDINGS AND RELATED IMPAIRMENTS

PHASE OF GAIT	GAIT DEVIATION	IMPAIRMENTS
Initial Contact	Contact with toes first	Plantar flexion contracture
		Painful heel
		Dorsiflexion weakness
		Knee flexion contracture
	Flat foot contact	Plantar flexion contracture
		Dorsiflexion weakness
		Short steps
Contact Response	Excessive pronation	Foot deformities
		Weakness of ankle inverters
	Inadequate pronation	Rigid foot and/or ankle
		Inadequate knee flexion
Mid-Stance	Inadequate dorsiflexion	Plantar flexion contracture
		Plantar flexion weakness
		Excessive supination
		Painful foot
		Claw/hammer toes and metatarsalgia
Terminal Stance	Early heel off	Plantar flexion contracture
		Inadequate knee extension
	Delayed heel off	Plantar flexion weakness
		Inadequate knee extension
Pre-Swing	Limited or absent push off	Plantar flexion weakness
		Painful foot
		Excessive pronation
		Claw toes and metatarsalgia
Swing	Toe drag	Dorsiflexion weakness

KNEE ARTHRITIS:
TYPICAL OGA FINDINGS AND RELATED IMPAIRMENTS

PHASE OF GAIT	GAIT DEVIATION	IMPAIRMENTS
Initial Contact	Inadequate extension	Knee flexion contracture
Contact Response	Inadequate flexion	Knee extension weakness
	Mediolateral instability	Knee instability
Mid-Stance	Inadequate extension	Knee flexion contracture
Terminal Stance	Inadequate flexion	Plantar flexion weakness
Pre-Swing	Inadequate flexion	Inadequate flexion ROM
Swing	Inadequate flexion	Inadequate flexion ROM
Late Swing	Inadequate extension	Knee flexion contracture

Table 3: Knee Arthritis: Typical OGA Findings and Related Impairments

However it may not be a reasonable goal—indeed it may be contraindicated—for individuals whose joint destruction and pain are so significant that increased walking speed would contribute to further joint destruction and pain.

INTERPRETATION OF OGA RESULTS

The original premise of this chapter was that the goal of treatment of gait dysfunction is to optimize gait, defining optimal gait as that which allows the individual to walk safely, comfortably, and efficiently so that the reason for walking can be accomplished. Faced with a patient who demonstrates a complex gait pattern of multiple, interrelated deviations, the clinician must reconsider the elemental tasks of gait. The clinician must first determine whether the primary difficulty in gait is related to the stance or swing phase. Treatment of the gait dysfunction, then, must be linked to the patient's own goals of ambulation as well as to the underlying pathology.

HIP ARTHRITIS:
TYPICAL OGA FINDINGS AND RELATED IMPAIRMENTS

PHASE OF GAIT	GAIT DEVIATION	IMPAIRMENTS
Initial Contact	Inadequate flexion	Hip flexor weakness
	Excessive flexion	Hip flexion contracture
		Forward lean of trunk
	Abnormal rotation	Hip contracture
	Abnormal abduction or adduction	Hip contracture
Contact Response	Abnormal abduction or adduction	Hip abductor weakness
		Hip pain
Mid-Stance	Excessive trunk lean	Hip abductor weakness to the stance side
		Hip pain
	Inadequate hip rotation	Hip contracture
	Inadequate hip extension	Hip contracture
Terminal Stance	Inadequate hip extension	Hip contracture
Pre-Swing	Inadequate hip extension	Hip contracture
Early Swing	Inadequate hip extension	Hip contracture
	Circumduction	Hip flexor weakness
		Hip pain
Late Swing	Inadequate flexion	Hip flexor weakness
		Hip pain
	Excessive flexion	Trunk forward lean

Difficulties in locomotion manifested by individuals with arthritis can be classified according to the basic elements. The primary tasks of the stance phase are support and propulsion. People with arthritis may have difficulty in this phase because of pain during weight bearing or inadequate joint stability for support. Pain and weakness also may lead to difficulty generating enough force for propulsion. Similarly, some patients may have greater difficulty during the swing phase. Joint pain and stiffness may limit the individual's ability to shorten the swing limb for foot clearance. Joint deformities may restrict foot placement. Pain and stiffness may also limit and slow joint excursions so that the angular momentum of the lower extremity is reduced. Winter has demonstrated that during gait considerable mechanical energy is transferred from thigh to leg and from foot to leg as well as between each lower extremity and even from upper to lower extremities (Winter, 1978). This transfer requires free movement between limb segments. Individuals whose movements are restricted by pain and stiffness are unable to transfer energy across segments and, consequently, may expend a great deal of additional energy to advance the limbs and body in space. This increased energy expenditure may contribute to the fatigue that people with arthritis experience.

Another clinical example may help to clarify application of these principles. The patient is a 48-year-old woman with traumatic arthritis in both knees. OGA has revealed that swing on the right was characterized by inadequate knee flexion in early and midswing, with inadequate extension in late swing. In general, the individual exhibited little knee motion throughout the gait cycle. Her walking speed was also slower than normal, and her gait pattern was consistent with someone who had severe ROM restrictions of the knee. Yet this individual had almost full ROM (0-120 degrees) of the knee as well as strength within functional limits (4/5 for quadriceps and hamstrings). Although this person could voluntarily increase walking speed, there was no corresponding increase in knee-joint excursion. She was able to increase knee flexion in early swing only by walking very slowly and actively moving the knee. If judged on the basis of joint excursions alone, as in OGA, the individual described in this scenario would be "improved" by the active knee flexion utilized during swing. However, Das and McCollum (1988) stated that transfer of momentum was an essential element of gait. Whether walking with little or no knee motion or actively flexing the knee while walking slowly, this person was unable to transfer momentum up and down the lower extremity. This individual's gait pattern was unsuccessful because it was inefficient. Treatment must then focus on the restoration of a freely swinging knee, which will allow transfer of momentum from thigh and foot to the leg rather than merely the restoration of normal knee-joint excursion.

OBJECTIVE MEASURES OF GAIT

Discussion to this point has focused on a qualitative assessment of gait. More objective measures may be suitable in some instances, particularly when documentation of progress toward a goal is required. Measurement of temporal and stride characteristics of gait is a common clinical assessment tool that provides objective data. These measurements include walking speed, step and stride length, stride width, and various temporal characteristics such as step and stride duration, double and single support time, and swing-stance time ratio. Average walking speed is easily derived by timing the subject's time to walk a known distance. Simple methods to derive the distance parameters of step and stride length are well known and generally consist of some method of marking each foot placement as the individual ambulates. The recording method may be merely ink marks on the soles of the shoes with a paper pathway, powdered shoes on a dark path, or carbon paper on an adhesive paper walkway (Walsh, 1995) These methods utilize relatively inexpensive materials, but data reduction is labor intensive and therefore increases the overall cost of the analysis. In addition, such systems do not allow timing of discreet periods or events of the gait cycle such as stance and swing times. Electronic walkways and shoe inserts offer an automated means of assessing the temporal and distance characteristics of these footfall variables. According to Walsh, the initial costs of such devices can be offset by the decrease in data reduction time when compared to the simpler systems. Several studies have demonstrated good reliability of walkway marking systems and the electronic systems (Boenig, 1977; Leiper & Craik, 1991). The value of these clinical measures is their objectivity and repeatability. However, as indicated in the preceding example, walking velocity or stride characteristics may not provide enough information to direct treatment to optimize the gait pattern. Although the patient was able to increase her walking speed, her walking efficiency remained inadequate.

Another clinically useful assessment tool is the ambulation profile, which is a system to describe an individual's ambulatory status (Malouin, 1995). Nelson's Functional Ambulation Profile (FAP) uses a series of timed tasks to assess static and dynamic stability as well as basic locomotor skills (Nelson, 1974). The GALS (gait, arms, legs, spine) locomotor screen uses a Likert score of 0-3 to evaluate gait and limb mobility (Plant, Linton, Dodd, Jones, & Dawes, 1993). Both tools have demonstrated moderate reliability. Such systems may be useful in classifying patients as well as identifying functional changes following intervention. However, neither system provides the sort of information that helps explain the mechanism of the deviation.

Finally, measures of cardiovascular fitness may be useful in assessing the locomotor abilities of individuals with arthritis. Although musculoskeletal pathology is the main limitation to ambulation in this population, locomotion also requires endurance. Many of the impairments found in arthritis lead to decreased efficiency of gait. As suggested earlier in this chapter, difficulty in limb clearance can lead to decreased efficiency in swing and make ambulation more strenuous. Thus an assessment of cardiovascular stress during gait may be helpful in assessing a patient's ambulatory status. Such a measure could be as simple as heart rate or blood pressure taken before and after a timed walk. While these measures will not indicate the source of the inefficiency, they do provide a simple indication of the change in efficiency with intervention.

In summary, there are many tools available to the clinician to assess the ambulatory status of persons with arthritis. The clinician's choice of the appropriate tool depends on the information sought. If the clinician wishes to identify the deviations and to determine the underlying mechanisms of the pathologies, OGA may be most useful, particularly when applied within the perspective of "optimal" rather than "visually correct" behavior. However, if the clinician needs to document improved functional performance, temporal and distance parameters, ambulation profiles, and heart and respiratory rates may be more useful.

GAIT ABNORMALITIES IN INDIVIDUALS WITH ARTHRITIS

The gait patterns of individuals with arthritis have been frequently studied and reported in the literature. These studies can be grouped by research parameters: temporal and stride characteristics, joint kinematics, joint kinetics, and energetics. A brief summary of these results will provide an overview of the commonly reported deviations.

Temporal and Stride Characteristics. Speed is decreased in those subjects with lower-extremity arthritis according to most reported studies comparing walking speeds in subjects with and without arthritis (Gyory et al., 1976; Murray et al., 1971; Quinn & Mote, Jr., 1992; Simkin, 1981; Smidt & Wadsworth, 1973; Stauffer et al., 1974; Wadsworth, Smidt, & Johnston, 1972). These findings have been observed in subjects with rheumatoid arthritis and those with osteoarthritis, with the former exhibiting a greater loss than the latter. Similarly, decreased walking speed has been reported regardless of the joints studied (Collopy et al., 1977; Simkin, 1981; Smidt & Wadsworth, 1973; Wadsworth et al., 1972).

Cadence (steps per minute), step length, and stride length are also reportedly diminished in persons with arthritis, regardless of which joints are studied or whether the subjects have OA or RA (Andriacchi, Ogle, & Galante, 1977; Murray et al., 1971; Simkin, 1981; Smidt & Wadsworth, 1973; Quinn & Mote, 1992). However, Andriacchi and colleagues reported that persons with arthritis of the knee demonstrated a shorter step length and a greater increase in cadence than the control participants even when walking speed was taken into account. In other words, changes in step length and cadence cannot be explained solely by decreased walking speed in persons with arthritis. Stauffer, Chao, and Gyory (1977) reported that patients who had greater joint involvement demonstrated a larger decrease in velocity, cadence, and stride length (Table 5).

These temporal and stride characteristics have been used frequently to evaluate the effectiveness of treatment, particularly surgery, for patients with arthritis (Andriacchi et al., 1977; Brown et al., 1980; Murray et al., 1971; Stauffer et al., 1974). These studies uniformly reported improvement toward normal following surgery. However, no author reported normalization of these parameters in periods of assessment ranging from 6 months to 4 years postoperatively.

These data demonstrate their usefulness as outcome measures. They also reflect the complexity of gait pathology in individuals with arthritis. Walking speed appears to be influenced by the severity of the disease. However, changes in stride characteristics cannot be totally explained by walking speed. Therefore the clinician must be cautious when using these measures clinically. These variables can be helpful in assessing response to treatment if applied in light of the overriding issues of safety, comfort, and efficiency. Improved walking speed with no concomitant increase in pain, or with decreased heart rate or respiratory rate may be better indicators of progress than walking speed alone.

Joint Kinematics. The effects of joint disease on joint excursions during locomotion in subjects with arthritis have also been investigated. A summary of these data is presented in Table 6. A brief comparison of these data with Tables 2-4 reveals significant similari-

TYPICAL CHANGES IN TEMPORAL AND STRIDE CHARACTERISTICS ASSOCIATED WITH ARTHRITIS

WALKING SPEED	Decreased
CADENCE	Decreased
STEP LENGTH	Decreased
STRIDE LENGTH	Decreased
STANCE TIME	Decreased

(Murray, Gore, & Clarkson, 1971; Simkin, 1981; Smidt & Wadsworth, 1973; Stauffer, Smidt, & Wadsworth, 1974)

Table 5: Typical Changes in Temporal and Stride Characteristics Associated With Arthritis

ties. The difference among these data is that the data in Table 6 were obtained from sophisticated, three-dimensional motion analysis, but the data reported in Tables 2-4 are derived from clinical observation.

Current data demonstrate the diversity of gait patterns exhibited by persons with arthritis. It is clear from these data that there is no single, predictable locomotor performance that can be attributed to arthritis. For example, although many authors reported similar abnormalities in the kinematics of the hip, Wadsworth and colleagues (1972) reported that 11 of 26 participants with hip disease had no abnormal hip motion. In individuals with hip disease, little or no correlation was found between joint excursion during gait and passive ROM (Murray et al., 1971; Stauffer et al., 1974). However, at the knee a strong relationship between knee extension during gait and active ROM of the knee was reported (Collopy et al., 1977). The data reinforce the complexity of the factors that influence joint excursions and serve to caution the clinician against the use of joint excursions alone as a measure of the quality of a gait pattern.

Joint Kinetics. Kinetic analysis of gait investigates the forces generated and energy expended during locomotion. The studies investigating changes in force can be divided into analyses of ground reaction forces (GRF) and joint reaction forces (JRF). A summary of these data is presented in Table 7. In general it is assumed clinically that a reduction in joint reaction force is a positive change resulting in a decrease in the destruction of the joint. Similarly, a reduced GRF is assumed to reduce pain and JRF, both positive changes for individuals with arthritis. Decreases in joint and ground reaction forces in these individuals are unsurprising, given the fact that walking speed is decreased in individuals with arthritis. However, studies have reported that speed alone is insufficient to explain the alterations in these forces (Andriacchi et al., 1977; Smidt & Wadsworth, 1973). In other words, other factors further reduce the forces to which the lower extremity is exposed during walking. Pain avoidance and muscular guarding may also affect the individual's

Typical Kinematic Changes Associated With Arthritis

Joint Affected	Phase	Deviation
Hip	Late stance	Decreased hip extension
	Late stance	Decreased ankle plantar flexion
	Swing	Decreased knee flexion
	Throughout	Decreased arm swing
	Unspecified	Increased anterior pelvic tilt
	Unspecified	Increased lateral plane motion of the head
	Unspecified	Increased transverse plane pelvic motion
Knee	Throughout	Decreased motions in all three planes
Ankle and Foot	Initial contact	Increased plantar flexion
		Compensatory excessive hip flexion
	Contact response	Decreased plantar flexion
		Compensatory inadequate knee flexion
	Late stance	Diminished roll off
		Compensatory excessive hip flexion

(Murray, Gore, & Clarkson, 1971; Smidt & Wadsworth, 1973; Stauffer, Smidt, & Wadsworth, 1974; Wadsworth, Smidt, & Johnston, 1972)

Table 6: Typical Kinematic Changes Associated With Arthritis

pattern of gait. Like the previous studies, these results emphasize the multifactorial nature of gait patterns in persons with arthritis.

Energetics. The metabolic cost of activity is frequently determined by the oxygen uptake measured during a task. Brown and colleagues (1980) assessed the oxygen uptake during free speed walking in 29 persons with OA of the hip before and after total hip replacement. The authors reported that these persons consumed more oxygen per distance walked than their age-matched controls without arthritis. These investigators stated that heart rate and oxygen uptake remained essentially unchanged following surgery up to 1 year postoperatively. However, the participants demonstrated increased walking velocity. Thus the authors concluded that the participants' walking efficiency was improved postoperatively. The authors also noted that despite improvements in temporal and distance parameters of gait, the participants walked more slowly, demonstrated a shorter stride, and utilized more oxygen per distance walked than age-matched control participants without arthritis.

Mechanical energy offers another means of assessing the efficiency of gait. There are two forms of mechanical energy, kinetic and potential. A limb segment such as the leg has kinetic energy, which is a function of its mass and velocity, and potential energy, which is a function of its weight and height from the ground. As the leg moves closer to and farther from the ground and more rapidly and then more slowly, its potential and kinetic energies increase and decrease. In the ideal situation, there is a perfect exchange of potential for kinetic energy and vice versa, so that no additional work is needed to continue the motion. Winter and colleagues (1976) investigated the flow between kinetic and potential energy within limb segments in healthy participants and reported approximately 50% transfer within the trunk and 33% transfer within the thigh. These levels suggest a relatively efficient motion that is somewhat self-sustaining. The investigators reported virtually no transfer within the leg. While there are no known studies assessing mechanical energy utilization in individuals with arthritis, it is reasonable to assume that mechanical energy, a function of velocity and displacement, is also altered since walking speed and joint kinematics are usually decreased in individuals with arthritis. The gait, therefore, is less efficient.

During walking, mechanical energy is also being transferred from one limb to another just as kinetic energy is transferred from a pole vaulter to his or her pole and then back to the vaulter. Robertson and Winter (1980) assessed the energy flow between segments in normal ambulation and reported that the transfer among the thigh, leg, and foot was substantial and could account for most of the energy changes in these limbs at the beginning and end of the swing phase of gait. This transfer means that movement of the thigh and foot actually contributes to the leg's movement and increases the efficiency of the

TYPICAL KINETIC CHANGES ASSOCIATED WITH ARTHRITIS		
JOINT AFFECTED	**PHASE**	**ABNORMALITY**
Hip*	Stance	Decreased vertical and anterior/posterior GRF Increased lateral GRF
Knee**	Stance	Decreased JRF Increased adduction moment
Foot and Ankle***	Stance	Decreased JRF Decreased local forces under heel, 1st and 2nd metatarsal heads, and toes

*(Andriacchi, Ogle, & Galante, 1977; Smidt & Wadsworth, 1973; Stauffer, Smidt, & Wadsworth, 1974)

**(Andriacchi, Ogle, & Galante, 1977; Quinn & Mote, Jr., 1992)

***(Simkin, 1981; Stauffer, Chao, & Gyory, 1977)

Table 7: Typical Kinetic Changes Associated With Arthritis

motion. This is consistent with Das and McCollum's (1988) essential task of "transfer of momentum" during swing. However, decreased walking speed, decreased step length, and decreased push-off will reduce the kinetic energy of the thigh and foot. In addition, without a freely swinging knee, transfer of even the decreased energy to the leg will be hampered and will require the individual to add energy during the swing, usually by active contraction of muscles such as the quadriceps and hamstrings. This will increase the overall energy cost of the gait. Recalling that one of the criteria for optimal gait is retaining adequate residual energy to accomplish the task for which the gait is intended, perhaps the temporal and kinematic parameters of gait can be made more functionally relevant by considering their effects on energy conservation.

It is essential to recognize that the factors most frequently studied as measures of locomotor performance, temporal and distance parameters, and kinematic and kinetic variables, are frequently in conflict with one another. That is, normalization of one factor such as walking speed may actually lead to negative changes in another factor such as the JRF. Similarly, improvement in joint excursion may be obtained at the expense of efficiency. Treatment goals must reflect an understanding of these relationships and frequently are compromises among maximal correction of any single factor. In other words the "target behavior" or optimal gait is that which is the most safe, most comfortable, and most efficient with the least negative effects.

TREATMENT OF GAIT DYSFUNCTIONS

Treatment plans will, of course, develop naturally from treatment goals. The preceding sections on optimal gait, evaluation and interpretation, and gait abnormalities provide the framework for acquiring data from which to establish treatment goals. It should be clear now that the goal of restoring a normal-appearing gait in an individual with arthritis is rarely achievable. Treatment goals must focus on minimizing discomfort and joint destruction and also maximizing safety and efficiency. These optimizing criteria can then be applied to each of the elemental tasks of the gait cycle. The basic tasks of the stance phase are support and propulsion. The basic tasks of swing are limb advancement and foot placement. The following discusses treatment considerations applied to each of these tasks (see Table 8).

SUPPORT

First consider the evidence one would obtain from a gait assessment that support was a significant problem for a subject. Of course, complaints obtained through interview suggesting support difficulties include reports of pain on weight bearing, difficulty climbing stairs, and a sense of "unsteadiness." Gait assessment might reveal decreased step length, increased double support time, and abnormalities in loading response at the knee (either inadequate or excessive knee flexion). There is an almost limitless list of possible causes for difficulties in support, but they generally can be organized into four categories: pain from weight bearing on severely eroded joints, joint deformities, joint instability, and muscle weakness. The association between difficulties in support and the underlying explanation can be identified by comparing the gait evaluation data with the data collected in the rest of the physical examination. Treatments can also be organized around these underlying explanations. Reduction of pain that arises from weight bearing on destroyed joints requires a reduction in the load on the joint. This may be achieved by simply instructing the patient to slow walking speed or shorten steps. These simple instructions are an example of choosing pain relief over normal appearance as the treatment goal.

Joint loading during the stance phase can be reduced further by the judicious use of walking aids such as crutches and canes. Blount's 40-year-old admonition still holds true, "Don't give up the cane!" (Blount, 1956). Canes have been estimated to diminish joint reaction forces at the hip by approximately 50%. Of course, principles of joint protection must be applied to the upper extremities using the assistive devices, particularly in polyarthropathies such as RA. Devices that allow weight bearing through the forearms and arms are particularly useful for individuals with hand involvement. However, the use of walking aids remains problematic for those with shoulder pain or instability. The clinician must choose the treatment that has the greatest positive effect and the least negative effect.

Some orthotic devices are also designed to unload painful joints. These are most commonly and, indeed most successfully, used at the knee for both the patellofemoral and tibiofemoral joints (Antich, 1997; Belyea, 1997).

Weight bearing on painful or deformed joints is frequently the underlying cause of difficulty with support. In arthritis, foot deformities are probably the most frequently occurring deformities resulting in pain on weight bearing. The techniques described above to reduce joint loading may also be beneficial in reducing pain during weight bearing on symptomatic joints. However, direct efforts to reduce the deformities or redistribute the load around them may prove more successful. Specifically, claw-toe deformities cause the metatarsal heads to be more exposed and result in increased pressures. These subjects also frequently have decreased and displaced soft tissue on the plantar surface. Metatarsal bars can be used to unload the metatarsal heads. However, soft shoe inserts or molded shoes may be more useful in reducing pressures on the plantar surface of the foot by providing a supplement to the soft tissue and by providing pressure relief for the protruding metatarsal heads (Lockard, 1988).

Support during stance is often compromised by joint instability in people with arthritis. Muscular support may be the first source of joint stability. Therefore the clinician must carefully assess joint strength to determine if active muscle contraction across an unstable joint can improve stability. In addition, improved strength at joints both proximal and distal to the unstable joint may improve the functional stability of the lower extremity. Winter (1980) has described a "support moment" that is defined as the sum of the muscular moments exerted at the hip, knee, and ankle during the stance phase. In healthy individuals, Winter noted considerable variance in the individual moments at the hip, knee and ankle but a significant constancy in the total supporting moment. Individuals with weakness may lack the variety of solutions to provide adequate support. Thus in the presence of quadriceps weakness, for example, additional strength at the hip and ankle must be relied upon to provide an adequate support moment. Clinicians can use this concept to justify strengthening joints surrounding the unstable joint.

Muscle weakness can be a direct cause of difficulties in support during stance. The quadriceps and gluteus medius are particularly important in providing support during the stance phase of gait. Weakness in these muscles produces rather stereotypical gait deviations, inadequate knee flexion at contact response in the case of quadriceps weakness, and a lateral lurch of the trunk during ipsilateral stance in the case of gluteus medius weakness.

Muscles also have been shown to be important shock absorbers. The shock-absorbing role of the quadriceps during weight acceptance is well known (Eberhart et al., 1947). Similarly, the simultaneous, controlled pronation of the foot is important for attenuating the impulses of rapid loading (Perry, 1992). Therefore improving strength while improving stability may actually reduce the joint stresses of the support task by absorbing the shock at impact and by helping to dissipate the loads across the joint. Thus muscle weakness can not only be a direct cause of decreased support but may also contribute to increased joint loads. Clinicians should carefully consider the benefits of increased strength. Of course, care must be taken during strengthening exercises to avoid high joint resultant forces that could further the joint destruction. Again, the choice of strengthening muscles as a treatment goal must be based on the benefits expected weighed against the possible risks.

PROPULSION

Evidence that a person is having difficulty with propulsion includes decreased step length and walking speed, and limited roll off and decreased hip extension in late stance. The task of propulsion is intimately related to the task of support. Propulsion requires the transmission of force through the lower extremities to the floor. Pain and joint instability may interfere with this task as well. Therefore, some of the means used to improve support (such as improved strength and orthotic intervention) may also help stabilize the limb for propulsion. The plantar flexors have been shown to be important in providing propulsive energy to the lower extremity (Winter, 1989). However, the ability of the plantar flexors to propel the body forward is also dependent upon the alignment of the body in space at the time of plantar flexion contraction. For example, contraction of the plantar flexors for propulsion normally occurs with the knee and hip extended so that the force exerted will be primarily a posterior force on the ground, which pushes the body anteriorly. The presence of a hip or knee flexion contracture would result in a more vertically applied force to the ground, which in turn would push the body more upward than forward. Therefore propulsion can be enhanced first by improving the propulsive force by strengthening the plantar flexors. Second, propulsion can be enhanced by improving the line of application of the force. This may require treatments designed to improve joint excursions of the hip and knee during mid and late stance. It may also require increased strength at the hip and knee to stabilize these joints adequately during push-off. Finally, propulsion forces are exerted through the forefoot. Therefore treatment to improve the patient's tolerance to forces through the forefoot may be beneficial. Treatment may require shoe inserts to relieve plantar pressures on the foot.

FOOT CLEARANCE AND LIMB ADVANCEMENT

Evidence for difficulty in swing includes a foot drag, short steps, inadequate knee extension at contact, and indications of increased workload such as elevated heart and respiratory rate. The tasks of swing are foot clearance and efficient limb advancement. Foot clearance requires shortening of the swing limb and usually occurs by dorsiflexion of the foot with flexion of the hip and knee. Again, data describing joint kinematics may be useful in identifying the cause of difficulties in limb clearance. A lack of knee-flexion ROM or dorsiflexion weakness could provide a direct explanation for difficulty in limb clearance. Treatment can then be directed specifically to reducing the impairment.

However, limb clearance and efficient limb advancement are also related to one another. Therefore, while there may be a temptation to encourage increased knee flexion to enhance limb clearance, such a kinematic change may actually decrease the efficiency of the swing. EMG data suggest that limb shortening in swing is the result of active hip flexion and passive knee flexion. The movement of the knee during swing is extremely rapid and requires a freely movable knee joint. Oligatti, Burgunder, and Mumenthaler (1988) reported a relationship between the metabolic cost of walking and the ability freely to flex and extend the knee in patients with multiple sclerosis. Similarly, the loss of freely swinging motion of the knee in individuals with arthritis may increase the metabolic cost of ambulation.

A person with arthritis who has knee pain and stiffness may exhibit decreased knee flexion during swing and therefore inadequate foot clearance. However, the increased stiffness also interrupts the interplay of the lower-extremity joints and prevents the transmission of energy among the joints. This loss of energy flow may actually contribute to the foot-clearance difficulty. Therefore, limb clearance may actually be improved by improving hip flexion during swing while facilitating relaxation at the knee joint. Proprioceptive neuromuscular facilitation (PNF) techniques can be particularly successful in enhancing hip flexion for swing. High velocity activities such as stationary bicycle exercise and relaxed oscillations may facilitate knee-joint relaxation during swing.

In conclusion, treatment of gait dysfunction in individuals with arthritis should originate from a clear understanding of the basic tasks of the gait cycle. Use of standard clinical evaluation tools such as observational gait analysis or devices to measure footfall parameters may be helpful in quantifying specific characteristics of the gait pattern. The clinician is cautioned that gait deviations rarely occur singularly and are often related to one another. The data derived from the various evaluation methods may be most enlightening to the clinician when considered from the perspective of the elemental tasks of support, propulsion, limb clearance, and transfer of momentum. By keeping these tasks in mind, the clinician can utilize a wide variety of interventions from exercise for motor learning or strengthening to orthoses and assistive devices to optimize the patient's gait. This approach recognizes that optimal gait may never be "normal" gait but may be the most successful means for the individual to transport himself or herself in order to accomplish the tasks of life.

TREATMENT SUGGESTIONS TO IMPROVE THE BASIC TASKS OF GAIT

TASK	TREATMENT
Support	Decrease joint loading by: • Decrease walking speed • Shorten steps • Use assistive devices • Use orthotic devices Relieve joint deformities • Use shoe modifications Support joint instabilities • Strengthen muscles • Use orthotic devices
	Increase muscle support • Strengthen muscles throughout the lower extremity
Propulsion	Strengthen the plantar flexors Improve the alignment of hip and knee during push off Increase the strength of the hip and knee
Limb Clearance/Limb Advancement	Improve knee flexion ROM Improve dorsiflexion strength Enhance active hip flexion Facilitate freely swinging knee motion

Table 8: Treatment Suggestions to Improve the Basic Tasks of Gait

SUMMARY

This chapter has presented a concept of optimal gait that is based on the elemental tasks of the gait cycle. Methods of clinical gait analysis were presented and interpretation of the results was discussed. Known data describing the gait patterns of individuals with arthritis were reviewed and suggestions offered for treatment of the gait dysfunctions associated with arthritis. These suggestions have illustrated how data can be gathered to evaluate the subject's ability to accomplish the task of ambulation and then how treatment plans can be based on criteria for optimizing the gait rather than attempting to make the gait pattern "look normal." Clinicians are reminded that safety and efficiency of ambulation may be the most important issues to consider when treating gait dysfunctions in individuals with arthritis.

REFERENCES

Andriacchi, T. P., Ogle, J. A., & Galante, J. O. (1977). Walking speed as a basis for normal and abnormal gait measurements. *Journal of Biomechanics, 10,* 261-268.

Antich, T. J. (1997). Orthoses for the knee: The tibiofemoral joint. In D. A. Nawoczenski & M. E. Epler (Eds.), *Orthotics in functional rehabilitation of the lower limb* (pp. 57-76). Philadelphia, PA: W. B. Saunders.

Belyea, B. C. (1997). The patellofemoral joint. In D. A. Nawoczenski & M. E. Epler (Eds.), *Orthotics in functional rehabilitation of the lower limb* (pp. 31-56). Philadelphia, PA: W.B. Saunders.

Blount, W. (1956). "Don't throw away the cane." *Journal of Bone and Joint Surgery, 38,* 695.

Boenig, D. D. (1977). Evaluation of a clinical method of gait analysis. *Physical Therapy, 57,* 795-798.

Brown, M., Hislop, H. J., Waters, R. L., & Porell, D. (1980). Walking efficiency before and after total hip replacement. *Physical Therapy, 60,* 1259–1263.

Collopy, M. C., Murray, M. P., Gardner, G. M., DiUlio, R. A., & Gore, D. R. (1977). Kinesiologic measurements of functional performance before and after geometric total knee replacement: One-year follow-up of twenty cases. *Clinical Orthopaedics and Related Research, 126,* 196-202.

Das, P., & McCollum, G. (1988). Invariant structure in locomotion. *Neuroscience, 25,* 1023-1034.

Eastlack, M. E., Arvidson, J., Snyder-Mackler, L., Danoff, J. V., & McGarvey, C. L. (1991). Interrater reliability of videotaped observational gait analysis assessments. *Physical Therapy, 71,* 465-472.

Eberhart, H. D., Inman, V. T., Saunders, J. B. et al. (1947). *Fundamental studies of human locomotion and other information relating to design of artificial limbs. A report to the National Research Council, Committee on Artificial Limbs, University of California, Berkeley.* Berkeley, CA: University of California, Berkeley.

Gyory, A. N., Chao, E. Y., & Stauffer, R. N. (1976). Functional evaluation of normal and pathological knees during gait. *Archives of Physical Medicine and Rehabilitation, 57,* 571-577.

Holt, K. G. (1993). Toward general principles for research and rehabilitation of disabled populations. *Physical Therapy Practice,* 1-18.

Krebs, D. E., Edelstein, J. E., & Fishman, S. (1985). Reliability of observational gait analysis. *Physical Therapy, 65,* 1027-1033.

Leiper, C. I., & Craik, R. L. (1991). Relationships between physical activity and temporal–distance characteristics of walking in elderly women. *Physical Therapy, 71,* 791-803.

Lockard, M. A. (1988). Foot orthoses. *Physical Therapy, 68,* 1866-1881.

Lundgren-Lindquist, B., Aniansson, A., & Rundgren, A. (1983). Functional studies in 79-year olds: III. Walking performance and climbing capacity. *Scandinavian Journal of Rehabilitation Medicine, 15,* 125-131.

Malouin, F. (1995). Observational gait analysis. In R. L. Craik & C. A. Oatis (Eds.), *Gait analysis: Theory and application* (pp. 112-124). St. Louis, MO: Mosby-Year Book.

Marshall, R. N., Myers, D. B., & Palmar, D. G. (1980). Disturbance of gait due to rheumatoid arthritis. *Journal of Rheumatology, 7,* 617–623.

Messier, S. P. (1994). Osteoarthritis of the knee and associated factors of age and obesity: effects on gait. *Medicine and Science in Sports and Exercise,* 1446-1452.

Messier, S. P., Loeser, R. F., Hoover, J. L., Semble, E. L., & Wise, C. M. (1992). Osteoarthritis of the knee: Effects on gait, strength and flexibility. *Archives of Physical Medicine and Rehabilitation, 73,* 29-36.

Murray, M. P. (1967). Gait as a total pattern of movement. *American Journal of Physical Medicine, 48,* 290-333.

Murray, M. P., Gore, D. R., & Clarkson, B. H. (1971). Walking patterns of patients with unilateral hip pain due to osteoarthritis and avascular necrosis. *Journal of Bone and Joint Surgery, 53-A*, 259-274.

Nelson, A. J. (1974). Functional ambulation profile. *Physical Therapy, 54*, 1059-1065.

Oligiatti, R., Burgunder, J. M., & Mumenthaler, M. (1988). Increased energy cost of walking in multiple sclerosis: Effect of spasticity, ataxia, and weakness. *Archives of Physical Medicine and Rehabilitation, 69*, 846-849.

Pathokinesiology Department & Physical Therapy Department. (1996). *Observational gait analysis handbook.* Downey, CA: Professional Staff Association of Rancho Los Amigos Medical Center.

Perry, J. (1992). Ankle foot complex. In J. Perry (Ed.), *Gait analysis: Normal and pathological function* (pp. 51-87). Thorofare, NJ: Slack.

Philbin, E. F., Groff, G. D., Ries, M. D., & Miller, T. E. (1995). Cardiovascular fitness and health in patients with end-stage osteoarthritis. *Arthritis Rheumatology, 38*, 799-805.

Plant, M. J., Linton, S., Dodd, E., Jones, P. W., & Dawes, P. T. (1993). The GALS locomotor screen and disability. *Annals of Rheumatic Disease, 52*, 886-890.

Quinn, T. P., & Mote, C. D., Jr. (1992). Prediction of the loading along the leg during snow skiing. *Journal of Biomechanics, 6*, 609-625.

Robertson, D. G. E., & Winter, D. A. (1980). Mechanical energy generation, absorption, and transfer amongst segments during walking. *Journal of Biomechanics, 13*, 845-854.

Shih, L. Y., Wu, J. J., & Lo, W. H. (1993). Changes in gait and maximum ankle torque in patients with ankle arthritis. *Foot and Ankle, 14*, 97-103.

Simkin, A. (1981). The dynamic vertical force distribution during level walking under normal and rheumatic feet. *Rheumatology and Rehabilitation, 20*, 88-97.

Smidt, G. L., & Wadsworth, J. B. (1973). Floor reaction forces during gait: Comparison of patients with hip disease and normal subjects. *Physical Therapy, 53*, 1056–1062.

Stauffer, R. N., Chao, E. Y. S., & Gyory, A. N. (1977). Biomechanical gait analysis of the diseased knee joint. *Clinical Orthopaedics and Related Research, 126*, 246-255.

Stauffer, R. N., Smidt, G. L., & Wadsworth, J. B. (1974). Clinical and biomechanical analysis of gait following Charnley total hip replacement. *Clinical Orthopaedics and Related Research, 99*, 70-77.

Wadsworth, J. B., Smidt, G. L., & Johnston, R. C. (1972). Gait characteristics of subjects with hip disease. *Physical Therapy, 52*, 829-838.

Walsh, J. P. (1995). Foot fall measurement technology. In R. L. Craik & C. A. Oatis (Eds.), *Gait analysis: Theory and application* (pp. 125-142). St. Louis, MO: Mosby-Year Book.

Winter, D. A. (1978). Calculation and interpretation of mechanical energy of movement. In R. S. Hutton (Ed.), *Exercise and Sport Sciences Reviews, Vol. 6* (pp. 183-201). Indianapolis, IN: American College of Sports Medicine.

Winter, D. A. (1980). Overall principle of lower limb support during stance phase of gait. *Journal of Biomechanics, 13*, 923-927.

Winter, D. A. (1989). Biomechanics of normal and pathological gait: implications for understanding human locomotor control. *Journal of Motor Behavior, 21*, 337-355.

Winter, D. A., Quanbury, A. O., & Reimer, G. D. (1976). Analysis of instantaneous energy of normal gait. *Journal of Biomechanics, 9*, 253-257.

PART THREE:
PATIENT MANAGEMENT

PATIENT EDUCATION FOR SELF-MANAGEMENT

Michele L. Boutaugh, BSN, MPH, and Teresa J. Brady, PhD, LP, OTR

INTRODUCTION

Despite advances in medical care, the course of rheumatic disease is often unpredictable, and chronic pain, disability, and reduced quality of life can persist. Nevertheless, changes in beliefs and behaviors within the control of the individual can achieve significant reduction in morbidity. Patient education that fosters positive health beliefs and self-management behaviors is a powerful adjunct to clinical care in enhancing health and quality of life.

Patient education has been defined as "planned, organized learning experiences designed to facilitate voluntary adoption of behaviors or beliefs conducive to health" (Burckhardt, 1994). The current trend in chronic illness management is on patient education with a self-management focus (Mahowald, Steveken, Young, & Ytterburg, 1988). Self-management is defined as "learning and practicing the skills necessary to carry on an active and emotionally satisfying life in the face of a chronic illness" (Lorig, 1993). Helping patients become self-managers requires moving beyond traditional didactic instruction of which the sole focus is on information transfer. Increasing patient knowledge is important, but rarely is it sufficient. Self-management requires acquisition of complex skills and attitudes. Some skills are related to adherence to prescribed treatments, a topic addressed in more detail in chapter 3 on adherence. In addition to treatment-related behaviors, people with rheumatic diseases need to learn generic skills such as how to communicate with their health care team, make informed decisions, and use problem-solving skills to adapt to changes in their symptoms, roles, and emotions. Helping patients acquire these skills and gain the confidence to apply them daily requires a multi-faceted, interactive educational approach (Lorig, 1996; Taal, Rasker, & Weigman, 1996). Table 1 contrasts the goals, content, and process of traditional patient instruction versus self-management education.

This chapter provides an overview of the why, what, and how of effective arthritis patient education for self-management. It begins with a summary of the large body of literature that documents why arthritis patient education has value. What constitutes effec- *219* tive education is defined through a review of the Arthritis and Musculoskeletal Patient Education Standards. The PRECEDE/PROCEED model is used as a framework for describing how occupational and physical therapy practitioners can plan a comprehensive one-to-one or small-group program. Key theories, samples of representative patient-education programs, and relevant educational interventions are also discussed.

WHY DO ARTHRITIS PATIENT EDUCATION?

THE STATE OF EDUCATION IN CLINICAL PRACTICE

Satisfaction with care is reported to increase as patients become more knowledgeable about their health problems and participate in decision making about their care (Bendtsen & Bjurulf, 1993; Lindner, 1992). However, numerous studies document that patients are often inadequately informed (Daltroy, 1993). In a community-based telephone survey of 645 people with musculoskeletal conditions, only 32% reported that they possessed a high level of knowledge about their conditions (Communication Technologies, 1993).

The value of minimal educational interventions within clinical practice is implied in an observational study of the exercise practices of elderly women with knee or hip osteoarthritis (Dexter, 1992). Of those who recalled receiving advice to exercise, 63% followed through, compared with only 23% of those never so advised. However, most of these exercisers did not exercise at a high enough frequency to receive therapeutic benefit. When the exercise recommendation was supplemented with instructional materials, exercise demonstration, and monitoring, not only did the percentage of participants exercising increase to almost 80%, but the frequency of exercise also increased to a therapeutic level. Similarly, studies of traditional joint-protection and energy-conservation instruction have usually shown improved knowledge but inconsistent behavior changes (Barry, Purser, Hazleman, et al., 1994; Gerber, Furst, Shulman, et al., 1987; Hammond, 1994a). Behavioral changes were achieved in a follow-up study in which joint-protection education was redesigned to include self-monitoring, guided practice and feedback, problem solving, modeling, goal setting, and self-reinforcement (Hammond, 1994b). In another pilot study in which one-to-one sessions were supplemented with a self-paced workbook, guided practice, and contracting, the experimental-group participants had significant changes in joint-protection practices and range-of-motion exercises, and positive but not significant health status changes (Neuberger, Smith, Black, & Hassenin, 1993).

IMPACT OF FORMAL PATIENT-EDUCATION PROGRAMS

As shown in Table 2, several literature reviews have been published about arthritis patient education, and some important observations have been noted in these reviews. First, arthritis-patient education can be effective in producing changes in knowledge, behaviors, psychosocial status, and health status. In the 45 studies reviewed by Hirano, Laurent, and Lorig (1994), knowledge improved in 50% of the studies, behavior changed in 35% of the studies, and psychosocial and health outcomes improved in 52% of the study interventions. Table 3 provides more detail on the reported types of significant changes in behaviors, psychosocial status, and health outcomes. Mullen, Laville, Biddle,

TRADITIONAL PATIENT INSTRUCTION VERSUS SELF-MANAGEMENT EDUCATION

	TRADITIONAL PATIENT INSTRUCTION	SELF-MANAGEMENT EDUCATION
ORIENTATION	Provider-centered	Patient-centered
EXPECTED OUTCOME	Knowledge increase; adherence to provider recommendations	Confidence and ability/skills to manage day-to-day care of condition; positive health outcomes (reduced pain, fatigue, dysfunction; maintained/improved health) and quality of life; appropriate health care utilization
CONTENT	Disease and treatment information	Cause, meaning, and how to deal with disease and its consequences; generalizable skills (e.g., problem-solving and decision-making, communicating with providers, assertiveness, self-monitoring)
PROCESS	Didactic instruction/lectures by professionals	Experiential methods (discussion, role modeling, brainstorming, demonstration/practice and feedback, goal-setting and contracting, peer support)

Table 1: Traditional Patient Instruction Versus Self-Management Education

SUMMARY OF ARTHRITIS PATIENT EDUCATION LITERATURE REVIEWS

REVIEW AUTHORS	DESCRIPTION
Lorig and Riggs (1983); Lorig et al. (1987); Hirano et al. (1994)	Review successively 145 articles and abstracts. Tabulate the percentage of studies that reported positive changes in knowledge, behavior, psychosocial status, and health status.
Holman and Lorig (1987)	Review arthritis and chronic disease patient education experiences; discuss possible problems and unresolved issues in patient education.
Mullen et al. (1987)	Use a meta-analysis to aggregate data across 15 controlled psycho-educational studies to examine the effects on pain, depression, and disability.
Feinberg (1988); Daltroy (1993)	Review the effects of doctor-patient communication and educational counseling techniques.
Tucker and Kirwan (1991)	Present the case for the therapeutic potential of patient education in RA; identifies the characteristics of those programs that positively influence health status: successful programs were based on patient needs and beliefs; targeted at outcomes like reducing pain and disability; used interactive teaching methods; developed self-management skills, problem solving, and self-efficacy; and incorporated exercise training.
Daltroy and Liang (1993)	Describe educational opportunities in prevention; reviews the results on knowledge, behaviors, health outcomes, post-surgical outcomes, and use of health services; describes areas for research.
DeVellis and Blalock (1993)	Review the most common components included in psychological and educational interventions aimed at preventing arthritis disability; discusses issues pertinent to assessing the efficacy of these various components.
Parker et al. (1993); Keefe and Van Horn (1993)	Review the results of studies utilizing cognitive behavioral therapy.
Mazzuca (1994)	Summarizes data on cost-benefits or cost-effectiveness of arthritis patient education.

Table 2: Summary of Arthritis Patient Education Literature Reviews

Hawley (1995)	Classifies and describes the "effect sizes" (i.e., a standardized measure of change) of psycho-educational interventions included in 34 studies with osteoarthritis and/or rheumatoid arthritis populations published between 1985-1994.
Taal et al. (1996)	Describe social learning theory and self-efficacy as an appropriate theoretical basis for self-management education. Summarizes eight studies on the impact of self-efficacy in arthritis patient education. Presents criteria for the development and evaluation of self-management education programs.
Superio-Cabuslay et al. (1996)	Compare impact on pain, disability, and tender joint counts of patient education interventions in OA and RA with nonsteroidal anti-inflammatory drug treatment by doing two meta-analyses: one of 19 patient education studies and one of 28 NSAID clinical trials.

Table 2: Summary of Arthritis Patient Education Literature Reviews (continued)

and Lorig (1987) found that experimental groups had an average of 16% improvement in pain, 22% improvement in depression, and 8% improvement in disability in comparison to control groups. Most of the studies reviewed by Hawley (1995) demonstrated positive "effect sizes" (a standardized measure of change) for knowledge, behavior, psychological status, pain, and/or functional status.

Second, most of the studies that reported significant changes in knowledge and health outcomes used participants who were already receiving medical care. The results of these studies suggest that considerable potential exists for improvement in the patient education routinely provided in clinical practice. More importantly, these results suggest that formal patient education programs can achieve clinically significant health outcomes over and above those of usual medical care. A meta-analytic comparison of patient-education studies in OA and RA with nonsteroidal anti-inflammatory drug treatment showed that patient-education interventions are 20-30% as efficacious as NSAID treatment for pain relief in OA and RA, 40% as efficacious for improvement in functional ability in RA, and 60-80% as efficacious in reducing tender joint counts (Superio-Cabuslay, Ward, & Lorig, 1996). These data provide strong support for considering patient education an integral part of quality clinical care.

Third, there is evidence, although limited, that arthritis patient education can have an impact on health care utilization and costs (Hawley, 1995; Mazzuca, 1994). Economic benefits have been reported for the Arthritis Self-Management Program (Lorig, Mazonson, & Holman, 1993); telephone support interventions (Maisiak, Austin, & Heck, 1996; Weinberger, Tierney, Cowper, Katz, & Booker, 1993), a mail-delivered, computer-tailored self-management program (Gale, Kirk, & Davis, 1994), and two small pilot tests of preoperative arthroplasty education programs (Graziano, Aronson, & Becerra, 1995; Orr, 1990). A recent cost-benefit study evaluated three experimental interventions (education, social support, and combined education and support) and found that participants in all three groups achieved significant health-status improvements as well as cost savings (Cronan, Groessl, & Kaplan, 1997).

QUALITY PATIENT EDUCATION: OVERVIEW OF STANDARDS

The Arthritis and Musculoskeletal Patient Education Standards were developed by a task force consisting of representatives of the Arthritis Foundation, the Association of Rheumatology Health Professionals, the American College of Rheumatology, the American Nurses Association, the American Occupational Therapy Association, and the American Physical Therapy Association (Burckhardt, 1994). The standards do not prescribe specific educational strategies or programs, but they describe the characteristics of a quality program as outlined in Table 4. The same criteria are also relevant to individual practice: assessment of the patient, followed by development of an individual educational plan with appropriate content, process, documentation, and outcome evaluation. The following section on the PRECEDE/PROCEED model describes how to put these standards into practice.

NEEDS-ASSESSMENT STANDARDS

A needs assessment should be the first step in development of a formal patient education program or when planning the education component of a treatment plan for an individual. Starting with a needs assessment helps assure that there is a better match between the patient's priorities and health professionals' interventions. There is frequent divergence of opinion between patients and health professionals about causes and the priority of problems, the choice of therapeutic and educational options, and definition of treatment success (Allegrante, Peterson, Kovar, & Gordon, 1990; Lorig, Cox, Cuevas, Kraines, & Britton, 1984; Potts & Silverman, 1990; Sotosky, McGrory, Metzger, & DeHoratius, 1992). These discrepancies can cause treatment refusal or failure.

PLANNING AND MANAGEMENT STANDARDS

Effective patient education is a planned process that utilizes input from health professionals and educators as well as from patients. Ensuring patients' involvement in the development of the teaching plan will increase the likelihood that they will assume responsibility for the plan's ultimate success. The program management criteria require that one person be assigned the role of coordinator with ultimate responsibility for ensuring clear communication among all who are involved in the education process. Within integrated health care systems, this coordinator can be a case manager, care coordinator, health educator, arthritis nurse specialist, or other rehabilitation professional.

TYPES OF SIGNIFICANT POSITIVE CHANGES REPORTED IN ARTHRITIS PATIENT EDUCATION STUDIES

BEHAVIORS	Exercise
	Adherence
	Self-care behavior
	General health behavior
	Pain behavior
	Relaxation
	Work simplification practices
	Sleep behavior
PSYCHOSOCIAL VARIABLES	Self-efficacy
	Helplessness
	Locus of control
	Depression
	Anxiety
	General attitude
HEALTH OUTCOMES	Pain
	Functional disability/ability
	Work capacity
	Work and exercise time
	Count of painful joints
	Physical activity level
	Disease activity
	General health score
	Grip strength
	Quality of life
	Stiffness level

Table 3: Types of Significant Positive Changes Reported in Arthritis Patient Education Studies. As summarized in the article by Hirano et al., 1994.

CURRICULUM STANDARDS

Self-management education should be a continuous process that considers the changing needs of the learner, crosses care settings, and covers a person's life-span. Protocols and teaching plans help outline the learning that a particular patient or target group may need, improve consistency and continuity of instruction, reduce duplication, and, if for-

OVERVIEW OF ARTHRITIS AND MUSCULOSKELETAL PATIENT EDUCATION STANDARDS AND REVIEW CRITERIA

A QUALITY PATIENT EDUCATION PROGRAM HAS THE FOLLOWING CHARACTERISTICS:

Program content and process is based on a **needs assessment** conducted with the target population (patients, family members, significant care providers) and as appropriate, with health care providers, administrators, and others who may impact the successful implementation of the program.

Program planning and management is a comprehensive process involving health professionals and educators, as well as people with rheumatic diseases and family members.

- Participation of a rheumatologist, health professionals, and patients in the program planning is documented.
- There is a designated program coordinator to oversee program quality and operation.

A written curriculum documents the program content and process. The curriculum is supported by professional consensus and research literature.

- Outcome objectives reflect the needs assessment results and patient goals.
- The curriculum plan includes content outlines, instructional methods, and materials that offer information and skills relevant to patient goals and needs.
- The curriculum and materials are appropriate for the specified target audience.
- The curriculum is reviewed and updated regularly (at least every 5 years).
- There is an assessment of appropriate community agency referral resources, which is updated at least every 2 years.

Instructors have recent training and experience in rheumatic disease and in educational principles and techniques.

- Instructors may be professionals or lay persons.
- Participation in regular continuing education is expected.
- There is documentation of regular contact between the instructors and the program coordinator.
- A resource person knowledgeable in program content and rheumatology is available to patients using a mediated program that does not require an instructor.

Program evaluation demonstrates effectiveness in maintaining or improving health status (i.e., pain, functional ability, psychological state, social functioning, and/or quality of life). Satisfaction data must also be collected and reviewed.
- Effectiveness is documented on standard, validated instruments.
- Evaluations must be done on all new, not previously approved programs and on approved programs that are used for a new patient group that differs from the population for which the program was designed.

Table 4: Overview of Arthritis and Musculoskeletal Patient Education Standards and Review Criteria. Adapted from Burckhardt (1994).

The program is documented, including the following aspects:

- The needs assessment methods and results
- Curriculum
- Instructor/resource person qualifications, training, supervision, and evaluation
- Program outcome evaluation and satisfaction data
- Number of participants entering and completing the program
- Any other documentation required by the standards

Table 4: Overview of Arthritis and Musculoskeletal Patient Education Standards and Review Criteria (continued).
Adapted from Burckhardt (1994).

matted as a checklist, can facilitate documentation of the teaching process. The standards also state the necessity for research-based educational programs. A later section in this chapter discusses theories and theory-based programs.

INSTRUCTOR STANDARDS

The fourth category of standards states the necessity for qualified instructors who may either be health professionals or lay persons. The effectiveness of lay persons, particularly to enhance self-efficacy and/or support, has been well documented. Lay persons have been used to provide telephone support (Rene, Weinberger, Mazzuca, Brandt, & Katz, 1992), as self-management course leaders (Lorig, Feigenbaum, Regan, Ung, & Holman, 1987; Cohen, Sauter, DeVellis, R., & DeVellis, B., 1986), as support-group facilitators (Cronan, Groessl, & Kaplan, 1997), and as peer educators providing education to low-income Hispanics and African Americans (Bill-Harvey et al., 1989). Occupational therapy and physical therapy practitioners and other rehabilitation professionals can play key roles in the education process, either by instructing in formal group programs or by integrating educational protocols into their individual treatment plans. They may have the opportunity to build relationships with patients over time and are trained to deal with the biological, psychological, and social aspects of health. As health care moves toward more managed care and integrated health care systems, the lines of responsibility for patient education may blur and heighten the need for flexibility in how each discipline defines their patient-education role.

DOCUMENTATION AND EVALUATION STANDARDS

The standards reinforce the necessity for documentation of the teaching process and evaluation of its results. Documentation can reduce duplication of effort when multiple providers are involved in the patient-education process. Documentation of patient teaching is also required to meet Joint Commission on Accreditation of Healthcare

Organizations (JCAHO) regulations for hospital patient-education programs (JCAHO, 1994).

To meet the evaluation criteria in the arthritis patient education standards, a program must demonstrate its outcome effectiveness. While not a specific criterion, in these times of rapid changes in health care delivery and financing, data collection on health care utilization and costs is also imperative if adequate third-party reimbursement and administrative support are to be realized.

THE PRECEDE/PROCEED MODEL AS A PLANNING TOOL

The PRECEDE/PROCEED model is useful for needs assessments and developing educational plans for individual patients or groups (Green & Kreuter, 1991). It helps practitioners avoid common errors in traditional patient instruction by emphasizing a systematic, comprehensive series of planning steps that produces a social, epidemiologic, behavioral, educational, and administrative diagnosis.

SOCIAL AND EPIDEMIOLOGIC DIAGNOSIS

Program planning begins with a comprehensive description of the needs and problems affecting the quality of life and health status of a target population. These data help to delineate desirable benefits or outcomes of a patient-education program and allow practitioners to fine-tune their content based on what patients really want and need to learn. One common mistake is to provide a lot of unnecessary information that wastes time that could be spent practicing needed skills and teaching strategies for maintaining the behavior. Hirano and colleagues (1994) reviewed nine need-assessment studies that documented that people with arthritis most commonly report problems such as pain, fatigue, disability and lifestyle changes, uncertainty about the future, and depression. Consequently, many of the successful arthritis-patient education programs have been designed specifically to address these problems. Needs assessment data can be collected via interviews, surveys, or focus groups. Within clinical practice, a simple way to assess the patient's key concerns is to ask: "What comes to mind when you think of arthritis?" See Lorig (1996) for descriptions of these techniques.

BEHAVIORAL DIAGNOSIS

This phase involves determining which behaviors should be the focus of the patient-education program. Since time is usually limited, it is necessary to set priorities. The PRECEDE model suggests listing the behaviors that might affect the key health problems and then prioritizing them based on which are most important in the health problem, and are the easiest to change. One or more behaviors are selected, depending upon the amount of available teaching time. It is essential to review what evidence exists in the literature to document that the behaviors are amenable to change and that such change will improve the health problem in question. Patients should be involved in priority selection since the more behaviors are chosen rather than prescribed, the higher the likelihood that they will be adopted (Lorig, 1996). The end product of this stage is the development of measurable behavioral objectives that specify what patients are expected to do as a result of participating in the educational session or program.

EDUCATIONAL DIAGNOSIS

The process continues with the listing of the predisposing factors (knowledge, attitudes, and beliefs that facilitate or hinder motivation to change), enabling factors (availability of skills and resources that allow a motivation to be realized), and reinforcing factors (consequences of behaviors and level of support) relevant to the selected behavior(s). This step helps to counter the tendency in traditional education to provide only didactic instruction to increase knowledge. Delineating the multideterminants of a behavior heightens awareness that a variety of educational strategies must be employed and helps to ensure selection of an appropriate mix of interventions. Table 5 lists sample questions that can be used to assess key beliefs and other factors relevant to behavior change and/or health status.

After selecting those factors with the highest importance and changeability, objectives should be written for each selected factor. Measurable objectives help clarify what the program should be accomplishing and serve as a basis for the program evaluation.

ADMINISTRATIVE DIAGNOSIS

Even well-planned and theoretically sound programs can fail because of logistical problems. The administrative diagnosis helps to identify the adequacy of economic and human resources and other critical factors that can help or inhibit a program. These findings also need to be considered in planning the program. The health care system continues to evolve, and it is wise to be open to new approaches. One major health facility started biweekly classes taught by a physical therapist for people with knee pain. There was initial concern about deviating from the traditional one-on-one appointments with a physical therapist, but experience has shown that patients and therapists are satisfied with the new system (Lorig, 1996).

PROGRAM PLANNING AND EVALUATION

After the diagnostic steps, the next step is to develop a teaching plan that outlines potential content and methods. Since the best combination of educational content and processes for one patient or group is not necessarily the best mix for another, those using a protocol need to be flexible, individualize instruction to match the priorities and progress of the learner, utilize teachable moments, and modify the amount and sequence of what is taught into manageable steps. For instance, a newly diagnosed patient is likely to be overwhelmed. Education at this time should focus on reducing anxiety and suggesting supportive resources. In addition to being able to adapt the content and sequencing, a protocol should provide a variety of different learning formats. Learners differ in the sources they prefer and learn best from, the learning conditions that are most effective, their information-processing style, and other personal abilities and characteristics. To

ASSESSMENT QUESTIONS

VARIABLE	SAMPLE ASSESSMENT QUESTIONS
Beliefs about disease and symptoms (models/attributions, severity, susceptibility)	• When you think of (condition), what comes to mind? • What do you think causes your (condition/symptoms)? • What are the greatest consequences (symptoms or problems) that have resulted from your condition?
Treatment models/attributions and goals	• What problem is the most important one to work on? • What change would you like to start on first (e.g., losing weight, starting an exercise program, regaining the ability to do a desired activity)? • What results are you expecting? • How long before you expect to see these results? • When do you expect to quit the treatment?
Behavioral capability (knowledge and skill to perform behavior)	• Tell me what you are going to do—what, how often, for how long, what intensity? • Tell me what you would do if you think the treatment isn't working or if (specific side effect) occurs. • Show me your exercises (or other skill).
Anticipated behavioral outcomes and outcome expectations	• What do you see as the advantages or benefits of (behavior)? • How valuable to you are these positive outcomes? Which benefit is the most important to you? • What do you see as the disadvantages (negative outcomes, costs, bad things that might happen)?
Barriers/environmental constraints	• Many people miss doing (behavior) sometimes—what could make it difficult for you to do (behavior) regularly?
Norms and social support	• What do most people who are important to you think about your doing (behavior)? • What family member or friend is most likely to help you do (behavior)? • How could they help you? What would you like them to do? Have you asked them to help?

	• What individuals or groups might oppose or disapprove of you doing (behavior)?
Self-efficacy	• How confident are you on a scale of 1 to 10, with 10 being very confident, that you can do (behavior) on a regular basis?
Stage of change/behavioral intention **Select which statement best matches you:**	• I do not (behavior) now and I don't intend to start in the near future (pre-contemplation). • I do not (behavior), but I am thinking of starting (contemplation). • I do (behavior) some, but not regularly (preparation). • I have been doing (behavior) regularly for the last 1-6 months and intend to continue (action). • I currently do (behavior) regularly and have done so for 6 months or longer and intend to continue (maintenance). (Adapted from Marcus et al., 1994)

Table 5: Assessment Questions (continued)

accommodate these differences, a mix of educational methods will allow patients to customize the educational program through goal setting and contracting for their at-home activities.

The objectives developed for the program serve as the basis for an evaluation plan. It is beyond the scope of this chapter to discuss appropriate evaluation methodology. DeVellis (1996) has outlined strategies for finding and evaluating measurement tools. Several good resources exist to help practitioners integrate evaluation into their programs (e.g., Green & Lewis, 1986; Lorig et al., 1996; Windsor, Baranowski, Clark, & Cutter, 1994).

Figure 1 summarizes the key steps of the PRECECE/PROCEED model, with deconditioning as the health problem and adoption of regular physical activity as the prioritized behavior. Table 6 displays how findings from the diagnosis of the predisposing, enabling, and reinforcing factors can target specific kinds of interventions within a formal group education program or the education component of an individual treatment plan. Appendix 1 contains a generic self-management education protocol adaptable for different patients or target groups.

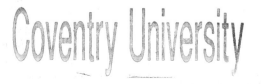

APPLICATION OF PRECEDE MODEL

STEP	SAMPLE FINDINGS
STEP 1 (SOCIAL DIAGNOSIS): Assess social/quality of life concerns of population.	Disability (Lost or restricted ability to fulfill work or other major roles/activities) Psychological distress (e.g., anxiety, depression)
STEP 2 (EPIDEMIOLOGIC DIAGNOSIS): Identify specific health problems that are relevant to the quality of life concerns.	Deconditioning effects (e.g., decreased flexibility, weakness, muscle atrophy, lack of cardiovascular fitness, fatigue, low pain threshold)
STEP 3 (BEHAVIORAL DIAGNOSIS): Identify the specific health-related behaviors that are causally linked to the health problems. Select the most important one(s) based on importance (relevance to changing the health problem) and changeability.	Engaging in an accumulated total of 30 minutes of moderate-intensity physical activity at least three times per week Range of motion/muscle strengthening exercises for affected joints, relevant to performance of valued activities/functions Joint protection techniques to decrease joint stress/maximize function (use of assistive devices; proper posture/biomechanics)
STEP 4 (EDUCATIONAL DIAGNOSIS): Identify the predisposing, enabling, and reinforcing factors relevant to the prioritized behavior(s) and select the most important ones based on their importance and changeability. (Note that this example only shows factors relevant to engaging in regular physical activity.)	Predisposing factors: • Perceived health status • Knowledge of effects of inactivity • Beliefs in benefits of physical activity and value placed on these beneficial outcomes • Belief that it is possible to affect health/quality of life outcomes • Perceived barriers/negative consequences (fear of injury/disease flare, costs, inconvenience) • Belief that important others (MD, therapist, family, peers, etc.) want person to exercise/motivation to comply with those opinions • Exercise self-efficacy • Current exercise level/status (Intention to exercise/stage of change) • Knowledge of appropriate exercise prescription (type, frequency, intensity, duration); precautions for exercise Enabling factors: • Availability/convenience of exercise facilities • Transportation • Skill in performing physical activity in safe manner • Time management and pacing skills Reinforcing factors: • Perceived improvement in symptoms, functional ability, psychosocial status and other intrinsic rewards • Negative consequences of exercising

STEP 5 (ADMINISTRATIVE/ ORGANIZATIONAL DIAGNOSIS): Assess organizational, administrative, managerial, and policy factors that can support or inhibit a program	• Adequacy of budget/ reimbursement • Sufficient personnel with appropriate training, time, and commitment • Administrative/institutional support • Adequacy of facilities/equipment • Territorial issues/ clear delineation of roles and responsibilities • Support from people with rheumatic diseases
STEP 6: PROGRAM DEVELOPMENT AND IMPLEMENTATION	
STEP 7: EVALUATION	

From Green, L. W., & Kreuter, M. W. (1991). *Health Education Planning: A Diagnostic Approach*. Mountain View, CA: Mayfield Publishing.

Figure 1: Application of PRECEDE Model (continued)

THEORETICAL BASIS

The current effective approaches to arthritis patient education have evolved from various theories. Table 7 presents some of the theories relevant to arthritis self-management education. Theories help practitioners identify factors that can affect patient behavior and health outcomes, and can also provide guidance for interventions. Of particular note is the self-efficacy construct within social learning theory (Bandura, 1991). Self-efficacy is the degree of confidence in one's ability to execute a behavior regularly. It is correlated with self-management behavior and positive health outcomes in arthritis (Taal et al., 1996). The model suggests several intervention strategies, including skills mastery, goal-setting, contracting, feedback, modeling, reinterpretation of symptoms, persuasion, and self-monitoring. When Lorig and colleagues evaluated the Arthritis Self-Management Program (ASMP), they found minimal correlation between increased exercise and relaxation behaviors and improvements in outcomes such as pain and depression. Further research documented that the addition of self-efficacy enhancing strategies to the ASMP increased the course's outcome effectiveness (Lorig & Gonzalez, 1992). Many of these self-efficacy enhancing strategies can easily be incorporated into clinical practice, as described in the section on building self-efficacy.

The Stress and Coping paradigm (Lazarus & Folkman, 1984) is commonly used as a framework for explaining adaptation and coping behaviors. Research suggests that the degree of impact that a functional impairment can have on psychological well-being depends on the importance attached to the activities that are impaired. This finding highlights the need to identify the patient's functional priorities as the basis for clinical recommendations (Blalock et al., 1992). Research has also suggested the value of providing

SAMPLE STRATEGIES BASED ON EDUCATIONAL DIAGNOSIS

DIAGNOSTIC FINDING	STRATEGY
PREDISPOSING FACTORS Lack of motivation for self-care	• Discuss one-to-one the causes of symptoms, benefits relevant to goals of doing behavior, and consequences of not doing behavior • Use group brainstorm and discussion led by positive role model • Use decision-analysis tool
Lack of understanding about recommended regimen	• Provide repetition; ask for recall • Supplement verbal instruction with audiovisual, computer aids, printed materials
Lack of confidence in ability to perform desired behavior	• Teach goal-setting and contracting • Build peer/family support; use role models as mentors • Give feedback/praise about progress towards goals
ENABLING FACTORS Lack of needed skills	• Train, starting with demonstration of simple to complex skills • Provide opportunity for repeat practice, return demonstration and feedback
Lack of available resources (transportation, facilities, costs, etc.)	• Problem-solve • Refer to resources
REINFORCING FACTORS Negative consequences of regimen	• Use one-to-one or group discussion: how to prevent/deal with side effects; modify regimen • Use one-to-one or group problem-solving discussion: how to increase positive consequences/rewards • Use one-to-one or group discussion of self-monitoring tools
Lack of support from significant others	• Involve significant others in clinical visits, educational program • Build peer support; refer to support groups; establish patient "mentors" • Refer to other health professionals as needed • Provide telephone calls in between visits to provide support, information, reminders

Table 6: Sample Strategies Based on Educational Diagnosis

individuals with a wide repertoire of cognitive and behavioral coping skills (Blalock, DeVellis, Holt, & Hahn, 1993). How to conceptualize and enhance perceived social support have also been the focus of much research (Lanza & Revenson, 1993; Roberts, Matecjyck, & Anthony, 1996). Many principles from the stress and coping paradigm are applied in cognitive behavioral treatment (CBT) programs, which are described in more detail in the next section.

SELECTED THEORIES RELEVANT TO ARTHRITIS PATIENT EDUCATION

THEORY/MODEL	KEY CONCEPTS
Classic Learning Theory (Skinner, 1953)	Learning a new complex behavior is facilitated by breaking it into smaller steps and then gradually increasing complexity (*shaping*); providing environmental cues to stimulate the behavior and positive *reinforcement* to motivate continuation.
Health Belief Model (Janz & Becker, 1984; Rosenstock, 1990)	Motivation to engage in appropriate health actions is determined by: (1) perceptions about the threats posed by a condition and/or its consequences, including the perceived *susceptibility* to a condition (or acceptance of a diagnosis) and *severity* (seriousness of the condition or of the consequences of not treating it); evaluation of the behavior in terms of its perceived *benefits* weighed against the costs or other *barriers* of all available alternatives; and the initiating stimulus of a *cue to action*. (Self-efficacy is a recent addition to this theory.)
Reasoned Action (Ajzen & Fishbein, 1980) & Planned Behavior (Ajzen, 1988)	*Reasoned Action: Behavioral intentions* are the immediate determinant of behaviors. The strength of one's intention to do a behavior is a function of: (1) attitudes toward the behavior (which include beliefs that particular outcomes will occur as a result of the behavior and evaluations of these outcomes); and (2) subjective norms, including a person's belief about what important others think and the person's motivation to comply with significant others' wishes. The theory of *Planned Behavior* adds to the Reasoned Action theory the concept of *perceived behavioral control* over opportunities, resources, and skills necessary to perform the behavior.
Multiattribute Utility theory (Carter, 1990); Decision-making models (Janis & Mann, 1977)	Behavior can be predicted directly from an individual's assessment of the benefits and barriers associated with performing and not performing a behavior. Decision-making can be facilitated through strategies like a Decision Balance Sheet to assess costs and benefits of behaviors to self and others.
Attribution theory (Lewis & Daltroy, 1990)	Individuals develop their own "models" or explanations of health-related events, including the causes and controllability of their illnesses and symptoms. These explanations in turn affect their thoughts, feelings, and behavior.
Learned Helplessness Theory (Seligman, 1975)	A type of attribution theory that helps to explain why people may react to fluctuating disease courses, in which there is not always a clear relationship between one's health actions and clinical outcomes, with feelings of hopelessness, lack of motivation for self-management, and giving up on treatment. Feelings of helplessness are generalized beliefs affecting multiple parts of a person's life, as opposed to self-efficacy, which is specific for certain behaviors.
Self Regulation (Leventhal, 1983); Learned Resourcefulness (Rosenbaum, 1988)	Individuals develop a plan for coping with their illness and its symptoms based on their disease models and then they regulate their behavior to maintain acceptable levels of health. Persons who acquire self-monitoring, problem-solving, emotion regulation, and other self-control skills are thought to develop a sense of *learned resourcefulness* i.e., the belief that they can effectively deal with manageable levels of stress.

Table 7: Selected Theories Relevant to Arthritis Patient Education

Social Cognitive Learning Theory (Bandura, 1986); Self-Efficacy (Bandura, 1991)	Explains behavior in terms of a continuous interaction among cognitive, emotional, behavioral, and environmental factors, all of which are to some extent causally related ("reciprocal determinism"). Actual performance of a behavior is influenced by one's *behavioral capability* (knowledge and skill to perform the behavior) as well as various cognitive factors including *self-efficacy* (degree of confidence in ability to perform a specific behavior), beliefs concerning the effects of the behavior (*outcome expectations*), and the value placed on these outcomes. Behavior can also be influenced by the reciprocal interaction among patients, their family members, and health care providers.
Stress and Coping paradigm (Lazarus & Folkman, 1984)	The impact of stressors such as pain, loss of function, feelings of helplessness, etc. are influenced by individuals' appraisal of the stressor and the amount of threat it creates ("primary appraisal"), as well as an assessment of whether the situation is controllable or changeable through one's coping strategies and resources ("secondary appraisal"). An individual will perceive a situation as stressful when it creates demands that exceed the person's abilities or resources.
Social Support (Israel & Shurman, 1990; Lanza & Revenson, 1993)	Social support can be defined in different ways. One categorization defines four types of support: *emotional* (empathy, caring), *instrumental* (provision of tangible aid), *informational* (advice, suggestions, information), and *appraisal* (feedback and other information useful for self-evaluation). Support may be positive or negative. Some types of support may work better in some situations than others.
Transtheoretical or Stages of Change model (Prochaska et al., 1992)	Individuals may go through several stages in their efforts to adopt and maintain a health behavior, including: *pre-contemplation* (don't yet perceive a problem; not yet considering possible change); *contemplation* (aware of a problem; thinking about change but no commitment to take action); *preparation* (have intention to take action; making small changes); *action* (actively engaging in the new behavior); and *maintenance* (working to sustain change and prevent relapse). Individuals may enter and exit the cycle at any stage, spend varying amounts of time in a stage, and may progress forward or relapse to earlier stages. With each stage, there are corresponding processes of change.
Relapse Prevention Theory (Marlatt and George, 1990)	Describes stages of change with a focus on how to utilize a wide range of self-management and self-control strategies for anticipating problems and for maintaining behavioral change over time. Factors that may lead to relapse include: negative emotional or physiologic states, beliefs about treatment outcomes, lack of coping skills, social pressure and lack of social support, interpersonal conflict, low motivation, high-risk situations, and perceived stress.

Table 7: Selected Theories Relevant to Arthritis Patient Education (continued)

The Transtheoretical or Stages of Change model (Prochaska, DiClemente, & Norcross, 1992) has not received much attention in the arthritis field but has been extensively utilized to explain processes of change relevant to exercise, smoking cessation, weight control, and other specific behaviors. This model outlines the stages an individual may move through to get ready for and undertake a behavior change, including precontemplation (not even thinking about a change), contemplation (thinking about a change), preparation (getting ready for change), action (actually doing the behavior), and maintenance (maintaining the behavior for 6 months or more). Many health professionals' recommendations are based on the assumption that a patient is ready and eager to change behavior or health habits. Low rates of adherence with treatment recommendations demonstrate that this assumption is faulty. By determining a patient's current stage of change, practitioners can direct interventions toward assisting the patient to progress along the change continuum. Success is measured in terms of movement along the stages, and not just in terms of whether they go into action or not. A type of stage model of change is being used as the basis for an osteoporosis project that is attempting to influence individuals' use of calcium and exercise (Blalock, DeVellis, R., Giorgino, & DeVellis, B., 1995).

Several researchers have described the practical application of theory-based interventions into arthritis patient education. Gonzalez, Goeppinger, and Lorig (1990) explain how to integrate strategies based on self-efficacy, stress and coping, social support, and learned helplessness theories into patient education and clinical practice. Daltroy (1993) describes principles derived from attribution and decision-making theory that have implications for improving doctor-patient communication. Allegrante, Kovar, MacKenzie, Peterson, and Gutin (1993) promoted regular physical activity through strategies based on self-efficacy and social-learning theory. Keefe and Van Horn (1993) fostered long-term maintenance of pain-coping skills through a cognitive-behavioral and relapse-prevention model. Gecht, Connell, Sinacore, and Prohaska (1996) used the Health Belief Model as the basis for examining the relationship between health beliefs and participation in exercise activities.

In addition to the individual and interpersonal theories listed in Table 7, a variety of broader theoretical frameworks recognize that individuals function within a social context. Particularly as providers try to reach underserved populations such as culturally diverse groups and/or try to provide community-based programs, it is imperative to have an understanding of principles derived from broader frameworks. Relevant theories and models include the biopsychosocial model of health (Parker et al., 1993), the social ecological approach (McLeroy, Bibeau, Steckler, & Glanz, 1988), the community empowerment and organizing model (Minkler, 1990), social marketing (Kotler & Andreason, 1987), communications for persuasion (McGuire, 1981), and the diffusion-of-innovations model (Rogers, 1983). Key concepts include involving the target population in needs assessment, using representatives of the target group in the planning and delivery of the interventions, involving the family and other significant others in the intervention, ensuring cultural relevance of the intervention's content and format, and taking the intervention out of the medical setting and into places that are familiar and comfortable to the target group.

RECENT EFFORTS

Psychoeducational interventions used for arthritis can be categorized in a variety of ways (DeVellis & Blalock, 1993; Hawley, 1995; Mullen et al., 1987). This section describes representative examples of five types of programs that have demonstrated effectiveness: (1) self-management education, (2) group exercise instruction, (3) cognitive-behavioral therapy (CBT), (4) mediated instruction, and (5) support and counseling programs including telephone programs and mutual-support programs. Also described in this section are recent efforts to serve special populations.

SELF-MANAGEMENT CLASSES

There are many self-management programs including the original Arthritis Self-Management Program developed by Lorig and colleagues (Lorig & Gonzales, 1992; Lorig, Mazonson, & Holman, 1993). This program was adopted by the Arthritis Foundation (AF), which disseminates it as the Arthritis Self-Help Course. Similar programs were developed and adopted by the AF for systemic lupus erythematosus (Braden, 1991; Braden, McGlone, & Pennington, 1993) and fibromyalgia (Johnson, Boutaugh, & Seikus, 1996). These programs are taught by trained professionals and/or lay leaders. There is an emphasis on interactive methods, experiential learning, and the use of self-efficacy enhancing techniques. Table 8 describes their content and format. Similar programs that have published evaluation data include self-management programs in the Netherlands (Taal et al., 1993) and in Australia (Lindroth, Bauman, Barnes, McCredie, & Brooks, 1989; Lindroth, Bauman, Brooks, & Priestly, 1995).

EXERCISE AND EDUCATION CLASSES

Educational classes that focus on exercise are a variation on the self-management class series. Typically they are taught by physical or occupational therapy professionals and fitness professionals. Content focuses on promoting the adoption of regular physical activity including range of motion, muscle strengthening, and low-impact aerobic activities. They often include self-efficacy enhancing strategies, problem-solving discussions, and other activities to promote long-term maintenance of exercise behavior. Examples of programs that have had positive health and psychological outcomes include the Arthritis Foundation's PACE® program (Doyle, Farrar, Ryan, & Sisola, 1990; Kennedy, Walker, Linnel, Johnson, & Socklear, 1992, the Educize® program (Connell, 1993; Perlman et al., 1990), which combines low-impact dance activities with problem-solving discussions; Minor and Brown's program (1993), which compared aerobic walking and aerobic aquatics to standard arthritis exercises, and a walking program for people with osteoarthritis (Allegrante et al., 1993; Kovar et al., 1992).

COGNITIVE BEHAVIORAL TREATMENT PROGRAMS

The cognitive behavioral treatment (CBT) approach has been used as the basis for several pain and stress management programs (Basler, 1993; Bradley et al., 1988; Buckelew & Parker, 1989; Calfas, Kaplan, & Ingram, 1992; Keefe et al., 1990; Keefe & Van Horn, 1993; O'Leary, Shoor, Lorig, & Holman, 1988; Parker, Iverson, Smarr, & Stucky-Ropp, 1993; Radojevic, Nicassio, & Weisman, 1992). CBT strategies can include helping patients learn to monitor the interactions among their thoughts, feelings, symptoms, behavior, and social environment; cognitive coping skill-training (e.g., problem-solving, relaxation skills, cognitive restructuring); behavioral coping skills (e.g., goal-setting, pacing, relapse prevention techniques); and strategies to promote social support. CBT programs typically are group sessions of 1-2 hours for 5-10 weeks, although one recently reported program included

ARTHRITIS FOUNDATION SELF-MANAGEMENT PROGRAMS

OFFERING NAME	KEY FEATURES	EVALUATION RESULTS
GROUP FORMAT		
Arthritis Self-Help Course (ASHC)	Format: 2 hours/week; 6 weeks Content: problem-solving; exercise; cognitive pain and stress management; managing fatigue; coping with depression; using medications wisely; evaluating unproven remedies; communicating with health care team/s.o.	• Increased knowledge • Increased frequency of exercise and relaxation • Increased self-efficacy • Decreased depression • Decreased pain (15-20%) • Decreased physician visits (43% decrease in 4 yrs.)
Systemic Lupus Erythematosus Self-Help Course	Format: 2.5 hours/week; 7 weeks Content: same as ASHC; also has stronger emphasis on fatigue management, coping with losses, depression, self-esteem issues; medications and treatments for complications; planning ahead for flare-ups; wellness issues, etc.	• Increased knowledge • Increased self-care (exercise, relaxation, etc.) • Decreased depression • Increased self-efficacy • Increased enabling skill • Improved life quality
Fibromyalgia Self-Help Course	Format: 2.5 hours/week; 7 weeks Content: same as ASHC; also has strong emphasis on pain, fatigue and sleep management; posture and body mechanics; coping strategies	• Increased confidence in managing condition • Decreased depression • Improved quality of life • Increased self-mastery
INDIVIDUAL FORMAT		
Bone-Up on Arthritis	Format: Self-paced; low-literacy; six lessons on audio cassettes and workbook Content: similar to ASHC	• Increased self-care behaviors • Decreased helplessness • Decreased pain • Decreased depression • Decreased disability
Arthritis Home Help[SM] (Healthtrac SMART)	Format: Quarterly health risk and arthritis status questionnaires; individualized, computer-tailored self-management plan; self-care books, relaxation audiotape Content: similar to ASHC	• Increased self-efficacy • Increased satisfaction with health care • Decreased pain • Improved ability to function • Improved affect • Decreased visits to MD/specialists

Table 8: Arthritis Foundation Self-Management Programs

computer-assisted one-on-one sessions (Parker et al., 1995). They are generally led by psychologists or specially trained professionals. Airth (1994) reports an occupational therapy treatment program that incorporated a cognitive-behavioral treatment approach into a 6-week class series on sleep, energy conservation, posture, assertive communication, stress management, and community resources.

MEDIATED PROGRAMS

Many alternative methods for program delivery have been tested in an effort to reach broader audiences and reduce costs. The Bone-Up on Arthritis program was evaluated as a small-group intervention versus a home-study version that incorporated audiocassettes, illustrated print materials, and telephone contacts by trained community coordinators. The home-study program achieved the same positive changes in self-care behavior and health outcomes when it was used as a small-group intervention (Goeppinger, Arthur, Baglioni, Brunck, & Brunner, 1989), and when disseminated through the Arthritis Foundation (Goeppinger, Macnee, Anderson, Boutaugh, & Stewart, 1995). However, when the Arthritis Foundation tried to reduce costs further by eliminating the trained community coordinators and supportive phone calls, behavioral changes were achieved but changes in health outcomes were not realized.

In an effort to increase utilization of the Arthritis Self-Management Program, Hawley (1994) compared the effectiveness of courses taught simultaneously to multiple sites via interactive television to traditional classes. Short-term changes in self-efficacy, self-care behavior, and depression were achieved in the studio and traditional classes, but there was minimal improvement among the remote-site participants.

Interactive computer programs were found effective in producing behavioral changes and some health outcomes with people with RA (Wetstone, Sheehan, & Votaw, 1985), an elderly population with osteoarthritis (Rippey, Bill, & Abeles,1987), and a group undergoing total joint arthroplasty (Reisine & Lewis, 1993; Tibbles, Lewis, Reisine, Rippey, & Donald, 1992). Computers are now being used to tailor the education provided to patients. In a program recently adopted by the Arthritis Foundation (Arthritis Home Help), patients complete a questionnaire and then are sent computer-tailored, individualized self-management materials (Gale et al., 1994). Computer-tailored messages are also being delivered via video discs. The Foundation for Informed Medical Decision Making has produced programs for use in the clinical setting to facilitate shared decision making on topics such as low back pain (Kasper, Mulley, & Wennberg, 1992).

TELEPHONE AND SOCIAL SUPPORT PROGRAMS

Telephone counseling programs have been found very effective in reducing pain and physical disability and/or improving psychological function. Rene and colleagues (1992) and Mazzuca and colleagues (1995) reported the effectiveness of using trained laypersons with an inner-city population. A program in Alabama using professional counselors was successful with a statewide sample of persons with RA or OA (Maisiak et al., 1996) and with lupus (Austin, Maisiak, Macrina, & Heck, 1996).

Support-group interventions that include family members and/or other persons with arthritis have had inconsistent results (DeVellis & Blalock, 1993). A recent, promising study (Cronan et al., 1997) compared the effectiveness of three interventions: a lecture series taught by health professionals that stressed how to use medical services appropriately, a social-support intervention that involved group discussions aimed at promoting empathy and sharing of coping techniques, and a combination in which the first hour of each meeting was lecture, followed by an hour of supportive discussion. All three groups showed a significant increase in well-being compared to the control group.

REACHING SPECIAL POPULATIONS

Most of the educational programs reported in the literature comprise primarily persons with osteoarthritis and rheumatoid arthritis. There is a need to do more to address the needs of those with osteoporosis, back pain, and less common forms of rheumatic disease as well as those with low literacy skills and culturally diverse populations. Community-based education and support programs have been developed for rural (Goeppinger et al., 1989) and inner-city low-literacy populations (Bill-Harvey et al., 1989); the First Nations population in Canada (McGowen, 1995); a Chinese-speaking population in the San Francisco area (Fung & Woo, 1995); and for African Americans and Latinos with lupus (Gonzalez et al., 1995; Robbins, 1994).

PRACTICAL APPLICATION

We have more to learn about what types or combinations of educational interventions are most effective and which mechanisms contribute to their efficacy. Nevertheless, there is a need to apply what is known into practice. This section reviews some theory-based principles and constructs that are relevant to arthritis patient education.

A PERSON-CENTERED, PROBLEM-BASED APPROACH

Person-centered care is based on eliciting and accommodating the patients' perspective: their definition of their problems, goals, beliefs about outcome, stage of change, and their preferences for education and treatment. Adults tend to be now-oriented and problem-focused in their learning activities. Therefore, by eliciting current concerns the therapist can capitalize on teachable moments, that is, when patients recognize that a problem need to be solved. Focusing on patients' symptoms or other concerns and what they want to accomplish allows the practitioner to tailor the educational messages and improve the chance for relevant behavioral change. The provider may want the patient to begin an exercise program, but framing the exercise recommendation as a way to achieve the patient's goals (e.g., to manage pain or to regain the ability to perform a desired activity) increases the likelihood that the patient will try exercising. Asking patients to explain the cause and meaning of their disease, its symptoms, and their expectations about treatment allows for correction of any misconceptions or false expectations and helps set priorities for treatment options.

The goal is to prioritize and negotiate a mutually acceptable education and treatment plan. As described in chapter 3, a positive atmosphere for negotiation is fostered by encouraging openness, by communicating acceptance and respect for the patient's perspectives and experiences, and by being flexible to negotiate the therapeutic regimen. The educator's role is simply to lay out the risks and benefits of various options to help the patient achieve an optimum balance between improved health status and quality of life.

USING CHANGE PROCESSES RELEVANT TO THE PATIENT'S STAGE OF CHANGE

Behavior changes such as adopting a regular exercise routine can be facilitated by beginning where the patient is on the stages-of-change continuum and selecting interventions relevant to the particular stage of change. Distinguishing among those who have not yet begun to contemplate a change, are just beginning to prepare for change, or are ready for action provides the opportunity to tailor the educational strategy to one that will facilitate movement toward the next stage of change. For example, it appears that most people are not in the action stage of doing at least a moderate level of exercising regularly. Marcus, Pinto, Simkin, Audrain, and Taylor (1994) studied working women and found that 39% of the sample were sedentary (precontemplative and contemplative), 34% were participating in irregular exercise (preparatory), and 27% were active (action and maintenance stage). Similarly, Ruggiero (1994) found that most of an HMO population were primarily inactive (36% precontemplative, 28% contemplative, 37% in preparation). Patients who are in the precontemplative stage will not respond well to traditional interventions such as self-help programs or action-oriented programs. They simply will not register for a program, or they will drop out. Verbal change processes such as consciousness raising about the value of a recommended behavior are appropriate for someone in the precontemplative stage. Contemplators can be helped to become determined to start exercising through such techniques as using a decision-making worksheet to weigh the pros and cons of continuing the same versus reasons to start a behavior. Once a person has moved into the action phase, behavioral control strategies become appropriate.

USING EFFECTIVE COMMUNICATION SKILLS

To promote understanding, practitioners need to provide specific instructions in lay language to inform patients about their diagnosis and why, what, how, and when to do a recommended treatment. Minor (1996) points out that exercise is dose-dependent: to achieve optimal benefit, patients must be given specific recommendations about type, intensity, duration, and frequency, as well as guidelines to prevent injury. Practitioners can help retention by summarizing conclusions and instructions at the end of visits and by distributing supplementary print material like Arthritis Foundation educational brochures. Patient understanding can be checked by having patients verbalize what, when, and how often they plan on doing the agreed regimen and by asking them to demonstrate any needed skills.

A MULTIFACETED APPROACH

Self-management for rheumatic conditions often requires learning a variety of information (cognitive), attitudes (affective), and skills (psychomotor), and these require different types of educational processes. Programs will be more effective if the learner is actively involved via multifaceted educational strategies—not just verbal instructions or distribution of print materials (Lorig, 1996). No single educational input should be expected to have a significant effect on health outcomes (Green & Kreuter, 1991). Posters and other audiovisuals can reinforce key messages. Each educational session should involve the patient's active participation and provide a variety of educational strategies such as discussion, brainstorming, problem solving, and guided practice. One effective formula for generating involvement is the activity-discussion-application approach. The patient (or small group) performs an activity (such as a demonstration of a relaxation technique). The activity is followed by a discussion of what good or bad happened and relevant feelings. The final step is to try to apply or generalize the experience to real life (Pike, 1989). This approach is frequently used in the Arthritis Self-Management Program. Class members are taught behaviors such as how to exercise, do relaxation techniques, and self-talk and are encouraged to practice these at home. Instead of doing a different topic every week, behavioral skills are taught over multiple sessions, and this allows time for repeated practice. During feedback sessions in subsequent classes, the group discusses problems and successes, and that helps make these activities an ongoing habit. Retention is improved when visual aids, recall of instructions, repetitive practice, and return demonstration are added to the educational protocol.

COGNITIVE-SKILLS TRAINING

Because maladaptive beliefs, feelings, and thoughts can play a significant role in behavior change and health status, it is important to teach patients various cognitive skills. For instance, explaining the many different possible causes for symptoms like pain and fatigue can help patients reinterpret the causes of their symptoms. When patients understand that their symptoms can be due to multiple causes beyond the disease process alone (e.g., deconditioning, stress, or depression), their motivation to consider other nonpharmacologic strategies and their sense of self-efficacy may increase (Lorig, 1996). Similarly, many CBT programs begin by helping patients reconceptualize their view of pain as a specific, addressable problem that is influenced by cognitions and behaviors.

A specific strategy for helping patients change maladaptive thoughts is called *cognitive restructuring* in CBT programs and *self-talk* in various self-management programs. Patients are encouraged to monitor when they have pain or other problems and to write down their associated thoughts and feelings. They also learn how to do a reality check on their beliefs and to change negative thoughts to positive statements (Allegrante et al., 1993; Lorig, 1996). Keeping a journal or diary or completing symptom-monitoring forms can help patients become more aware of their thought patterns.

BEHAVIORAL TECHNIQUES

Various reports have estimated that adherence rates for people with arthritis range from 16% to 84% for medications; from 39% to 65% for exercise; and 25% to 65% for splint usage (Rapoff, 1996). Expecting strict adherence is often not appropriate in rheumatic diseases because disease fluctuations can necessitate changes in the treatment regimen, and some prescribed modalities such as medications can have significant side effects. Nevertheless, coaching patients to achieve their desired behavior changes is an important role for rehabilitation professionals. A variety of behavioral techniques can facilitate and help maintain changes in behavior.

Practitioners can help ensure that patients have the behavioral capability by providing clear demonstrations of any necessary skills and allowing adequate opportunities for guided practice, feedback, and discussion of barriers to continuing the behavior at home. Skill mastery is enhanced by beginning with simple, easily mastered tasks and gradually building in complexity.

As described in chapter 3, another important strategy is to increase the number of positive consequences while decreasing the negative consequences or drawbacks of doing a behavior. Complex regimens should be simplified as much as possible, and the therapist and patient should work together to problem-solve any barriers. Positive reinforcements can include token reinforcements such as achievement awards (e.g., certificates of achievement, tee-shirts, sample assistive or exercise aids). Patients can be encouraged to develop their own reward systems and/or involve their significant others in providing praise and other types of support.

New habits can be built by using environmental cues to prompt and motivate behaviors, for example, linking a new behavior such as use of a stationary bicycle to an old behavior like watching a favorite TV show. Self-monitoring tools such as an exercise or food diary can serve both to remind and reinforce behaviors. Reviewing such tools during clinical visits serves to reinforce progress.

Various relapse-prevention strategies can also be taught. Patients can be reassured that missing an exercise session and other lapses are often inevitable and should be treated as only temporary setbacks and not reasons for stopping the behavior altogether. Anticipating what problems or conditions might precipitate a relapse is essential so that alternative responses for coping with these situations can be developed.

PROBLEM-SOLVING AND DECISION-MAKING SKILLS

Practitioners can help their patients become more active partners in their care by teaching them how to solve problems rather than providing the solution (Gonzalez et al., 1990). Patients who present a problem can be asked to generate a list of potential solutions, including any they have used in the past to deal with the problem. The next step is to examine the pros and cons of each option before selecting which one to try. To help people make decisions about their treatment, a decision-making or "force-field analyses" worksheet can help in listing out the pros and cons of their options (see Figure 2 for an example).

BUILDING SELF-EFFICACY

Self-efficacy can be increased by breaking down skills and behaviors into easily mastered components and helping patients reinterpret their symptoms. Other key strategies are short-term goal setting and contracting, feedback, persuasion, and modeling (Lorig & Gonzalez, 1992). Patients can be helped to set realistic short-term goals by identifying what they are doing now and then suggesting that they set a goal to just do a little more. Once patients have experienced success with one treatment component, other components can gradually be added. Commitment can be strengthened by having patients write

---

PROS AND CONS OF EXERCISING WORKSHEET

Action	*Inaction*
Benefits of exercising	Benefits of not exercising
Drawbacks of exercising	Drawbacks of not exercising

Figure 2: Pros and Cons of Exercising Worksheet

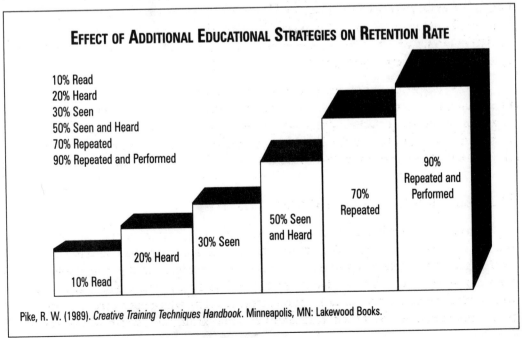

EFFECT OF ADDITIONAL EDUCATIONAL STRATEGIES ON RETENTION RATE

10% Read
20% Heard
30% Seen
50% Seen and Heard
70% Repeated
90% Repeated and Performed

10% Read
20% Heard
30% Seen
50% Seen and Heard
70% Repeated
90% Repeated and Performed

Pike, R. W. (1989). *Creative Training Techniques Handbook*. Minneapolis, MN: Lakewood Books.

Figure 3: Effect of Additional Educational Strategies on Retention Rate

down their goals in a contract that states a clear description of the activity, how long it will be done, how many times, and how often. Therapists should ask patients about their level of confidence in their ability to carry out their contract. When they do not feel confident, the goal should be modified so that it is achievable, and any perceived barriers should be addressed. Follow-up contacts should include monitoring progress on goals and providing praise and positive feedback.

A powerful way to influence patients' level of self-efficacy and motivate behavior change is to provide positive role models, for example, people with arthritis who are successfully managing their condition. Modeling can be achieved by using people with arthritis as lay instructors or mentors. The effectiveness of print and audiovisual materials can be increased by visuals and real-life vignettes of people who are representative of the target population's age and ethnic diversity. Practitioners also need to be aware that they will be observed and should practice what they preach about exercise, weight control, smoking, and other behaviors.

Credible people can be used to persuade patients to change specific behaviors. Peer educators can be very influential. Often the opinion of the physician and other health professionals is also judged important. Practitioners can build their persuasive ability by showing respect, providing factual information about recommendations, and being flexible to negotiation (Jensen & Lorish, 1994).

BUILDING CAPACITY TO GIVE AND RECEIVE SUPPORT

Natural support networks can be nurtured by asking patients what family members or significant others are most likely to help them with their self-management and then clarifying what kind of help is desired. This may vary from doing the recommended behavior with the patient to providing praise or other positive consequences, giving reminders, etc. Important significant others should be encouraged to participate in clinical visits and patient-education activities. The effectiveness of self-management classes and support groups is enhanced when they are structured to encourage participants to help each other. Patients who are successfully managing their disease can also provide support to new patients, for example, by linking up people who have had successful joint-replacement surgery with those considering such surgery. As described in an earlier section, telephone counseling programs also appear to be very effective in reinforcing information and providing support. (See the section on telephone and social support programs for program descriptions.)

REFERRAL

As described in chapter 17, there are a variety of appropriate referral sources including other health professionals and community resources. The Arthritis Foundation is a source for printed and audiovisual materials, exercise classes, support groups and self-management programs (see Table 8). Potential referral sources should be contacted in advance to ensure that their services are appropriate and to obtain a contact person's name and phone number.

Summary

Patient education can produce changes in knowledge, behavior, and health status; and there is preliminary evidence that patient education can also influence health care utilization and cost. It is remarkable that these changes were observed in patients who were already receiving medical care. Ample opportunities are available to improve outcomes with appropriate patient-education programs.

Arthritis patient-education programs with documented effectiveness can take a variety of forms such as self-management classes, cognitive behavioral treatments, and telephone support programs. While program formats may vary, high-quality programs share similar characteristics. Key psychoeducational theories provide the theoretical underpinnings of self-management enhancing patient-education programs. Theory-based practical applications include using a patient-centered, multifaceted approach, processes that match the patient's readiness to change, and behavioral techniques such as teaching cognitive skills, including problem solving and decision making; and building both self-efficacy and the capacity to give and receive support.

Because of their functional orientation and understanding of biopsychosocial factors, occupational and physical therapy practitioners are well positioned to provide self-management enhancing education to help individuals with rheumatic diseases improve their health and quality of life.

REFERENCES

Airth, T. (1994). Occupational therapy treatment of fibromyalgia: Efficacy of a cognitive-behavioral group in clinical study. *Arthritis Care and Research, 7,* S11.

Ajzen, I. (1988). *Attitudes, personality, and behavior.* Chicago: Dorsey Press.

Ajzen, I., & Fishbein, M. (1980). *Understanding attitudes and predicting social behavior.* Englewood Cliffs, NJ: Prentice Hall.

Albrecht, M., Goeppinger, J., & Anderson, M. K. (1993). The Albrecht nursing model for home healthcare. Predictors of satisfaction with a self-care intervention program. *Journal of Nursing Administration, 23,* 51-54.

Allegrante, J. P., Kovar, P. A., & MacKenzie, C. R. (1993). A walking education program for patients with osteoarthritis of the knee: Theory and intervention strategies. *Health Education Quarterly, 20,* 63-81.

Allegrante, J. P., Peterson, M. G., Kovar, P. A., & Gordon, A. (1990). Beliefs held by physicians and patients regarding compliance with treatment and educational needs in arthritis and musculoskeletal diseases. *Arthritis Care and Research, 3,* S10.

Austin, J., Maisiak, R., Macrina, D., & Heck, L. (1996). Health outcome improvements in patients with systemic lupus erythemarosus using two telephone counseling interviews. *Arthritis Care and Research, 9,* 391-399.

Bandura, A. (1986). *Social foundations of thoughts and action.* Englewood Cliffs, NJ: Prentice Hall.

Bandura, A. (1991). Self-efficacy mechanism in psychological activation and health promoting behavior. In J. Madden, IV (Ed.), *Neurobiology of learning, emotion, and affect.* New York: Raven Press.

Barry, M. A., Purser, J., & Hazleman, R. (1993). Effect of energy conservation and joint protection education in rheumatoid arthritis. *British Journal of Rheumatology, 33,* 1171-1174.

Bartholomew, L. K., Koenning, G., Dahlquist, L., & Barron, K. (1994). An educational needs assessment of children with juvenile rheumatoid arthritis. *Arthritis Care and Research, 7,* 136-143.

Basler, H. D. (1993). Group treatment for pain and discomfort. *Patient Education and Counseling, 20,* 167-175.

Bendtsen, P., & Bjurulf, P. (1993). Perceived needs and patient satisfaction in relation to care provided in individuals with rheumatoid arthritis. *Quality Assur. Health Care, 5,* 243-253.

Berry, S. L., Hayford, J. R., & Ross, C. K. (1993). Conceptions of illness by children with juvenile rheumatoid arthritis: A cognitive developmental approach. *Journal of Pediatric Psychology, 1,* 83-97.

Bill-Harvey, D., Rippey, R., & Abeles, M. (1989). Outcome of an osteoarthritis education program for low-literacy patients taught by indigenous instructors. *Patient Educ Couns, 20,* 167-175.

Blalock, S. J., DeVellis, B. M., & DeVellis, R. F. (1992). Psychological well-being among people with recently diagnosed rheumatoid arthritis: Do self-perceptions of abilities make a difference? *Arthritis and Rheumatism, 35,* 1267-1272.

Blalock, S. J., DeVellis, R. F., Giorgino, K. B., & DeVellis, B. M. (1995). Osteoporosis prevention: Using a stage-model approach to examine the predictors of exercise activity and calcium consumption. *Arthritis and Rheumatism, 38,* S311.

Blalock, S. J., DeVellis, B. M., Holt, K., & Hahn, P. M. (1993). Coping with rheumatoid arthritis: Is one problem the same as another? *Health Education Quarterly, 20,* 119-132.

Braden, C. J. (1991). Patterns of change over time in learned response to chronic illness among participants in a systemic lupus erythematosus self-help course. *Arthritis Care and Research, 4,* 158-167.

Braden, C. J., McGlone, K., & Pennington, F. (1993). Specific psychosocial and behavioral outcomes from the Systemic Lupus Erythematosus Self-Help Course. *Health Education Quarterly, 20,* 29-41.

Bradley, L. A., Young, L. D., & Anderson, K. O. (1988). Effects of cognitive-behavior therapy on rheumatoid arthritis pain behavior: One year follow-up. In R. Dubner, G. Gebhart, & M. Bond (Eds.), *Pain research and clinical management, 3 (Proceedings of the 5th World Congress on Pain)*, 310-314. Amsterdam: Elsevier.

Buckelew, S. P., & Parker, J. C. (1989). Coping with arthritis pain: A review of the literature. *Arthritis Care and Research, 2*, 136-145.

Burckhardt, C. S. (1994). Arthritis and musculoskeletal patient education standards. *Arthritis Care and Research, 7*, 1-4.

Calfas, K. J., Kaplan, R. M., & Ingram, R. E. (1992). One-year evaluation of cognitive-behavioral intervention in osteoarthritis. *Arthritis Care and Research, 5*, 202-209.

Carter, W. B. (1990). Health behavior as a rational process: Theory of reasoned action and multiattribute utility theory. In K. Glanz, F. M. Lewis, & B. K. Rimer (Eds.), *Health behavior and health education: Theory, research, and practice*, (pp. 63-91). San Francisco, CA: Jossey-Bass.

Clanton, D., & Petri, M. (1995). Importance of a health educator in SLE: A clinical trial (abstract). *Arthritis and Rheumatism, 8*, S381.

Cohen, J. L., Sauter, S., DeVellis, R. F., & DeVellis, B. M. (1986). Evaluation of arthritis self-management courses led by laypersons and by professionals. *Arthritis and Rheumatism, 29*, 388-393.

Communication Technologies. (1993). *A study of help-seeking among individuals with musculoskeletal conditions in San Mateo County, California.* San Francisco, CA: Communication Technologies.

Connell, K. J., Gecht, M. R., & Grosso, P. C. (1993). Multi-media dissemination of Educize for arthritis [abstract]. *Arthritis Care and Research, 6*, S22.

Cronan, R. A., Groessl, E., & Kaplan, R. M. (1997). The effects of social support and education interventions on health care costs. *Arthritis Care and Research, 10*, 99-110.

Daltroy, L. H. (1992). Arthritis patient education. *Bulletin on the Rheumatic Diseases, 41*, 2-4.

Daltroy, L. H. (1993). Doctor-patient communication in rheumatological disorders. *Baillieres Clinical Rheumatology, 7*, 221-239.

Daltroy, L. H., Katz, J. N., & Liang, M. H. (1992). Doctor-patient communication and adherence to arthritis treatments. *Arthritis Care and Research, 5*, S19.

Daltroy, L. H., & Liang, M. H. (1993). Arthritis education: Opportunities and state of the art. *Health Education Quarterly, 20*, 3-16.

Davis, P., Busch, A. J., & Lowe, J. C. (1994). Evaluation of a rheumatoid arthritis patient education program: Impact on knowledge and self-efficacy. *Patient Educ Couns, 24*, 55-61.

DeVellis, R. F. (1996). A consumer's guide to finding, evaluating, and reporting on measurement instruments. *Arthritis Care and Research, 9*, 239-245.

DeVellis, R. F., & Blalock, S. J. (1993). Psychological and educational interventions to reduce arthritis disability. *Baillieres Clinical Rheumatology, 7*, 397-416.

Dexter, P. A. (1992). Joint exercises in elderly persons with symptomatic osteoarthritis of the hip or knee. *Arthritis Care and Research, 5*, 36-41.

Doyle, M. A., Farrar, V., Ryan, S., & Sisola, S. (1990). An evaluation of PACE (abstract). *Arthritis Care and Research, 3*, S7.

Feinberg, J. (1988). The effect of patient-practitioner interaction on compliance: A review of the literature and application in rheumatoid arthritis. *Patient Educ Couns, 11*, 171-187.

Fung, L. C., & Woo, J. (1995). Arthritis education and support program in Chinese (abstract). *Arthritis and Rheumatism, 38*, S306.

Gale, F. M., Kirk, J. C., & Davis, R. (1994). Patient education and self-management: Randomized study of effects on health status of a mail-delivered program (abstract). *Arthritis and Rheumatism, 37*, S197.

Gecht, M. R., Connell, K. J., Sinacore, J. M., & Prohaska, T. R. (1996). A survey of exercise beliefs and exercise habits among people with arthritis. *Arthritis Care and Research, 9,* 82-88.

Gerber, L., Furst, G., & Shulman, B. (1987). Patient education program to teach energy conservation behaviors to patients with RA: A pilot study. *Archives of Physical Medicince and Rehabilitation, 68,* 442-445.

Giorgino, K. B., Blalock, S. J., & DeVellis, R. F. (1994). Appraisal of and coping with arthritis-related problems in household activities, leisure activities, and pain management. *Arthritis Care and Research, 7,* 20-28.

Goeppinger, J., Arthur, M. W., & Baglioni, A. J. (1989). A reexamination of the effectiveness of self-care education for persons with arthritis. *Arthritis and Rheumatism, 32,* 706-716.

Goeppinger, J., Macnee, C., & Anderson, M. K. (1995). From research to practice: The effects of the jointly sponsored dissemination of an arthritis self-care nursing intervention. *Applied Nursing Research, 8,* 106-113.

Gonzalez, I., Sher, N., & Horton, R. (1995). Charla de lupus: A multipurpose community-based program to provide peer support and education to underserved populations with SLE [abstract]. *Arthritis Care and Research, 8,* S13.

Gonzalez, V. M., Goeppinger, J., & Lorig, K. (1990). Four psychosocial theories and their application to patient education and clinical practice. *Arthritis Care and Research, 3,* 132-143.

Graziano, S., Aronson, S., & Becerra, J. (1995). A multidisciplinary preoperative arthroplasty education program [abstract]. *Arthritis and Rheumatism, 38,* S154.

Green, L. W., & Kreuter, M. W. (1991). *Health education planning: A diagnostic approach.* Mountain View, CA: Mayfield Publishing.

Green, L. W., & Lewis, F. M. (1986). *Measurement and evaluation in health education and health promotion.* Palo Alto, CA: Mayfield Publishing.

Hammond, A. (1994a). Joint protection behavior in patients with rheumatoid arthritis following an education program: A pilot study. *Arthritis Care and Research, 7,* 5-9.

Hammond, A. (1994b). Helping rheumatoid arthritis patients adopt hand protection behaviors [abstract]. *Arthritis Care and Research, 7,* S8.

Hawley, D. (1994). Increasing the dissemination of the Arthritis Self-Management Course: A controlled experiment with interactive television: Follow-up results at 1 year (abstract). *Arthritis Care and Research, 7,* S11.

Hawley, D. (1995). Psycho-educational interventions in the treatment of arthritis. *Baillieres Clinical Rheumatology, 9,* 803-823.

Hirano, P. C., Laurent, D. D., & Lorig, K. (1994). Arthritis patient education studies, 1987-1991: A review of the literature. *Patient Educ Couns, 24,* 9-54.

Holman, H., & Lorig, K. (1987). Patient education in the rheumatic diseases: Pros and cons. *Bulletin on the Rheumatic Diseases, 37,* 36-43.

Israel, B. A., & Schurman, S. J. (1990). Social support, control, and the stress process. In K. Glanz, F. M. Lewis, & B. K. Rimer (Eds.), *Health behavior and health education: Theory, research, and practice,* (pp. 187-215). San Francisco, CA: Jossey-Bass.

Janis, I. L., & Mann, L. (1977). *Decision making.* New York: Free Press.

Janz, N. K., & Becker, M. H. (1984). The health belief model: A decade later. *Health Education Quarterly, 11,* 1-47.

Jensen, G. M., & Lorish, C. D. (1994). Promoting patient cooperation with exercise programs. *Arthritis Care and Research, 7,* 181-189.

Johnson, D. A., Boutaugh, M., & Seikus, P. (1996). Effectiveness of the Arthritis Foundation Fibromyalgia Self-Help Course [abstract]. *Arthritis and Rheumatism.*

Joint Commission on Accreditation of Healthcare Organizations. (1994). *1995 Comprehensive Accreditation Manual for Hospitals.* Oakbrook Terrace, IL: Author.

Kaspar, J. F., Mulley, A. G., & Wennberg, J. E. (1992). Developing shared decision-making programs to improve the quality of health care. *QRB, 18,* 183-190.

Keefe, F. J., Caldwell, D. S., & Williams, D. A. (1990). Pain coping skills in the management of osteoarthritic knee pain II: Follow-up results. *Behavioral Therapy, 21,* 435-444.

Keefe, F. J., & Van Horn, Y. (1993). Cognitive-behavioral treatment of rheumatoid arthritis pain: Maintaining treatment gains. *Arthritis Care and Research, 6,* 213-222.

Kennedy, C., Walker, K., & Linnel, S. (1992). Effect of exercise on social activity and health status in women with RA. *Research Quarterly for Exercise and Sport, 63* (Suppl. A 91).

Kotler, P., & Andreason, A. R. (1987). *Strategic marketing for nonprofit organizations* (3rd ed). Englewood Cliffs, NJ: Prentice Hall.

Kovar, P. A., Allegrante, J. P., & MacKenzie, R. (1992). Supervised fitness walking in patients with osteoarthritis of the knee. *Annals of Internal Medicine, 116,* 529-534.

Lanza, A. F., & Revenson, T. A. (1993). Social support interventions for rheumatoid arthritis: The cart before the horse? *Health Education Quarterly, 20,* 97-118.

Lazarus, R. S., & Folkman, S. (1984). *Stress appraisal and coping.* New York: Springer.

Leventhal, H., Safer, M. A., & Panagis, D. M. (1983). The impact of communications on the self-regulation of health beliefs, decisions, and behavior. *Health Education Quarterly, 10,* 3-29.

Lewis, F. M., & Daltroy, L. H. (1990). How causal explanations influence health behavior: Attribution theory. In K. Glanz, F. M. Lewis, & B. K. Rimer (Eds.), *Health behavior and health education: Theory, research, and practice* (pp. 92-114). San Francisco, CA: Jossey-Bass.

Lindner, K. (1992). Encourage information therapy. *Journal of the American Medical Association, 267,* 2592.

Lindroth, Y., Bauman, A., & Barnes, C. (1989). A controlled evaluation of arthritis education. *British Journal of Rheumatology, 28,* 7-12.

Lindroth, Y., Bauman, A., Brooks, P. M., & Priestly, D. (1995). A 5-year follow-up of a controlled trial of an arthritis education programme. *British Journal of Rheumatology, 34,* 647-652.

Lorig, K. (1993). Self-management of chronic illness: A model for the future. *Generations,* 11-14.

Lorig, K. (1996). *Patient education: A practical approach* (2nd ed.). Thousand Oaks, CA: Sage Publications.

Lorig, K., Cox, T., Cuevas, Y., Kraines, & Britton (1984). Converging and diverging beliefs about arthritis: Caucasian patients, spanish speaking patients, and physicians. *Journal of Rheumatology, 11,* 76-79.

Lorig, K., Feigenbaum, P., & Regan, C. (1987). A comparison of lay-taught and professional-taught arthritis self-management course. *Journal of Rheumatology, 13,* 763-767.

Lorig, K., & Gonzalez, V. (1992). The integration of theory with practice: A 12-year case study. *Health Education Quarterly, 19,* 355-368.

Lorig, K., & Holman, H. (1993). Arthritis self-management studies: A twelve-year review. *Health Education Quarterly, 20,* 17-28.

Lorig, K., Konkol, L., & Gonzalez, V. (1987). Arthritis patient education: A review of the literature. *Patient Education and Counseling, 10,* 207-252.

Lorig, K., Mazonson, P., & Holman, H. (1993). Evidence suggesting that health education for self-management in patients with chronic arthritis has sustained health benefits while reducing health care costs. *Arthritis and Rheumatism, 36,* 439-446.

Lorig, K., & Riggs, G. (1983). *Arthritis patient education: Biblioprofile no. 1.* Arlington, VA: Arthritis Information Clearinghouse.

Lorig, K., Stewart, A., & Ritter, P. (1996). *Outcome measures for health education and other health care interventions.* Thousand Oaks, CA: Sage Publications.

Mahowald, M., Steveken, M., Young, M., & Ytterburg, S. (1988). The Minnesota arthritis training program: Emphasis on self-management, not compliance. *Patient Educ Couns, 11,* 235-241.

Maisiak, R., Austin, J., & Heck, L. (1996). Health outcomes of two telephone interventions for patients with rheumatoid arthritis or osteoarthritis. *Arthritis and Rheumatism 1996, 39*, 1391-1399.

Marcus, B. H., Pinto, B. M., & Simkin, L. R. (1994). Application of theoretical models to exercise behavior among employed women. *American Journal of Health Promotion, 9*, 49-55.

Marlatt, G. A., & George, W. H. (1990). Relapse prevention and the maintenance of optimal health. In S. A. Shumaker & E. B. Schron (Eds.), *The handbook of health behavior change* (pp. 44-63). New York: Springer Publishing.

Mazzuca, S. A. (1994). Economic evaluation of arthritis patient education. *Bulletin on the Rheumatic Diseases, 43*, 6-8.

Mazzuca, S. A., Brandt, K. D., Katz, B. P., Chambers, M., Stewart, K. D., Byrd, D. J., & Hanna, M. (1995). Self-care education improves the health status of inner-city patients with osteoarthritis of the knee [abstract]. *Arthritis and Rheumatism, 38*, S269.

Mazzuca, S. A., Brandt, K. D., Katz, B. P., Chambers, M., Stewart, K. D., Nayee, H., & Byrd, D. J. (1994). Initial effects of self-care education on the quality of life of inner-city patients with OA of the knee [abstract]. *Arthritis Care and Research, 7*, S16.

McGowen, P. (1995). Qualitative evaluation: First nations arthritis self-management program [abstract]. *Arthritis and Rheumatism, 38*, S306.

McGuire, W. (1981). Theoretical foundations of campaigns. In R. E. Rice & W. J. Paisley (Eds.), *Public communication campaigns*, 41-70.

McLeroy, K. R., Bibeau, D., Steckler, A., & Glanz, K. (1988). An ecological perspective on health promotion programs. *Health Education Quarterly, 15*, 351-377.

Minkler, M. (1990). Improving health through community organization. In K. Glanz K, F. M. Lewis, & B. K. Rimer (Eds.), *Health behavior and health education: Theory, research, and practice* (pp. 257-287). San Francisco, CA: Jossey-Bass.

Minor, M. A. (1996). Arthritis and exercise: The times they are a-changin. *Arthritis Care and Research, 9*, 79-81.

Minor, M. A., & Brown, J. D. (1993). Exercise maintenance of persons with arthritis after participation in a class experience. *Health Education Quarterly, 20*, 83-95.

Mullen, P. D., Laville, E. A., Biddle, A. K., & Lorig, K. (1987). Efficacy of psychoeducational interventions on pain, depression, and disability in people with arthritis: A meta-analysis. *Journal of Rheumatology, 14* (Supp. 15), 33-39.

Neuberger, G. B., Smith, K. V., Black, S. O., & Hassanein, R. (1993). Promoting self-care in patients with arthritis. *Arthritis Care and Research, 6*, 141-148.

O'Leary, A., Shoor, S., Lorig, K., & Holman, H. R. (1988). A cognitive-behavioral treatment for rheumatoid arthritis. *Health Psychology, 7*, 527-544.

Orr, P. M. (1990). An educational program for total hip and knee replacement patients as part of a total arthritis center program. *Orthopedic Nursing, 9*, 61-9, 86.

Orr, P. M., & Bratton, G. N. (1992). The effect of an inpatient arthritis rehabilitation program on self-assessed functional ability. *Rehabilitation Nursing, 17*, 306-310.

Parker, J. C., Smarr, K. L., Buckelew, S. P., Stuckey-Ropp, R. C., Hewett, J. E., Johnson, J. C., Wright, G. E., Irvin, W. S., & Walker, S. E. (1995). Effects of stress management on clinical outcomes in rheumatoid arthritis. *Arthritis and Rheumatism, 38*, 1807-1818.

Parker, J. C., Bradley, L. A., DeVellis, R. M., Gerber, L. H., Holman, H. R., & Keefe, F. J. (1993). Biopsychosocial contributions to the management of arthritis disability. *Arthritis and Rheumatism, 36*, 885-888.

Parker, J. C., Iverson, G. L., Smarr, K. L., & Stucky-Ropp, R. C. (1993). Cognitive-behavioral approaches to pain management in rheumatoid arthritis. *Arthritis Care and Research, 6*, 207-212.

Perlman, S. G., Connell, K. J., & Clark, A. (1990). Dance-based aerobic exercise for rheumatoid arthritis. *Arthritis Care and Research, 3*, 29-35.

Pike, R. W. (1989). *Creative training techniques handbook*. Minneapolis, MN: Lakewood Books.

Potts, M. K., & Silverman, S. L. (1990). The importance of aspects of treatment for fibromyalgia: Differences between patient and physician views. *Arthritis Care and Research, 3*, 11-18.

Prochaska, J. O., DeClemente, C. C., & Norcross, J. (1992). In search of how people change: Applications to addictive behaviors. *American Psychologist, 49*, 1102-1114.

Radojevic, V., Nicassio, P. M., & Weisman, M. H. (1992). Behavioral intervention with and without family support for rheumatoid arthritis. *Behavioral Therapy, 23*, 13-30.

Rapoff, M. (1996). Adherence to regimens for rheumatic diseases. In S. Wegener, B. Belza, & E. Gall (Eds.), *Clinical care in the rheumatic diseases*. Atlanta, GA: American College of Rheumatology.

Reisine, S., & Lewis, C. (1993). Impact of a structured computer assisted patient education program in total joint arthroplasty [abstract]. *Arthritis Care and Research, 6*, S3.

Rene, J., Weinberger, M., & Mazzuca, S. A. (1992). Reduction of joint pain in patients with knee osteoarthritis who have received monthly telephone calls from lay personnel and whose medical treatment regimens have remained stable. *Arthritis and Rheumatism, 35*, 511-515.

Rippey, R. M., Bill, D., & Abeles, M. (1987). Computer-based patient education for older persons with osteoarthritis. *Arthritis and Rheumatism, 30*, 932-935.

Roberts, B. L., Matecjyck, M. B., & Anthony, M. (1996). The effects of social support on the relationship of functional limitations and pain to depression. *Arthritis Care and Research, 9*, 67-73.

Robbins, L. (1994). Results from a pilot study of a translated, culturally sensitive SLE self-help course for Latino lupus patients [abstract]. *Arthritis Care and Research, 7*, S6.

Rogers, E. M. (1983). *Diffusion of innovations*. New York: Free Press.

Rosenbaum, M. (1988). Learned resourcefulness, stress and self-regulation. In S.Fisher & J. Reason (Eds.), *Handbook of life stress, cognition and health*. John Wiley and Sons.

Rosenstock, I. M. (1990). The health belief model: Explaining health behavior through expectancies. In K. Glanz, F. M. Lewis, & B. K. Rimer (Eds.), *Health behavior and health education: Theory, research, and practice* (pp. 39-62). San Francisco, CA: Jossey-Bass.

Ruggiero, L. (1994). Accelerating progress toward behavior change: Overview of the transtheoretical model. Vail, CO: Rocky Mountain Cardiovascular Disease Conference.

Seligman, M. (1975). *Helplessness: On depression, development and death*. San Francisco, CA: W. H. Freeman.

Skinner, B. F. (1953). *Science and human behavior*. New York: Free Press.

Sotosky, J. R., McGrory, C. H., Metzger, D. S., & DeHoratius, R. J. (1992). Arthritis problem indicator: preliminary report on a new tool for use in the primary care setting. *Arthritis Care and Research, 5*, 157-162.

Superio-Cabuslay, E., Ward, M. E., & Lorig, K. (1996). Patient education interventions in OA and RA: A meta-analytic comparison with non-steroidal anti-inflammatory drug treatment. *Arthritis Care and Research, 9*, 292-301.

Taal, E., Rasker, J. J., & Wiegman, O. (1996). Patient education and self-management in the rheumatic diseases: A self-efficacy approach. *Arthritis Care and Research, 9*, 229-238.

Taal, E., Riemsma, R. P., & Brus, H. L. (1993). Group education for patients with rheumatoid arthritis. *Patient Education and Counseling, 20*, 177-187.

Tibbles, L., Lewis, C., & Reisine, S. (1992). Computer assisted instruction for preoperative and postoperative patient education in joint replacement surgery. *Computers in Nursing, 10*, 208-212.

Tucker, M., & Kirwan, J. R. (1991). Does patient education in rheumatoid arthritis have therapeutic potential? *Annals of Rheumatic Disease, 50* (Suppl. 3), 422-428.

Weinberger, M., Tierney, W. M., Cowper, P. A., Katz, B. P., & Booker. (1993). Cost-effectiveness of increased telephone contact for patients with osteoarthritis. *Arthritis and Rheumatism, 36*, 243-246.

Weinberger, M., Tierney, W. M., Booher, P. A., & Katz, B. P. (1989). Can the provision of information to patients with osteoarthritis improve functional status? A randomized controlled trial. *Arthritis and Rheumatism, 32*, 1577-1583.

Wetstone, S. L., Sheehan, T. J., & Votaw, R. G. (1985). Evaluation of a computer based education lesson for patients with rheumatoid arthritis. *Journal of Psychology, 12*, 907-912.

Windsor, R. A., Baranowski, T., Clark, N., & Cutter, G. (1994). *Evaluation of health promotion and education programs.* Palo Alto, CA: Mayfield Publishing.

SAMPLE SELF-MANAGEMENT EDUCATION PROTOCOL

LEARNING OBJECTIVES After participation in educational session(s), the client will:	CONTENT	PROCESS AND MATERIALS	DATE COVERED Initials	DATE MET Initials	N/A *
1. State own type of rheumatic condition	• Ask client to name the diagnosis and to describe the causes of the condition and its symptoms • Reinforce understanding and correct any misconceptions • Provide written and/or audiovisual information on diagnosis • Provide reassurance and/or refer to support resources as needed for maladaptive responses to the diagnosis	1:1 discussion Supplementary print, AV, or computer-based materials on condition Referral as needed			
2. Express concerns and problems relevant to arthritis	• Encourage client to bring list • Ask about concerns and legitimize psychosocial issues • Identify which concerns are highest priority • Refer to other caregivers as needed	1:1 or peer group discussion			
3. Identify treatment goals	• Ask client to state his/her treatment goals (e.g., what symptom, activity does client want most to impact?) • Brainstorm/describe multiple causes of symptoms • Explain purpose, risks, costs, and benefits of various treatment options. Frame recommendations as ways to achieve client goals and explain how NOT doing the behavior will negatively affect client goals • Assess and clarify any unrealistic expectations about treatment options • Assist client in prioritizing goals and selecting mutually agreed-upon treatment option(s)	1:1 or peer group brainstorm and discussion; written or AV aids on symptoms and treatment options, e.g., Arthritis Foundation booklets: *Managing Your Pain, Managing Your Fatigue, Managing Your Stress, Managing Your Activities*			

4. State intention to perform specific behavior(s) relevant to goals	• Assess stage of change/readiness to perform behavior • Use persuasion and/or positive role models to encourage behavior change • Build commitment to do behavior through Pros-Cons Worksheet • Tailor treatment recommendation to fit client needs, lifestyle and resources • Simplify and/or negotiate changes in regimen if client is uncommitted	1:1 or peer group discussion			
5. Recall specific treatment recommendation	• State specific recommendation, including purpose, dosage/amount/intensity, frequency and duration, when not to do behavior, common risks/side effects and how to handle these, how to judge treatment efficacy, when to return for follow-up • Ask client to summarize what was heard • Provide written materials	1:1 discussion; client recall; written materials			
6. State confidence in ability to do behavior regularly	• Break behavior down into small steps • Demonstrate behavior; have client return demonstration; provide corrective feedback; schedule return visits to allow for repeat practice opportunities; encourage at-home practice • Guide client in developing written contract with short-term goals, specifying what, how much, when, and how often he or she will do behavior • Ask level of confidence in ability to achieve short-term goal; if not confident, assist client in adapting goal and problem-solve barriers • Provide feedback upon return visit: ask client what he or she did at home and positive and negative results; examine any completed diaries/journals; praise progress	Demonstration; guided practice/return demonstration; short-term goal-setting and contracting; feedback; problem-solving			
7. Maintain behavior on regular basis	• Ask client to state factors affecting behavior (potential problems/barriers) • Discuss other potential barriers which client may not have anticipated (e.g., costs, inconvenience, time, lack of support from family) • Assist client in identifying possible	1:1 or peer group discussion; problem-solving discussion; decision making practice; discussion; demonstration, practice of cognitive-behavioral			

	solutions for barriers; teach problem-solving process
	• Provide decision rules for modifying treatment recommendations; practice with "What if" situations to assess understanding
	• Train and/or refer for training in cognitive-behavioral skills relevant to maintaining the behavior:
	   – self-talk
	   – environmental cueing/building behavior into daily routine
	   – self-monitoring
	   – establishing positive consequences/rewards
	• Ask about missed treatments; problem solve or change treatment if needed
		skills; referral to other professionals, self-help classes, CBT programs			

8. State that has adequate level of support to achieve desired goals	• Ask client to identify individuals and groups that may help or hinder behavioral change • Ask client to identify what type of support is needed • Role-play how to ask for needed help • Problem-solve how to deal with negative support • Train and/or refer for training in communication skills • Invite significant others to participate in clinical visit/educational sessions • Involve client with positive role models • Refer to support groups and peer-led self-management classes • Provide supportive telephone calls • Increase level of supervision if necessary	1:1 or peer group discussion; role-play; problem-solving discussion; communication skills demonstration and practice; support groups; telephone counseling			
9. State that behavioral relapses/setbacks are not failures.	• Explain that relapses are temporary setbacks that are often inevitable and should be viewed as valuable learning opportunities and not as failures or as reasons to stop the behavior • Ask the client to predict possible risk situations or causes for relapse • Assist client in developing contingency plan	1:1 or peer group brainstorm and discussion			

Appendix 1: Sample Self-Management Education Protocol (continued)

10. Utilize health care system and community resources appropriately	• Describe client's role and responsibilities as active member of health care team • Describe role and responsibilities of health professionals • Describe when and how to access members of health care team and the health care system • Refer to other health care team members and community resources as appropriate • Train and/or refer for assertiveness skills training	1:1 or peer group discussion; assertiveness training; Arthritis Foundation booklets: *Managing Your Health Care; Services of the Arthritis Foundation;* community resource directory			
11. Demonstrate ability to make informed decision about unproven remedies	• Define unproven remedies • List five questions for clients to ask when evaluating an unproven remedy or research report • Roleplay how to deal with significant other who is pushing an unproven remedy	1:1 or peer group discussion; roleplay; Arthritis Foundation booklet: *Unproven Remedies*			

* Not applicable to client

Appendix 1: Sample Self-Management Education Protocol (continued)

PAIN MANAGEMENT INTERVENTIONS FOR PATIENTS WITH RHEUMATIC DISEASES

Laurence A. Bradley, PhD

Patients with rheumatic diseases view pain as a major challenge and as one of the most important consequences of their illnesses (Bradley, 1996). Indeed, it has been found that pain is more important than physical or psychological disability in explaining medication usage among patients with rheumatoid arthritis (RA)(Kazis, Meenan, & Anderson, 1983). Pain is also a significant predictor of patient and physician assessments of the patients' general health status as well as future levels of pain and disability (Kazis et al., 1983). Moreover, despite advances in the medical management of the rheumatic diseases, patients rarely experience complete pain relief (Bradley, 1996).

Psychological and social variables influence patients' pain experiences (Bradley, 1994). Thus, management of pain may be enhanced if treatment providers recognize these psychosocial factors and can use psychological interventions that effectively reduce pain in patients with rheumatic disease. This chapter will review the relationships that have been established between psychosocial factors and pain and describe effective psychological and behavioral methods for pain management.

PSYCHOSOCIAL FACTORS AND PAIN

DEPRESSION AND ANXIETY

Depression and anxiety are negative psychological states frequently found in patients with rheumatic disease. For example, the frequency with which depression and anxiety disorders are diagnosed among RA patients ranges from 14% to 42% (Ahles, Khan, Yunus, et al., 1991; Blalock, DeVellis, Brown, et al., 1994; Frank, Beck, Parker, et al., 1988). Similarly, the frequency of lifetime diagnoses of major depression and anxiety disorders in patients with the fibromyalgia syndrome (FMS) ranges from 26% to 71% (Aaron et al., 1996; Hudson, Goldenberg, Pope, Keck, & Schlesinger, 1992; Hudson, Hudson, Pliner, Goldenberg, & Pope, 1985). Clinically significant levels of depression are found in 14% to 23% of patients with osteoarthritis (OA) (Dexter & Brandt, 1994); little is known regarding the frequency of anxiety disorders in these patients. Although there are large differences in the frequency of depression and anxiety among patients with various rheumatic diseases, all of the frequency rates noted above are substantially greater than the population base rates for these psychological disorders (Frank & Hagglund, 1996).

Depression and anxiety are associated with several other clinical variables in patients with rheumatic disease. For example, patients with RA who experience depression, compared to those who are not depressed, report higher levels of pain, greater numbers of painful joints, poorer functional ability, and more days spent in bed (Katz & Yelin, 1993). Depression also is associated with higher levels of pain and functional disability in patients with OA and FMS (Bradley & Alarcón, 1996; Summers, Haley, Reveille, & Alarcón, 1988). Moreover, psychological distress is associated with high levels of medical service use among patients with RA and FMS. For example, it has been found that over a 5-year period, RA patients with elevated scores on a geriatric depression scale reported significantly more physician visits and hospitalizations related to their disease than patients whose depression scores were within normal limits (Katz & Yelin, 1993). Both cross-sectional and longitudinal studies of persons with FMS have revealed that the frequency of lifetime psychiatric diagnoses is strongly associated with seeking medical treatment for their pain and other symptoms (Aaron et al., 1996; Aaron et al., in press). In addition, FMS patients who report that psychological trauma preceded or coincided with the onset of their pain more frequently obtain medical consultations than patients without trauma (Aaron et al., 1997). These findings suggest that early identification and effective treatment of psychological distress might reduce patients' health care costs as well as improve overall health.

Some effort has been devoted to identifying the predictors of depression and anxiety in patients with rheumatic disease. Most of this work has been performed using patients with RA. There is evidence that measures of disease activity such as the number of tender or painful joints are associated with anxiety and depression (Parker, Smarr, Anderson, et al., 1992; Parker, Smarr, Walker, et al., 1991). However, pain severity, age, neuroticism, lack of satisfaction with current lifestyle, and degree of functional impairment are better predictors of psychological distress than are joint counts and other measures of disease activity (Affleck, Tennen, Urrows, et al., 1992; Frank et al., 1988; Hawley & Wolfe, 1988). It has been suggested that disease activity might be a more powerful predictor of depression or anxiety if patients were studied intensively over short periods. This hypothesis was tested in a study that required RA patients to make daily multiple ratings of mood status over 75 consecutive days (Affleck, Tennen, Pfeiffer, et al., 1992). Consistent with the findings noted above, disease activity did not predict daily mood. Instead, the most powerful predictors of daily mood states were age, neuroticism, and chronic pain.

STRESS

Rheumatologic disorders produce numerous stressors in addition to psychological distress that may influence pain. These stressors include activity limitations and functional impairments in the home and workplace as well as financial hardships produced by loss of income and high health care costs (Clarke et al., 1993; Felts & Yelin, 1989; Liang, Larson, Thompson, et al., 1984; Pincus, Mitchell, & Burkhauser, 1989; Yelin, 1992). Another important source of stress is changes in patients' social relationships and in their appearance. It has been found, for example, that between 43% and 52% of patients with RA report dysfunction in the areas of social interaction, communication with others, and emotional behavior (Deyo, Inui, Leininger, et al., 1982). In addition, two independent studies have reported that about 60% of patients with RA experience at least one major psychosocial change related to family functioning such as increased arguments with spouses, changes in the health of family members, and sexual dysfunction (Liang, Rogers, Larson, et al., 1984; Yelin, Feshbach, Meenan, et al., 1979).

Most of the research concerning stress and pain has been performed with patients with RA. It has been found that these persons frequently report that stress tends to precede flare-ups in disease activity (Affleck et al., 1987). Indeed, there is evidence that the hypothalamus and other neural structures involved in stress responses are also involved in the inflammatory process in RA (Chikanza, Petrou, Kingsley, et al., 1992). Abnormal function of the hypothalamic-pituitary-adrenal axis also may be involved in abnormal pain perception among patients with FMS (Crofford et al., 1992). Finally, there is evidence that daily stressors and mood are both involved in immune system responses and pain among patients with RA. It has been shown that daily stresses are associated with mood disturbances that, in turn, are related to decreases in soluble interleukin-2 receptor levels and increases in joint pain (Harrington, Affleck, Urrows, et al., 1993).

SLEEP DISTURBANCE

High frequencies of disturbances have been documented in patients with a variety of rheumatologic disorders including RA, OA, and Sjögren's syndrome (Wegener, 1996). However, sleep disturbance is most consistently found among patients with FMS. These patients frequently show a specific anomaly characterized by intrusion of alpha waves during non-REM sleep (Branco, Atalaia, & Paiva, 1994). This "alpha-delta" sleep anomaly, which is associated with local tenderness, pain, and stiffness in patients with FMS, may be induced by emotionally arousing events (Moldofsky, 1986). It also has been demonstrated in healthy persons that noise-induced disruption of Stage 4 non-REM sleep directly leads to the appearance of the alpha-delta sleep anomaly as well as to onset of musculoskeletal pain and negative mood changes (Moldofsky & Scarisbrick, 1976). A return to undisturbed sleep in these healthy persons is followed by normalized sleep physiology and alleviation of symptoms. However, patients with FMS who display alpha-delta sleep anomaly do not report greater symptom severity than those without the anomaly. Moreover, the anomaly does not respond to a low-dosage (25 mg) nightly regimen of amitriptyline (Carette, Oakson, Guimont, & Steriade, 1995). Thus, disturbed sleep plays a role in symptom production and amplification in FMS, but the precise mechanism has not yet been identified.

BELIEFS AND COPING STRATEGIES

There is consistent evidence that patients' beliefs about their abilities to control or influence their symptoms are associated with pain. Two beliefs that have been studied extensively in patients with rheumatologic disorders are learned helplessness and self-efficacy. These beliefs also may influence patients' abilities to use various coping strategies to reduce or adapt to their pain and other symptoms.

LEARNED HELPLESSNESS

This term refers to a phenomenon characterized by emotional, motivational, and cognitive deficits in adaptive coping with stressful situations. The deficits are produced by the belief that no viable solutions are available to eliminate or reduce the stress (Garber & Seligman, 1980). It has been hypothesized that learned helplessness may underlie a portion of the psychological distress and pain experienced by patients with RA and other rheumatologic disorders (Bradley, 1985). Many patients may develop the belief that their diseases are beyond their effective control because they tend to be characterized by causes that are not well understood, chronic and unpredictable courses, and variable responses to medical treatments. These patients tend to perceive that, regardless of their actions, they will not be able to substantially reduce the pain or other symptoms associated with their conditions. This perception of uncontrollability may cause patients to experience depression and anxiety (i.e., emotional deficits) that, in turn, may lead to increased pain and reduced attempts either to engage in activities of daily living (i.e., motivational deficits) or to develop new means of adapting to their pain, disabilities, and distress (i.e., cognitive deficits). These deficits may be particularly profound and resistant to change among patients who view the consequences of their conditions as relatively stable over time and global in nature (i.e., adversely affecting numerous vocational, recreational, social, and marital or sexual activities).

The importance of helplessness beliefs in adaptation to rheumatologic disorders has been demonstrated in many studies (Bradley, 1993). For example, high levels of helplessness are associated with high levels of pain, depression, and functional disability among patients with RA both at baseline and over follow-up periods of up to 3 years (Lorish, Abraham, Austin, Bradley, & Alacón, 1991; Smith, Peck, & Ward, 1990). These studies have led many health professionals to believe that perception of control over pain and other symptoms (low helplessness) is desirable for patients with rheumatologic illnesses. It should be noted, however, that patients with RA who believe they can control their symptoms tend to suffer psychological distress in response to flares in disease activity and pain unless they are able cognitively to restructure their pain experiences (Tennen, Affleck, Urrows, et al., 1992). One example of this cognitive restructuring would be the adoption of the belief that pain has allowed one to appreciate the preciousness of life. These findings have led psychological therapists to focus upon enhancing both perceptions of control and coping with flare-induced losses of control among patients with rheumatologic disorders (Keefe & Van Horn, 1993). This topic will be addressed in greater detail in the section on psychological and behavioral therapies for pain management.

SELF-EFFICACY

This construct is closely related to belief in one's level of symptom control or help-lessness. However, in contrast to perceptions of control over symptoms, self-efficacy (SE) represents a belief that one can perform specific behaviors to achieve specific health-relat-ed goals. Thus, whereas control tends to represent a relatively consistent belief regarding a wide array of symptoms, an individual may vary with respect to SE beliefs concerning dif-ferent behaviors. An individual with RA, for example, may have high SE for pacing daily activities to reduce pain and fatigue but also may have low SE for performing water-based exercise to improve physical function (Lorig, Chastain, Ung, et al., 1989).

The importance of SE is that it tends to predict pain and other dimensions of health status if individuals believe that the relevant behaviors will lead to improved health (Bradley, 1994). Indeed, it has been reported that high SE for pain is correlated with low frequencies of observable displays of pain behavior among patients with RA and FMS even after controlling for demographic factors and disease activity (Buckelew et al., 1994; Buescher et al., 1991). Given these findings, psychological and behavioral interventions for patients with rheumatologic disorders emphasize the development of high levels of SE for pain through rehearsal of adaptive behaviors in the home, social, and work envi-ronments. Many of these adaptive behaviors may be considered as coping strategies.

COPING STRATEGIES

Coping is defined as behavior performed to manage environmental and internal demands (i.e., stressors and conflicts among them) that tax or exceed a person's resources (Bradley, 1994). The coping process actually consists of several stages. These are (a) appraising the threat associated with a particular stressor, (b) performing the adaptive behaviors or coping strategies that may control the effects of the stressor, and (c) evalu-ating the outcomes produced by the behavior and, if necessary, performing alternative coping responses. It should be noted that coping strategies may be categorized as either direct action or palliative strategies (Burish & Bradley, 1983). Direct action strategies consist of behaviors that contribute to the removal of the stressor whereas palliative strategies are responses that diminish the negative impact of the stressor. For example, a patient with RA who experiences a flare in disease activity may seek treatment from her physician (direct action) and use relaxation or other distractors (palliative) to control the impact of pain associated with the flare.

Numerous studies have been performed on the coping responses of patients with rheumatologic disorders. Although a variety of instruments has been used to evaluate coping, there has been remarkable consistency in the findings reported across investiga-tions and across disorders. For example, it has been shown repeatedly that passive coping strategies, such as catastrophizing (e.g., believing that no coping strategy will effectively control pain and other symptoms) and escapist fantasies (e.g., hoping that pain will get better someday) are correlated with high levels of pain (Brown & Nicassio, 1987; Martin et al., 1996) and psychological distress (Keefe, Brown, Wallston, et al., 1989; Martin et al., 1996) in patients with RA, OA, and FMS. Conversely, psychological adjustment and relatively low levels of pain tend to be associated with strategies such as attempts to derive personal meaning from the illness experience, seeking information about arthritis, focusing on positive thoughts during pain episodes, and infrequent use of catastrophizing (e.g., Affleck, Urrows, Tennen, et al., 1992).

PSYCHOLOGICAL AND BEHAVIORAL INTERVENTIONS FOR PAIN MANAGEMENT

Given the relationships that have been documented between pain and patient beliefs and coping strategies, several psychological and behavioral interventions have been developed to alter patients' perceptions of control, SE beliefs, and coping strategies and thereby improve pain and other health status variables. The following section reviews these interventions and presents a detailed examination of one intervention that may be adapted for use by clinicians.

All of the psychological and behavioral interventions reviewed below tend to share similar treatment components. These include education, training in relaxation and other coping skills, and rehearsal of these newly learned skills in home and work environments. The effects of nearly all of the interventions have been assessed relative to those produced by waiting-list or attention-placebo control conditions administered while patients are receiving conventional medical therapies from their physicians. Thus, the effects produced by these interventions represent improvements attained by patients in addition to those produced by physician-prescribed therapies. The following discussion examines the interventions developed for patients with RA, OA, and FMS.

RHEUMATOID ARTHRITIS

One of the first psychological therapies was a biofeedback-assisted group therapy intervention that trained patients with RA and their family members in relaxation and behavioral coping skills (Bradley et al., 1987). Relative to a credible attention-placebo (i.e., social support group meetings) and no adjunct treatment conditions, the intervention produced significant reductions in patients' displays of pain behavior (e.g., guarded movement during walking) and number of painful or tender joints. Indeed, the joint count reduction produced by this relaxation-based therapy has been replicated by several other investigators (e.g., O'Leary, Shoor, Lorig, et al., 1988). Moreover, during a 1-year follow-up period, patients who received the intervention reported significantly lower usage of outpatient health care services and incurred lower medical service costs than patients in the other two study conditions (Young, Bradley, & Turner, 1995). The former patient group also reported significantly lower pain intensity and depression than patients who received no adjunct treatment. However, posttreatment reductions in pain behavior and joint counts produced by the group therapy intervention were not maintained at 1-year follow-up.

Unpublished post hoc analyses of the data from this study suggested that treatment gains on all variables, including pain behavior and joint counts, were best maintained at follow-up by patients who reported good compliance with at least two of the major treatment components (i.e., relaxation, biofeedback, practice of other behavioral and cognitive coping skills). Similar observations by other investigators have led to increased interest in developing methods to enhance maintenance of patient improvement after formal treatment has been terminated. The most detailed model for enhancing outcome maintenance has been termed *relapse prevention* (Keefe & Van Horn, 1993). This model suggests that relapse tends to occur when patients' symptoms increase in intensity and their perceptions of symptom control are diminished. Indeed, these circumstances can be expected to occur relatively often given the unpredictable courses of most of the rheumatologic diseases. At these times, patients are likely to experience psychological distress, reduce their efforts to cope with their symptoms, and thus experience a relapse in pain, emotional distress, and functional ability. It is suggested, then, that psychological and behavioral interventions might produce better long-term improvements if they include components designed to help patients respond effectively to potential relapse situations. Specifically, all phases of treatment should include (a) identification of high-risk situations that are likely to tax coping resources, (b) identification of the early signs of relapse, such as increases in pain or depression, (c) rehearsal of cognitive and behavioral skills for coping with these early relapse signs, and (d) provision of self-rewards for effective performance of coping responses to potential relapse. Indeed, a recent study of a stress management intervention that incorporated the relapse prevention model showed that, relative to attention-placebo and no adjunct treatment conditions, stress management produced significant improvements in RA patients' pain ratings, reports of helplessness, and coping strategy usage that persisted for 15 months following treatment (Parker, Smarr, Buckelew, et al., 1995).

OSTEOARTHRITIS

Two investigations have examined the effects of a coping skills training intervention on patients with OA of the knee (Keefe et al., 1990a, b). This training program, relative to arthritis education without adjunct treatment, produced significant reductions in patients' ratings of pain and psychological disability that generally were maintained at 6 month follow-up. The coping skills intervention also produced significant improvements in patients' reports of physical disability from posttreatment to follow-up.

The Arthritis Self-Management Program (ASMP) is a standardized intervention designed to enhance patients' perceptions of SE for pain, disability, and other arthritis symptoms. It has been evaluated primarily with large groups of patients with OA and RA. The most recent study of the effectiveness of the ASMP with these patients showed that it produced significant increases in SE for pain and other symptoms as well as significant reductions in pain ratings and arthritis-related physician visits that persisted up to 4 years after treatment (Lorig, Mazonson, & Holman, 1993).

Provision of counseling by telephone represents a new, inexpensive method for improving patients' health status. The first of these interventions, developed for patients with OA, reviewed educational information, medications, and clinical problems identified by the patients. Moreover, it taught them strategies for increasing their involvement in their encounters with their physicians (Weinberger, Tierney, Cowper, Katz, & Booher, 1993). The intervention produced significant reductions in patients' reports of pain and functional ability and did not substantially increase their health care costs.

Recently, telephone-based counseling interventions have been tested with patients with RA and systemic lupus erythematosus (Maisiak, Austin, West, & Heck, 1996). However, the results of these interventions have not been uniformly positive. It remains to be determined whether the promising initial results of telephone-based counseling can be consistently reproduced in OA patients as well as in patients with other rheumatologic diseases.

FIBROMYALGIA

The use of psychological and behavioral interventions for patients with fibromyalgia (FM) is a relatively recent development. Two studies have shown that these interventions produce significant improvements in patient reports of pain, psychological distress, and psychological disability (Goldenberg, Kaplan, Nadeau, et al., 1994; Nielson, Walker, & McCain, 1992). An additional study found that education regarding stress management, behavior change, and aerobic fitness altered the frequency of tender point counts from abnormal (> 11) to normal (< 11) in 70% of the patients at posttreatment (Bennett et al., 1996). It also produced significant reductions in patient reports of pain, physical disability, psychological distress, and catastrophizing. Although none of these investigations used attention-placebo comparison groups to control for the nonspecific effects of treatment, the effects of one intervention were maintained for 1 year following treatment (Neilson et al., 1992). It is unlikely, then, that the positive effects of the intervention were due solely to nonspecific or placebo factors.

One recent investigation examined the effects of an intervention designed to enhance perceptions of SE among patients with FMS relative to those produced by an attention placebo and a waiting-list control condition (Goosens et al., 1996; Vlaeyen et al., 1996). The SE intervention produced no significant effects on patient ratings of pain and depression or their pain behavior at either posttreatment or 1-year follow-up. Moreover, the direct medical costs of the patients who received the SE intervention showed a significant increase during follow-up relative to those of patients who received the attention placebo. Note, however, that the SE intervention patients showed very poor compliance with the instructions to practice their newly learned skills outside of the treatment setting. Thus, one must conclude that the efficacy of psychological and behavioral interventions for FMS patients has not yet been adequately assessed.

SUMMARY

There is consistent evidence that psychological and behavioral interventions produce significant improvements in ratings of pain and other dimensions of health status among patients with RA and OA. The effects of these therapies for patients with FMS appear to be promising, but a rigorous, well-executed controlled trial has not yet been performed with this patient population.

Although the evidence reviewed above is encouraging, only a few resources are available to clinicians who wish to incorporate psychological and behavioral principles in their work with patients with rheumatologic illnesses (e.g., Gatchel & Turk, 1996). Therefore, the following section describes in detail the psychological, relaxation-based intervention that was shown by this author and colleagues to be effective for patients with RA (Bradley et al., 1987).

TREATMENT COMPONENTS OF A PSYCHOLOGICAL INTERVENTION FOR PATIENTS WITH RHEUMATOID ARTHRITIS

This intervention has been carefully described in a previously published manual for pain clinicians (Bradley, 1996). It should be noted that the intervention, which is outlined in Table 1, included four components typically found in psychological and behavioral therapies for pain. These are (a) education, (b) skills acquisition, (c) cognitive and behavioral rehearsal, and (d) generalization and maintenance. The intervention also required spouses or significant others to meet in a series of ten 90-minute small-group sessions with the patients and the therapist. Spouse participation is not common to all interventions; however, it has been shown that the participation of spouses tends to enhance treatment outcomes among patients with RA (Radojevic, Nicassio, & Weisman, 1992).

EDUCATION

The primary purposes of the educational component are to present a credible rationale for the treatment intervention, to elicit the active collaboration of patients and spouses with the therapist, and to help patients and spouses begin to alter negative perceptions regarding their abilities to manage the pain and other consequences of RA. It is especially important during the educational component to encourage patients and spouses to believe that they can learn the skills necessary to cope better with pain and other illness-related problems. Therefore, we devoted the first week's treatment session to a discussion of the medical and psychosocial consequences that are often associated with RA.

Throughout this discussion, we attempted to help patients and spouses recognize that unpredictable variations in pain and other symptoms of RA have negative effects on their psychological status, as well as on their perceived abilities to control their painful symptoms and function effectively. These negative consequences, in turn, may lead patients to fail to adhere to their prescribed medication or exercise regimens and thus may further exacerbate disease activity and pain. We then described the major components of the psychological intervention to the patients and spouses and explained how the components of the intervention were designed to help them maintain better control of their pain, psychological reactions, and health-related behavior.

One important component of the intervention is relaxation training. We explained that nearly all persons can learn to induce a relaxed state. We also explained that we ulti-

A PAIN MANAGEMENT INTERVENTION FOR PATIENTS WITH RA

EDUCATION

WEEK 1. EDUCATION AND RATIONALE
 A. Discuss the medical and psychosocial consequences of RA.
 B. Provide a credible rationale for use of the intervention for pain and psychological distress.

WEEK 2. DISCUSSION OF PATIENTS' AND SPOUSES' BEHAVIORS
 A. Develop a consensus that patients may learn to control their pain better and that spouses may learn to respond appropriately to patients' displays of high and low pain levels.
 B. Review the components of the intervention and discuss how this intervention may help patients and spouses achieve their pain control goals.

SKILLS ACQUISITION: COGNITIVE AND BEHAVIORAL REHEARSAL

WEEK 3. FIRST THERMAL BIOFEEDBACK TRAINING SESSION
 A. Identify target joint or muscle, and provide visual and auditory feedback regarding increases in skin surface temperature at the target.
 B. Give instruction in use of home thermal biofeedback unit and in daily practice of temperature control skills.

WEEK 4. FIRST RELAXATION TRAINING SESSION
 A. Provide progressive muscle relaxation training in group session.
 B. Give instruction in deep breathing and relaxation imagery.
 C. Provide relaxation audiocassettes and instructions for home practice of relaxation by patients and spouses.

WEEK 5. SECOND THERMAL BIOFEEDBACK TRAINING SESSION
 A. Continue practice of skin surface temperature control skills in the clinic and home environments.

WEEK 6. SECOND RELAXATION TRAINING SESSION
 A. Instruct patients and spouses to provide progress reports on successes and difficulties in using relaxation, imagery, and biofeedback skills.
 B. Instruct group members to provide reinforcements for success and to assist one another in solving problems related to usage of their skills.
 C. Provide instruction in relaxation and deep breathing, as well as relaxation and pain relief imagery.
 D. Assist patients and spouses in identifying arthritis-related problems, behavioral goals and strategies, and rewards for patients' use of their strategies.

WEEK 7. THIRD THERMAL BIOFEEDBACK TRAINING SESSION
    A.   Continue practice of skin surface temperature control skills in the clinic and home environments.
    B.   Decrease visual and auditory feedback in the clinic environment.

WEEK 8. RELAXATION AND BEHAVIORAL GOAL SETTING
    A.   Instruct patients and spouses to provide progress reports on successes and difficulties in using relaxation, imagery, biofeedback, and behavioral goal-setting skills.
    B.   Instruct patients to place relaxation cues in their home and work environments.
    C.   Assist patients and spouses in modifying behavioral goals and strategies, as well as rewards for patients' use of their strategies.

WEEK 9. FOURTH THERMAL BIOFEEDBACK TRAINING SESSION
    A.   Continue practice of skin surface temperature control skills in the clinic and home environments.
    B.   Decrease visual and auditory feedback in the clinic environment.

WEEK 10. RELAXATION AND BEHAVIORAL GOAL SETTING
    A.   Instruct patients and spouses to provide progress reports on successes and difficulties in using relaxation, imagery, biofeedback, and behavioral goal-setting skills.
    B.   Assist patients and spouses in modifying behavioral goals and strategies, as well as rewards for patients' use of their strategies.
    C.   Instruct patients and spouses to identify additional arthritis-related problems, behavioral goals and strategies, and rewards for patients' use of their strategies.

WEEK 11. RELAXATION AND BEHAVIORAL GOAL SETTING
    A.   Instruct patients and spouses to provide progress reports on successes and difficulties in using relaxation, imagery, biofeedback, and behavioral goal-setting skills.
    B.   Assist patients and spouses in modifying behavioral goals and strategies, as well as rewards for patients' use of their strategies.

WEEK 12. RELAXATION AND BEHAVIORAL GOAL SETTING
    A.   Instruct patients and spouses to provide progress reports on successes and difficulties in using relaxation, imagery, biofeedback, and behavioral goal-setting skills.
    B.   Assist patients and spouses in modifying behavioral goals and strategies, as well as rewards for patients' use of their strategies.
    C.   Instruct patients and spouses to identify additional arthritis-related problems, behavioral goals and strategies, and rewards for patients' use of their strategies.
    D.   Instruct patients to remove relaxation cues from their home and work environments.

WEEK 13. FIFTH THERMAL BIOFEEDBACK TRAINING SESSION
    A.   Continue practice of skin surface temperature control skills in the clinic and home environments.
    B.   Eliminate visual and auditory biofeedback in the clinic environment.

Table 1: A Pain Management Intervention for Patients with RA (continued)

GENERALIZATION AND MAINTENANCE

WEEK 14. PROGRESS REPORTS AND PLANNING FOR TREATMENT TERMINATION

    A.   Instruct patients and spouses to provide progress reports on successes and difficulties in using relaxation, imagery, biofeedback, and behavioral goal-setting skills.

    B.   Assist patients and spouses in modifying behavioral goals and strategies, as well as rewards for patients' use of their strategies.

    C.   Ask patients and spouses to identify arthritis-related problems they expect to encounter after treatment is completed, and to describe behavioral goals and strategies as well as rewards that may help them cope with these problems.

WEEK 15. PROGRESS REPORTS AND PLANNING FOR TREATMENT TERMINATION

    A.   Instruct patients and spouses to provide progress reports on successes and difficulties in using relaxation, imagery, biofeedback, and behavioral goal-setting skills.

    B.   Assist patients and spouses in modifying behavioral goals and strategies, as well as rewards for patients' use of their strategies.

    C.   Ask patients and spouses to identify arthritis-related problems they expect to encounter after treatment is completed, and to describe behavioral goals and strategies as well as rewards that may help them cope with these problems.

    D.   Make plans to telephone each patient once a month during the next 6 months to provide assistance in maintaining relaxation, imagery, biofeedback, and behavioral goal-setting skills.

Table 1: A Pain Management Intervention for Patients with RA (continued). Source: Adapted from Bradley, 1996.

mately wished to teach the patients and spouses to use "short cuts" such as deep breathing and mental imagery to induce a relaxed state quickly during periods of high stress or pain. This will allow them to reduce their stress and pain in many circumstances and thus cope in an adaptive manner with these unpleasant states.

We devoted the beginning of the second week's treatment session to a brief review of the issues noted above. We especially encouraged the patients and spouses to ask questions that had occurred to them in discussing the previous week's session. This allowed us to correct any misperceptions about RA or the intervention and to engage the participants further in the treatment. We then led an intensive discussion of the spouses' reactions to the patients' behavioral displays of pain. The first purpose of this discussion was to elicit the active participation of the spouses in the intervention, since many spouses tend to believe that they play a minor role in the medical treatment of the patients' conditions. Moreover, we used this discussion to begin a process of reconceptualization about the role of spouse-patient interactions in the patients' pain experiences. We used experiences reported by spouses to demonstrate that their reactions to the patients' pain may reinforce either adaptive or maladaptive coping responses. The discussion allowed us to lead the participants to agree that the major treatment goals should be to help patients learn to control their pain better, and to help both the patients and spouses learn methods that they can use together to cope better with pain and the other medical and psychosocial problems associated with RA. We also conveyed to the participants that achieving these goals would help them to live more fulfilling and active lives within the limitations imposed by the disease.

SKILLS ACQUISITION: COGNITIVE AND BEHAVIORAL REHEARSAL

The purpose of the skills acquisition component is to help patients and spouses engage actively in the process of learning new behaviors and cognitions that will help them better manage pain and other RA-related problems. The purpose of the rehearsal component is to help patients and spouses practice and consolidate new pain management behaviors and cognitions and to apply these effectively in their home and work environments.

Table 1 shows that these components were implemented in group and individual sessions conducted from the 3rd through the 13th weeks' sessions. With regard to skills acquisition, we first devoted attention to helping patients learn self-regulation techniques that may enable them to reduce their pain. We dedicated the 3rd and 4th weeks' treatment sessions to training in thermal biofeedback and progressive muscle relaxation. During the 3rd week, patients met individually with one of the treatment team members for the first of five thermal biofeedback training sessions. Each patient began the initial biofeedback session by identifying a joint or muscle for which he or she wished to develop improved pain control. The patient then engaged in a 60-minute training protocol in which he or she received auditory and visual feedback regarding increases in skin surface temperature at the target joint or muscle. We implemented cognitive and behavioral rehearsal of the biofeedback instruction in two ways. First, at the end of the initial training session, the patient learned to operate a small battery-powered biofeedback unit for home practice that provided visual feedback concerning changes in skin surface temperature. We instructed the patient to practice with the home biofeedback unit at least once each day. In addition, all patients engaged in additional individualized thermal biofeedback training in 60-minute sessions at the 5th, 7th, 9th, and 13th weeks. During the course of these sessions, we gradually decreased the frequency of feedback to help patients learn to control skin temperature in the absence of visual or auditory cues outside of the laboratory.

We conducted the initial relaxation training session at the 4th week in a group meeting with patients and spouses. Both patients and spouses performed a progressive muscle relaxation protocol. It should be noted that nearly all patients with RA will experience increased pain if they attempt to tense and relax some muscle groups. Therefore, we instructed the participants that if they experienced increased pain while tensing a muscle, they should immediately relax that muscle and not attempt to tense it again during future exercises. With this precautionary procedure, we find that almost all of our patients can achieve a relatively relaxed state, even if they cannot exert control over all muscles. Once a state of relaxation was achieved, all participants engaged in the first of several cognitive and behavioral rehearsal exercises. We instructed the patients and spouses to breathe deeply and vividly imagine a scene from their life histories that they associate with deep relaxation or feelings of serenity. We also asked them to focus their attention on the experience of enhanced relaxation when they imagined their respective scenes. This instruction assists the participants in diverting their attention from pain or other unpleasant feelings or thoughts, and it reaffirms that they are very capable of controlling internal events. At the end of the session, we gave the patients an audiocassette of the relaxation and deep breathing instruction and asked them to practice their newly learned relaxation and imagery skills at least twice each day. Finally, we instructed the spouses to practice relaxation at home with the patients. Our rationale is that spouses who experience the benefits of relaxation will tend to encourage the patients to participate actively in treatment and to adhere to home practice of biofeedback, relaxation, and future assignments for practicing coping skills.

At the 6th week, patients and spouses participated in a second group relaxation training session. We first asked the patients to provide progress reports on the successes and difficulties they encountered in practicing their relaxation, imagery, and biofeedback skills. We focused particular attention on their thoughts and feelings during these successes and failures. We also asked the patients to describe any environmental events that may have interacted with their thoughts, feelings, and behaviors. Moreover, we encouraged the patients and spouses to provide verbal reinforcement to each other and to the other group members for their successes, as well as to suggest strategies that may help the group members resolve their practice difficulties.

After the patients gave their progress reports, we led the group members through the relaxation protocol and asked them to use their imagery and deep breathing to enhance their perceptions of relaxation. We also asked them to develop and use another image drawn from their life histories this time, an image involving warmth and relief from arthritis pain (e.g., lying in the sand at the seashore during the summer). We instructed the patients to focus on their images of warmth and pain relief as they performed relaxation and deep breathing during the group session and their home practices.

We continued to provide patients and spouses with cognitive and behavioral rehearsal instructions for relaxation throughout the remaining group sessions. In addition, we suggested at the 8th week that patients place cues such as Post-It Notes® at various sites in their home and work environments. We instructed the patients that whenever they saw a cue, they were to scan their bodies for areas of muscle tension. If patients found one or more tension areas, they were to breathe deeply and use their imagery for 1-2 minutes in order to relax. The purpose of this procedure is to help patients learn to evoke feelings of relaxation quickly in multiple situations outside the treatment setting that are associated with increases in pain or muscle tension. The patients reported their successes and difficulties in performing these procedures as well as the interactions among thoughts, feelings, and environmental events at the 10th and 12th weeks' group meetings. At the end of the 12th week's session, we instructed the patients to continue the tension monitoring and breathing/imagery procedures in their home and work environments without the use of cues.

In addition to the biofeedback and relaxation training procedures described above, we devoted part of the 6th week's session to teaching behavioral goal-setting or coping skills to the patients and spouses. We required each patient and spouse to agree to work together to help the patient cope better with a specific arthritis-related problem. Once the agreement was reached, we instructed the patient and spouse to formulate the problem in terms of observable behaviors. For example, nearly all participants agreed that fatigue is an important problem affecting the patients and their relationships with their family members or friends. The participants identified many behavioral manifestations of fatigue; the most common involved bed rest and withdrawal from family activities.

After the problem behaviors were identified, we instructed the patients and spouses to agree upon a goal that the patients could attain during the week that might help them reduce the frequencies of these behaviors. We also asked them to agree upon a series of strategies the patients could use to achieve their goals, as well as upon rewards that could be provided to patients for using each strategy. These goals, strategies, and rewards were recorded in a written contract between each patient and spouse. For example, patients and spouses who reported fatigue as a problem frequently identified spending more time together in leisure activities as a behavioral goal. Therefore, they usually developed written daily schedules for patients' activity and rest periods, in an attempt to reduce patients' fatigue behaviors and to create more opportunities for shared leisure activities. The rewards for following these schedules often included verbal self-reinforcement as well as allowing the patients to choose the leisure activities they desired.

At the conclusion of the meeting, we instructed the participants to use their behavioral strategies during the subsequent 2 weeks. We emphasized that patients should attempt to avoid negative thoughts and feelings about themselves when they had difficulty in achieving their goals. We also pointed out that all patients would experience some problems in performing the desired behaviors. At these times, the patients should attempt to replace negative thoughts with this cognition: "I can think of another behavior that I can perform to receive my reward and achieve my goal."

At the 8th week's group meeting, we asked the patients and spouses to discuss the successes and difficulties they encountered in performing their behavioral goal-setting skills. We encouraged them to modify their goals, behavioral strategies, and rewards with our help and with assistance from the other group members. At the conclusion of the meeting, we reminded the patients to avoid negative cognitions and feelings as they attempted to implement their behavioral strategies during the next 2 weeks.

We repeated this procedure at the 10th, 11th, and 12th weeks' group meetings. At the 10th and 12th weeks' meetings, we also required the patients and spouses to identify new arthritis-related problems and to develop and implement appropriate goals, behavioral strategies, and rewards for coping with these problems. Thus, the patients actively rehearsed strategies for three personal goals and were assisting one another with a variety of goals and behavioral strategies as they entered the final phase of the intervention.

GENERALIZATION AND MAINTENANCE

The purpose of the generalization and maintenance component is to help patients retain their learned skills and avoid increases in pain following treatment. Therefore, at the 14th and 15th weeks' group meetings, we asked the patients and spouses to discuss their beliefs and feelings regarding new problems they might encounter after the termination of the treatment intervention. These problems often were associated with possible increases in disease activity or disability with advancing age. Therefore, we asked them to describe possible goals, behavioral strategies, and rewards for coping with their anticipated problems. We also frequently encouraged them to use their newly learned skills to cope with problems unrelated to RA that they might confront in the future. These strategies are consistent with the relapse prevention model described earlier in this chapter.

FUTURE DIRECTIONS FOR PAIN MANAGEMENT

Clinicians and investigators should focus their attention on three major issues in order to enhance the benefits of the pain management interventions described above. First, increased emphasis should be placed on the prevention of patient relapse following treatment. For example, clinicians might wish to modify the intervention described by emphasizing relapse prevention throughout the cognitive and behavioral rehearsal component. Second, due to the changes that are occurring in the health care system in the United States, attention should be focused on measuring changes in health care costs produced by management interventions. It is necessary to collect accurate data concerning changes in both the direct (e.g., physician charges) and indirect (e.g., lost income or disability payments) costs produced by pain management therapies. There is an especially great need to examine the cost-effectiveness of "minimal" interventions such as telephone-based counseling. Finally, little effort has been devoted thus far to assessing the effects of pain management interventions delivered early after the diagnosis of a rheumatologic disease is made. It is necessary to examine this issue as one might anticipate greater long-term success if patients are taught effective strategies for pain management before they develop maladaptive pain-related beliefs and behaviors.

REFERENCES

Aaron, L. A., Bradley, L. A., Alarcón, G. S., Alexander, R. W., Alexander, M. T., Martin, M. Y., & Alberts, K. R. (1996). Psychiatric diagnoses are related to health care seeking behavior rather than illness in fibromyalgia. *Arthritis and Rheumatism, 39,* 436-445.

Aaron, L. A., Bradley, L. A., Alarcón, G. S., Triana-Alexander, M., Alexander, R. W., Martin, M. Y., & Alberts, K. R. (1997). Perceived physical and emotional trauma as precipitating events in fibromyalgia: Associations with health care seeking and disability status but not pain severity. *Arthritis and Rheumatism, 40,* 453-460.

Aaron, L. A., Bradley, L. A., Alexander, M. T., Alexander, R. W., Alberts, K. R., Martin, M. Y., & Alarcón, G. S. (In press). Work stress, psychiatric history, and medication usage predict initial use of medical treatment for fibromyalgia symptoms: a prospective analysis. In T. S. Jensen (Ed.), *Proceedings of the VIIIth World Congress on Pain, Progress in Pain Research and Management,* Vol. 5. Seattle, WA: IASP Press.

Affleck, G., Tennen, H., Pfeiffer, C., et al. (1987). Appraisals of control and predictability in adapting to a chronic disease. *Journal of Personality and Social Psychology, 53,* 273-279, 1987.

Affleck, G., Tennen, H., Urrows, S., et al. (1992). Neuroticism and the pain-mood relation in rheumatoid arthritis: insights from a prospective daily study. *Journal Consult Clinical Psychology, 60,* 119-126.

Affleck, G., Urrows, S., Tennen, H., et al. (1992). Daily coping with pain from rheumatoid arthritis: Patterns and correlates. *Pain, 51,* 221-230.

Ahles, T. A., Khan, S., Yunus, M. B., et al. (1991). Psychiatric status of patients with primary fibromyalgia, patients with rheumatoid arthritis, and subjects without pain: a blind comparison of DSM-III diagnoses. *American Journal of Psychiatry, 148,* 1721-1726.

Bennett, R. M., Burckhardt, C. S., Clark, S. R., O'Reilly, C. A., Wiens, A., & Campbell, S. M. (1996). Group treatment of fibromyalgia: a 6 month outpatient program. *Journal of Rheumatology, 23,* 521-528.

Blalock, S. J., DeVellis, R. F., Brown, G. K., et al. (1989). Validity of the Center for Epidemiologic Studies-Depression scale in arthritis populations. *Arthritis and Rheumatism, 32,* 991-997.

Bradley, L. A. (1985). Psychological aspects of arthritis. *Bulletin of Rheumatic Diseases, 35,* 1-12, 1985.

Bradley, L. A. (1993). Psychosocial factors and arthritis. In H. R. Schumacher, J. H. Klippel, & W. J. Koopman (Eds.), *Primer on the rheumatic diseases* (10th ed., pp. 319-322). Atlanta, GA: The Arthritis Foundation.

Bradley, L. A. (1994). Psychological dimensions of rheumatoid arthritis. In F. Wolfe & T. Pincus (Eds.), *Rheumatoid arthritis: Critical issues in etiology, assessment, prognosis, and therapy.* New York: Marcel Dekker.

Bradley, L. A. (1996). Pain. In S. T. Wegener, B. L. Belza, & E. P. Gall (Eds.), *Clinical care in the rheumatic diseases.* Atlanta, GA: Association of Rheumatology Health Professionals.

Bradley, L. A. (1996). Cognitive-behavioral therapy for chronic pain. In R. J. Gatchel, & D. C. Turk (Eds.), *Psychological approaches to pain management.* New York: Guilford Press.

Bradley, L. A., & Alarcón, G. S. (1996). Fibromyalgia. In W. J. Koopman (Ed.), *Arthritis and allied conditions* (13th edition). New York: Lippincott.

Bradley, L. A., Young, L. D., Anderson, K. O., Turner, R. A., Agudelo, C. A., McDaniel, L. K., Pisko, E. J., Semble, E. L., & Morgan, T. M. (1987). Effects of psychological therapy on pain behavior of rheumatoid arthritis patients: treatment outcome and six-month follow-up. *Arthritis and Rheumatism, 30,* 1105-1114.

Branco, J., Atalaia, A., & Paiva, T. (1994). Sleep cycles and alpha-delta sleep in fibromyalgia syndrome. *Journal of Rheumatology, 21,* 1113-1117.

Brown, G. K., & Nicassio, P. M. (1987). Development of a questionnaire for the assessment of active and passive coping strategies in chronic pain patients. *Pain, 31*, 53-64.

Buckelew, S. P., Parker, J. C., Keefe, F. J., Deuser, W. E., Crews, T. M., Conway, R., Kay, D. R., & Hewett, J. E. (1994). Self-efficacy and pain behavior among subjects with fibromyalgia. *Pain, 59*, 377-384.

Buescher, K. L., Johnston, J. A., Parker, J. C., Smarr, K. L., Buckelew, S. P., Anderson, S. K., & Walker, S. E. (1991). Relationship of self-efficacy to pain behavior. *Journal of Rheumatology, 18*, 968-972.

Burish, T. G., & Bradley, L. A. (1983). Coping with chronic disease: Definitions and issues. In T. G. Burish, & L. A. Bradley (Eds.), *Coping with chronic disease: Research and applications.* New York: Academic Press.

Carette, S., Oakson, G., Guimont, C., & Steriade, M. (1995) Sleep electroencephalography and the clinical response to amitryptyline in patients with fibromyalgia. *Arthritis and Rheumatism, 38*, 1211-1217.

Chikanza, I. C., Petrou, P., Kingsley, G., et al. (1992). Defective hypothalamic response to immune and inflammatory stimuli in patients with rheumatoid arthritis. *Arthritis and Rheumatism, 35*, 1281-1288.

Clarke, A. E., Esdaile, J. M., Bloch, D. A., Lacaille, D., Danoff, D. S., & Fries, J. F. (1993). A Canadian study of the total medical costs for patients with systemic lupus erythematosus and the predictors of costs. *Arthritis and Rheumatism, 36*, 1548-1559.

Crofford, L. F., Pillemer, S. R., Kalogeras, K. T., Cash, J. M., Michelson, D., Kling, M. A., Sternberg, E. M., Gold, P. W., Chrousos, G. P., & Wilder, R. L. (1994). Hypothalamic-pituitary-adrenal axis perturbations in patients with fibromyalgia. *Arthritis and Rheumatism, 37*, 1583-1592.

Dexter, P., & Brandt, K. (1994). Distribution and predictors of depressive symptoms in osteoarthritis. *Journal of Rheumatology, 21*, 279-286.

Deyo, R. A., Inui, T. S., Leininger, J., et al. (1982). Physical and psychosocial function in rheumatoid arthritis: clinical use of a self-administered health status instrument. *Archives of Internal Medicine, 142*, 879-882.

Felts, W., & Yelin, E. H. (1989). The economic impact of the rheumatic diseases in the United States. *Journal of Rheumatology, 16*, 867-884.

Frank, R. G., Beck, N. C., Parker, J. C., et al. (1988). Depression in rheumatoid arthritis. *Journal of Rheumatology, 15*, 920-929.

Frank, R. G., & Hagglund, K. J. (1996). Mood disorders. In S. T. Wegener, B. L. Belza, & E. P. Gall (Eds.), *Clinical care in the rheumatic diseases.* Atlanta, GA: Association of Rheumatology Health Professionals.

Garber, J., & Seligman, M. E. P. (Eds.). (1980). Human helplessness: Theory and applications. New York: Academic Press.

Gatchel, R. J., & Turk, D. C. (Eds.). (1996). *Psychological approaches to pain management.* New York: Guilford Press.

Goldenberg, D. L., Kaplan, K. H., Nadeau, M. G., et al. (1994). A controlled study of a stress-reduction, cognitive-behavioral treatment program in fibromyalgia. *Journal of Musculoskeletal Pain, 2*, 53-66.

Goossens, M. E. J. B., Rutten-van Molken, M. P. M. H., Leidl, R. M., Bos, S. G. P. M., Vlaeyen, J. W. S., & Teeken-Gruben, N. J. G. (1996). Cognitive-educational treatment of fibromyalgia. II. Economic evaluation. *Journal of Rheumatology, 23*, 1246-1254.

Harringon, L., Affleck, G., Urrows, S., et al. (1993). Temporal covariation of soluble interleukin-2 receptor levels, daily stress, and disease activity in rheumatoid arthritis. *Arthritis and Rheumatism, 36*, 199-203.

Hawley, D. J., & Wolfe, J. (1988). Anxiety and depression in patients with rheumatoid arthritis: a prospective study of 400 patients. *Journal of Rheumatology, 15*, 932-941.

Hudson, J. I., Goldenberg, D. L., Pope, H. G., Keck, P. E., & Schlesinger, L. (1992). Comorbidity of fibromyalgia with medical and psychiatric disorders. *American Journal of Medicine, 92,* 363-367.

Hudson, J. I., Hudson, M. S., Pliner, L. F., Goldenberg, D. L., & Pope, H. G. (1985). Fibromyalgia and major affective disorder: A controlled phenomenology and family history study. *American Journal of Psychiatry, 142,* 441-446.

Katz, P. P., & Yelin, E. H. (1993). Prevalence and correlates of depressive symptoms among persons with rheumatoid arthritis. *Journal of Rheumatology, 20,* 790-796.

Kazis, L. E., Meenan, R. F., & Anderson, J. J. (1983). Pain in the rheumatic diseases: investigation of a key health status component. *Arthritis and Rheumatism, 26,* 1017-1022.

Keefe, F. J., Brown, G. K., Wallston, K. A., et al. (1989). Coping with rheumatoid arthritis pain: catastrophizing as a maladaptive strategy. *Pain, 37,* 51-56.

Keefe, F. J., Caldwell, D. S., Williams, D. A., Gil, K. M., Mitchell, D., Robertson, C., Martinez, S., Nunley, J., Beckham, J. C., Crisson, J. E., & Helms, M. (1990a). Pain coping skills training in the management of osteoarthritic knee pain: a comparative study. *Behavior Therapy, 21,* 49-62.

Keefe, F. J., Caldwell, D. S., Williams, D. A., Gil, K. M., Mitchell, D., Robertson, C., Martinez, S., Nunley, J., Beckham, J. C., Crisson, J. E., & Helms, M. (1990b). Pain coping skills training in the management of osteoarthritic knee pain: II. Follow-up results. *Behavior Therapy, 21,* 435-447.

Keefe, F. J., & Van Horn, Y. (1993). Cognitive-behavioral treatment of rheumatoid arthritis pain: Maintaining treatment gains. *Arthritis Care Resources, 6,* 213-222.

Liang, M. H., Larson, M, Thompson, M., et al. (1984). Costs and outcomes in rheumatoid arthritis and osteoarthritis. *Arthritis and Rheumatism, 27,* 522-529.

Liang, M. H., Rogers, M., Larson, M., et al. (1984). The psychosocial impact of systemic lupus erythematosus and rheumatoid arthritis. *Arthritis and Rheumatism, 27,* 13-19.

Lorig, K., Chastain, R. L., Ung, E., et al. (1989). Development and evaluation of a scale to measure perceived self-efficacy in people with arthritis. *Arthritis and Rheumatism, 32,* 37-44.

Lorig, K. R., Mazonson, P. D., & Holman, H. R. (1993). Evidence suggesting that health education for self-management in patients with chronic arthritis has sustained health benefits while reducing health care costs. *Arthritis and Rheumatism, 36,* 439-446.

Lorish, C. D., Abraham, N., Austin, J., Bradley, L. A., & Alarcón, G. S. (1991). Disease and psychosocial factors related to physical functioning in rheumatoid arthritis patients. *Journal of Rheumatology, 18,* 1150-1157.

Maisiak, R., Austin, J. S., West, S. G., Heck, L. (1996). The effect of person-centered counseling on the psychological status of persons with systemic lupus erythematosus or rheumatoid arthritis: A randomized controlled trial. *Arthritis Care Resources, 9,* 60-66.

Martin, M. Y., Bradley, L. A., Alexander, R. W., Alarcón, G. S., Triana-Alexander, M., Aaron, L. A., & Alberts, K. R. (1996). Coping strategies predict disability in fibromyalgia. *Pain, 68,* 45-53.

Moldofsky, H. (1986). Sleep and musculoskeletal pain. *American Journal of Medicine, 81*(Suppl. 3A), 85-89.

Moldofsky, H., & Scarisbrick, P. (1976). Induction of neurasthenic musculoskeletal pain syndrome by selective sleep stage deprivation. *Psychosomatic Medicine, 38,* 35-44.

Nielson, W., Walker, G., & McCain, G. A. (1992). Cognitive-behavioral treatment of fibromyalgia syndrome: Preliminary findings. *Journal of Rheumatology, 19,* 98-103.

O'Leary, A., Shoor, S., Lorig, K., et al. (1988). A cognitive-behavioral treatment for rheumatoid arthritis. *Health Psychology, 7,* 527-544.

Parker, J., Smarr, K., Anderson, S., et al. (1992). Relationship of changes in helplessness and depression to disease activity in rheumatoid arthritis. *Journal of Rheumatology, 19,* 1901-1905.

Parker, J. C., Smarr, K. L., Buckelew, S. P., et al. (1995). Effects of stress management on clinical outcomes in rheumatoid arthritis. *Arthritis and Rheumatism, 38,* 1807-1818.

Parker, J. C., Smarr, K. L., Walker, S. E., et al. (1991). Biopsychosocial parameters of disease activity in rheumatoid arthritis: a prospective study of 400 patients. *Arthritis Care Resources, 4,* 73-80.

Pincus, T., Mitchell, J., Burkhauser, R. V. (1989). Substantial work disability and earnings losses in individuals less than age 65 with osteoarthritis: comparisons with rheumatoid arthritis. *Journal of Clinical Epidemiology, 42,* 449-457.

Radojevic, V., Nicassio, P. M., & Weisman, M. H. (1992). Behavioral intervention with and without family support for rheumatoid arthritis. *Behavior Therapy, 23,* 13-30.

Smith, T. W., Peck, J. R., & Ward, J. R. (1990). Helplessness and depression in rheumatoid arthritis. *Health Psychology, 9,* 377-389.

Summers, M. N., Haley, W. E., Reveille, J. D., & Alarcón, G. S. (1988). Radiographic assessment and psychologic variables as predictors of pain and functional impairment in osteoarthritis of the knee or hip. *Arthritis and Rheumatism, 31,* 204-209.

Tennen, H., Affleck, G., Urrows, S., et al. (1992). Perceiving control, construing benefits, and daily processes in rheumatoid arthritis. *Canadian Journal of Behavioral Sciences, 24,* 186-203.

Vlaeyen, J. W. S., Teeken-Gruben, N. J. G., Goosens, M. E. J. B., Rutten-van Molken, M. P. M. H., Pelt, R. A. G. B., van Eek, H., & Heuts, P. H. T. G. (1991). Cognitive-educational treatment of fibromyalgia: a randomized clinical trial. I. Clinical effects. *Journal of Rheumatology, 23,* 1237-1245.

Wegener, S. T. (1996). Sleep disturbance. In S. T. Wegener, B. L. Belza, & E. P. Gall (Eds.), *Clinical care in the rheumatic diseases.* Atlanta, GA: Association of Rheumatology Health Professionals.

Weinberger, M., Tierney, W. M., Cowper, P. A., Katz, B. P., & Booher, P. A. (1993). Cost-effectiveness of increased telephone contact for patients with osteoarthritis: a randomized controlled trial. *Arthritis and Rheumatism, 36,* 243-246.

Yelin, E. (1992). Arthritis: The cumulative impact of a common chronic condition. *Arthritis and Rheumatism, 35,* 489-497.

Yelin, E., Feshbach, D. M., Meenan, R. F., et al. (1979). Social problems, services, and policy for persons with chronic disease: the case of rheumatoid arthritis. *Social Science and Medicine, 13,* 13-20.

Young, L. D., Bradley, L. A., & Turner, R. A. (1995). Decreases in health care resource utilization in patients with rheumatoid arthritis following a cognitive-behavioral intervention. *Biofeedback and Self-Regulation, 20,* 259-268.

JOINT PROTECTION AND FATIGUE MANAGEMENT

Joy Cordery, OTR, and Mary Rocchi, PT

INTRODUCTION

Joint protection (JP) is a concept underlying all rehabilitation of persons whose joints are at risk from arthritis. It is a way of looking at a person's activities to see if the manner in which the joints are used contributes to pain and deformity. Originally, JP was directed to reducing pain and inflammation and protecting the fragile joint capsules and ligaments of patients with rheumatoid arthritis (RA) and other inflammatory arthritides (Cordery, 1962, 1965). In this chapter, JP has been expanded to include patients with osteoarthritis (OA) by addressing how to lessen microtrauma to articular cartilage and subchondral bone. In all cases, JP aims to reduce loading through vulnerable joints (Chamberlain, Ellis, & Hughes, 1984) and then develop strategies to help preserve the integrity of joint structures, relieve pain in the joints during activities, and help reduce local inflammation.

Fatigue management designates self-management training to reduce fatigue. For people with rheumatic disease, this approach incorporates not only energy-conservation training but also physical fitness and lifestyle behavior to help the person improve functional endurance and accomplish more in life despite fatigue and illness (Melvin, 1989; Tack, 1990).

Joint protection, energy conservation, and fatigue management are serious undertakings: They involve changing behavior, and those of us who struggle with bad habits know how hard that is.

ORIGINS OF JOINT PROTECTION

The need to consider protecting joints became evident to one of the authors (Cordery, 1962) after one of her patients, an active 30-year-old woman with a 5-year history of moderate RA, had lifted her heavy topcoat by her fingers and ruptured the radial collateral ligament of her index finger. Ligamentous and capsular structures can be elongated by chronic joint inflammation, and their attachment to bone can be weakened by underlying bone erosion; placing force on them greater than their residual strength can result in injury or rupture.

The injury to this woman was not inevitable. There are ways of lifting a coat (using a fist in the shoulder or using the palms of both hands on a hanger) that do not place undue force on vulnerable small joints. Another woman continued to embroider a cushion during a flare-up of her thumb interphalangeal (IP) joint. Repetitive strong pinch resulted in the elongation or rupture of the thumb IP ulnar collateral ligament. The patient no longer had an effective pinch. This injury was not inevitable either; a small plastic or leather cylinder slipped over the IP joint would have distributed the force along the phalanges and protected the ligament. And she would have had less pain while sewing. But how were these women to know these things? At that time, patients were encouraged to disregard their disabilities, but for those with a rheumatic disease, such disregard could be disastrous.

These and other observations on the hand led to the development of a set of principles of joint protection (Cordery, 1965) to guide occupational therapists in their work with patients with RA (see Table 1). These principles were stimulated by the author's previous anatomical research with E. M. Smith at the University of Michigan and were based on the anatomy and physiology of joints and the biomechanical analyses of Smith, Juvinal, Bender, and Pearson (1966). Smith and colleagues were the first to propose that the force of normal muscular activity acting on diseased joint restraints was an important factor in the development of rheumatoid hand deformity, and that deformities occur dynamically and not solely because of disease. They identified the pull of the flexor ten-

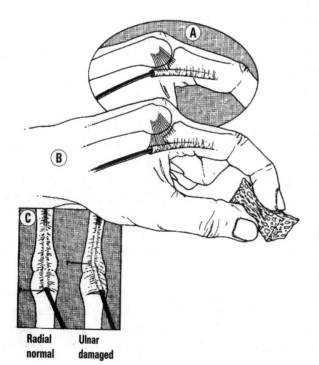

Radial normal   Ulnar damaged

Figure 1. Influence of the long flexors in metacarpophalangeal ulnar drift deformity. (A) MCP joint with normal ligamentous stability. (B) When the collateral ligaments are weakened and stretched by synovitis, 'bowstringing" of the flexor tendons across the joint occurring in strong pinch and grasp elongates the ligaments further, resulting in ulnar drift and volar subluxation of the proximal phalanx. (C) Volar view of the MCP joint showing the ulnar component of force of the long flexors as they pass through the fibrous tunnel. After the accessory collateral ligament has elongated, the pull of the flexors moves the fibrous tunnel ulnarly. Flexor force is directed to the proximal phalanx resulting in ulnar drift. From Melvin, 1989, with permission.

PRINCIPLES OF JOINT PROTECTION

FOR RA AND INFLAMMATORY JOINT DISEASES

1. Respect pain.
2. Maintain muscle strength and joint range of motion.
3. Use each joint in its most stable anatomic and/or functional plane.
4. Avoid positions of deformity and forces in their direction.
5. Use strongest joints available for the job.
6. Use correct patterns of movement.
7. Avoid staying in one position for long periods.
8. Avoid starting an activity that cannot be stopped immediately.
9. Balance rest and activity.
10. Reduce the force.

FOR OSTEOARTHRITIS

1. Increase muscle strength and fitness.
2. Maintain joint range of motion.
3. Reduce excessive loading on joints.
4. Avoid pain in activities.
5. Balance activity and rest.
6. Avoid staying in one position for long periods.

Table 1: Principles of Joint Protection. From Cordery, 1996.

dons as a primary deforming force for MCP ulnar drift and volar subluxation (Figure 1). Prior to their research, the leading theory of the cause of ulnar drift was the ulnar dislocation of the extensor tendons, but now it is realized that this is a consequence, not a cause, of MCP ulnar drift. Smith and colleagues (1966) were the first to apply engineering principles to analyzing the dynamics of hand deformity. They saw deformity as a new dynamic equilibrium following capsuloligamentous elongation and tendon shifts. Once such a deformity in the hand had occurred, no conservative measure could reverse it. Smith proposed that treatment must be preventive and consider everyday use of the joints.

A joint-protection approach analyzes the patient's activities of daily living and devises strategies that attempt to ensure that forces applied to joints are no greater than the joints involved can absorb. This approach is used in the active phase of disease or where joint instability is present (Brewerton & Lettin, 1973; Cordery, 1965; Kay, 1979; Melvin, 1989.

EVIDENCE FOR THE VALUE OF JOINT PROTECTION AND ENERGY CONSERVATION APPROACHES

Many years have passed since the protective approach was proposed. What evidence exists that it is effective? A review of the literature related to the major premises of the theory suggests answers.

JP HELPS PRESERVE THE INTEGRITY OF JOINT STRUCTURES

Research into prevention of anything is extremely difficult, particularly in a fluctuating, unpredictable disease such as RA. The nearest approach has been to compare the dominant hand of a person with RA with the nondominant one. Assuming that the dominant hand is subject to more stress than the nondominant one, Hasselkus, Kshepaharan, and Safrit (1981) studied 51 patients but found no difference between the dominant and nondominant hands in clinically observable joint changes.

Others have questioned the assumption that the dominant hand experiences more stress. Feinberg and Trombly (1995) pointed out that whereas the dominant hand is used more for dexterous tasks involving pinch and grasp, the nondominant hand is used for stabilization and is equally subjected to deforming, static pinch-and-grasp forces. This has also been a finding in a study into osteophyte formation in hands with osteoarthritis (OA) of the carpometacarpal (CMC) joint. Using microfocal radiography, Buckland-Wright, Macfarlane, and Lynch (1991) found a pattern of osteophyte formation in the dominant hand related to precision handling, power grip, and pulp pinch, and a pattern in the CMC joint of the nondominant hand probably related to forces exerted in power grip. In a comparison of handedness and hand use in OA of the hand, Lane, Bloch, Jones, Simpson, and Fries (1989) could not find radiologic or clinical differences between the dominant and nondominant hands. They suggested that it was possible that dominant activities (e.g., writing, eating, hammering) were not as different from nondominant hand use as was commonly supposed. A number of the participants in the study of Hasselkus and colleagues (1981) commented that persons with RA tend to shift much of their activity from a painful dominant hand to a less painful, nondominant one, thus somewhat equalizing the resulting stress during joint use. Hasselkus also pointed out that the use or nonuse of a cane was not recorded and might have proved another important variable.

In a radiographic study of 208 patients with RA, Mody, Meyers, and Reinbach (1989) did not find a significant difference in the proportions of patients who had swan-neck deformity, boutonnière, or uncorrectable ulnar drift in the dominant hand compared with the nondominant. They did find, however, that there were statistically significant greater radiographic changes of the dominant hand, and the index and middle fingers were more severely involved. Hand function was more severely impaired in the dominant hand.

Since there has been little research, use of JP principles is still based on understanding the anatomy of normal joints, the disease processes, the pathomechanics of deformity, and clinical experience. "Although it is probably impossible to prove that JP actually prevents deterioration in a particular joint, it is reasonable to apply sound bioengineering principles to joint functioning in arthritis in an attempt to conserve joint function" (Chamberlain, 1994, section 8, 7.6).

JP RELIEVES PAIN AND REDUCES LOCAL INFLAMMATION

The effectiveness of JP methods in reducing pain can be demonstrated easily in the occupational therapy clinic (Melvin, 1989). Have a patient identify an activity that causes pain, then let him or her perform the activity and rate the pain. Next, have the patient perform the activity using JP principles and reassess the pain. The reduction in pain is quite dramatic. For example, a cook who is used to lifting a saucepan with one hand can be shown how to slide the pan or use an oven mitt and lift with both hands (see Figure 2). A craftsperson can be shown different uses of a vise to stabilize tools. "The reduction of inflammation is variable and may take 1 to 5 days to be noticeable to the patient, depending upon the activities eliminated and the amount of stress reduced in the joint. When patients are taught how to monitor the signs and symptoms of inflammation and rate their pain and swelling on an analogue scale, they are able to appreciate the benefits of joint-protection methods" (Melvin, 1989, p. 420).

Hammond (1994a) studied JP behaviors in 11 people with RA following an education program. Ten participants were videotaped incorporating four JP behaviors while performing meal preparation tasks. She found that although participants reported that they were paying increased attention to joint care since education, that the education was relevant, and that they altered hand movements in daily tasks, only one subject showed an increase in JP behavior using this specific educational approach. One possible reason for the disappointing outcome could have been that her subjects knew the techniques but not the principles and their specific application.

Hammond did find a positive correlation to the presence of hand pain and the implementation of JP behavior. This indicates that those in pain may be more receptive to changing patterns.

Hammond (1994b) later designed an improved education program that included 5 hours of practical training in JP methods, guided practice and feedback, modeling, problem solving, goal setting, and self-reinforcement. Using the Joint Protection Behavioral Assessment (Hammond, 1994c), she found that JP behaviors increased significantly.

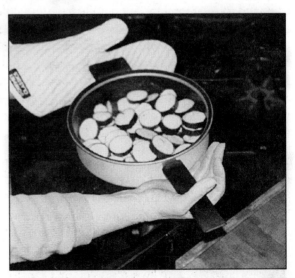

Figure 2. When it is not possible to slide a saucepan, using two hands to lift it reduces the force on each and allows the weight to be carried on the palms instead of by the fingers.

Nordenskiöld (1994) studied 53 women with RA and demonstrated that occupational therapy (OT) in a standardized JP course for 13 hours over 3 weeks managed by a team (OT for 6 hours; PT for 4 hours; MD for 1 hour; SW for 2 hours) resulted in a statistically significant reduction in pain using assistive devices (upright-handled bread knife (see Figure 3) and cheese slicer, a broad-handled potato peeler, spring-assisted scissors) compared with using ordinary household tools. Pain was similarly reduced when using a wrist orthosis and when using two hands instead of one in daily activities. "The benefit to the subjects was increased function, decreased pain, a better possibility of maintaining roles and the possibility that work at home, on the job, and in leisure activities will be easier to perform" (Nordenskiöld, 1994, p. 303).

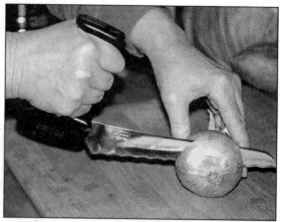

Figure 3. Using a straight-bladed knife requires strong grip and wrist ulnar deviation. An angled knife allows cutting to be done with minimal grip from the fingers and the wrist in a more neutral position.

ENERGY CONSERVATION INCREASES FUNCTIONAL ENDURANCE

The first prospective, randomized trial of energy conservation and JP for patients with RA was organized on a multicenter basis by the National Institutes of Health, United States Department of Health and Human Services. Twenty-eight patients entered the study and 25 completed the 3-month follow-up. Gerber, Furst, Smith, and colleagues (1987) compared a 6-week workbook-based program for teaching energy conservation behavior with a program of standard occupational therapy techniques. After 3 months both groups showed similarly improved levels of pain and fatigue. An increased level of physical activity was found in 11% of the control group and 50% of those having the experimental workbook approach ($p = .10$). A better balance of rest and physical activity was found in 22% of the control group and in 50% of the experimental workbook group ($p = .07$). In the control group, only one patient had increased the time spent physically active, whereas there were seven in the workbook-based group. Although significance was not achieved in this study, the authors believe the study provided preliminary data on an important connection between the practice of energy conservation behaviors, defined as breaking up physically active periods with rest periods, and increased amounts of physical activity. Furst, Gerber, Smith, Fisher, and Shulman (1987) suggested that traditional energy conservation training techniques in occupational therapy may not be optimally effective.

TEACHING JOINT PROTECTION

Changing work methods and attitudes requires more engagement than just to understand; therefore, the most important goal is to build a basis for the individual's creative thinking that will enable them to find their own solutions to their problems.

Nordenskiöld (1994, p. 303)

Central to the JP approach is the therapist's facilitation of the patient's abilities to analyze his or her problems and find the best solutions. Methods and devices should be presented as "something positive you can do to help your joints." A person who feels there is something he or she can do to affect the situation has a greater sense of self efficacy and is more likely to follow through with the solution (see chapter 10, Patient Education, and chapter 3, Adherence.) Most patients have already devised some methods for reducing pain and forces on joints (Hammond, 1994a). Therapists can enhance a person's self-esteem by finding out what the person has done on his or her own, assess and reinforce self-management techniques that are effective, and focus instruction on areas not yet mastered (Poole, 1995).

Many clinics have their own methods for teaching JP and may have lists of *do's* and *don'ts* based on the initial Cordery principles. This is not recommended because *teaching must be individualized to the person*. Every person's pattern of involvement is different, and each person's way of life and needs are different. Each person's way of learning is different: some learn by reading, others by hearing, and still others by doing.

Education has the best chance of succeeding when it makes the patient's joints feel better, when it uses tasks that the person has identified as significant, and when the teaching style matches the patient's learning style (Sliwa, 1983). The program most likely to help change behavior allows the person to discuss and practice, permits change to evolve as a product of experience, and lets the patient see positive outcomes.

The programs of Nordenskiöld (1994), Furst and colleagues (1987), and Hammond (1994b), which found that patients' behavior had been affected in a positive way, were based on cognitive, behavioral, learning theories (Furst et al. used the PRECEDE model; see chapter 10). Methods included the use of workbooks, the patient's own needs and experiences as the starting point, small groups (about five participants), two-way communication, theory, and practice sandwiched together and repeated, extended learning time (3-6 weeks), practical home tasks after every meeting, and the ultimate goal of stimulating the participants to find their own solutions.

CONTRACTING AND DEMONSTRATING EFFICACY

On the first contact, (Melvin, personal communication, 1996) uses a few key techniques and avoids focusing on the person as having a chronic disease for life. She has found that persons with early RA are terrified of deformity and very eager to protect joints, especially when the techniques are presented in a self-empowerment format and kept simple. She finds that it is very difficult to get patients to change behavior unless they can see fairly immediate benefits. She creates verbal contracts with clients in which she teaches them methods for reducing pain, inflammation, and damage to their joints if they, in turn, agree to implement the techniques for 2 days. If they agree, she teaches them the techniques and methods for self-assessment of pain and swelling at baseline and at the end of each day, using a 10-point analog scale. For example, for MCP synovitis she teaches them to use the palms of their hands as much as possible (see discussion of JP for MCP synovitis.) Her professional goal is not to achieve compliance, over which she feels she has no control, but to teach the techniques in such a way that persons can see the benefit of implementing the techniques and make informed decisions to use the methods. She reports that all of her patients taught these methods were able to perceive a reduction in hand pain and stiffness at the end of the second day. On follow-up visits, patients taught in this manner reported that they used the techniques and found them helpful.

Sliwa (1983) emphasizes that learning can be activated only by and inside the learner—"We have to turn them on, stimulate all the senses"—and that a successful learning experience facilitates mastery of the material on both an intellectual and emotional level. Shumway-Cook and Wollacott (1995) emphasize that the person has to develop a kinesthetic sense of the pattern you want him or her to use.

Assessing the patients' learning style and adapting patient education to it are essential to effective teaching. Learning style can be determined by asking the patient how he or she learns best: written instruction, spoken instruction, demonstration, or practice. A helpful question is, "When you prepare packaged food for the first time, do you read the instructions or learn by doing?" (Melvin, personal communication, 1996). Because of cognitive, emotional, or other problems, not everyone is able to learn or to solve problems. Learning is promoted by repeatedly altering the way the message is presented, giving the individual extensive practice with positive reinforcement from the therapist, and arranging regular follow-up (Cynkin, personal communication, 1996). Follow-up with the therapist is most important so that when the need becomes apparent, new measures can be introduced to counteract the effects of disease progression (Agnew, 1987).

JOINT PROTECTION FOR INFLAMMATORY JOINT DISEASES: RATIONALE AND TREATMENT IMPLICATIONS

The following principles apply to persons with RA, psoriatic arthritis, systemic lupus erythematosus (SLE) with joint swelling, and juvenile rheumatoid arthritis (JRA). All of these are conditions in which swelling and inflammation elongate and damage joint capsules and ligaments. (Note: Many persons with SLE only have mild arthritis or arthralgias. See disease-specific chapters in Volume 2.) These principles apply to all joints.

1. RESPECT PAIN

The pain-sensitive structures in the joint are the fibrous capsule, ligaments, fat pads, and periosteum. Pain receptors are absent in the synovium, intraarticular fibrocartilage (e.g., menisci) and articular cartilage (Hertling & Kessler, 1996). Persons with inflammatory arthritis need to respect pain and to recognize when pain is an indicator of joint harm. Pain is the best protection we have against abuse of inflamed and damaged joints (Bennett, 1965). Although fear of joint pain can lead to unnecessary inactivity, total disregard for joint pain can lead to unnecessary joint damage and increased pain. When pain is present at rest, it is likely to stem from joint synovitis and activity should then be scaled back (Sliwa, 1986). *Patients should carry out activities and exercise only up to the point of pain.* A person with acute synovitis who reports doing strenuous activity without proportional pain (from a high pain threshold, medication, or psychological denial) should use swelling and warmth as the guideline for monitoring activity (Melvin, personal communication, 1989).

Some authorities state that pain or discomfort lasting more than a certain time (Melvin, 1 hour for RA; Leonard, 2 hours for RA; Moskowitz, 30 minutes for OA) shows the activity was excessive. While discomfort lingering after activity or exercise should be limited, an exact time has not been established.

2. MAINTAIN MUSCLE STRENGTH AND JOINT RANGE OF MOTION

Efficient, strong muscles are fundamental to the support and stability of joints, and for most joints they are their best protection against injury to the capsule, ligament, and cartilage. *The exceptions in rheumatoid and psoriatic arthritis, SLE, and JRA are the wrists and hands, where strong muscles and fragile joints are a formula for deformity* (Melvin, personal communication, 1996; see Hands with Inflammatory Joint Disease). JP during therapeutic exercise includes ensuring that muscle pull does not accentuate deformity.

Joint range of motion (ROM) should be maintained so that a loss of range at one joint will not allow force to be transmitted (unduly) to another. For example, loss of knee extension will affect the hip, loss of ankle dorsi flexion will affect the knee, and loss of MCP extension will affect PIP flexion. Normal ROM maintains joint mobility through lubrication of the joint, maintains the health of the cartilage and capsule, is important for maintenance of muscle function, and enables the joint to work at biomechanical advantage. Joint position and ROM are critical for optimum functioning of muscles (Maehlums, 1994).

To allow coordinated use of the hand, extension, radial and ulnar deviation of the wrist, extension of the MCP, and flexion of PIP need to be preserved. Alternative methods of using the hands that protect small, vulnerable joints (e.g., by carrying objects on the palms of the hands instead of by the fingers; see Figure 2) are usable only if motion has been maintained at the shoulder and elbow, and if pronation and supination of the forearm and extension of the wrist are possible.

In the presence of acute joint inflammation, joint protection includes avoiding strong muscular effort or moving into joint end ranges, as this raises intra-articular pressure to the point it can drive synovial fluid into bone and contribute to its erosion (Castillo, El Sallab, & Scott, 1965).

3. USE EACH JOINT IN ITS MOST STABLE ANATOMIC AND/OR FUNCTIONAL PLANE

The most stable anatomic and/or functional plane is one in which resistance to the motion is provided by *muscle*, not ligament. This is especially important in protecting knees, wrists, MCP joints, thumbs, and back. For example, rising from a chair should be done while maintaining a bilaterally symmetrical trunk, not leaning over to one side. This allows muscle power to be used to greatest advantage and avoids forces stressing ligaments of the knee. Pinch should be against the pad of the thumb, slightly flexed at the IP to prevent hyperextension, and not against its side, to avoid external load on the ulnar collateral ligament.

4. AVOID POSITIONS OF DEFORMITY AND FORCES IN THEIR DIRECTION

The person with arthritis should avoid external loads (such as using fingers to push out of a chair) and internal forces (such as strong grip and pinch) that facilitate deformity. *However, this principle applies only to patients whose involvement puts them at risk.* For example, the person with RA whose fingers have not been affected has no need for instruction about those joints. The exact loads and forces to avoid depend upon the joints affected and the disease being treated. For the person with involvement of the cervical spine, review posture at work, during leisure activities, and resting in bed. For persons with knee involvement, avoiding excessive thigh adduction will decrease forces into valgus deformity.

5. USE THE STRONGEST JOINTS AVAILABLE FOR THE JOB

Large joints are "stronger" than small ones. Using the strongest joints is one of the tenets of body mechanics; for example, use the knees for lifting, not the back. When the knees are affected by arthritis, however, a modification of this technique is needed such as moving the object to where the person can sit to lift it, or asking others to help (Furst et al., 1985). When sliding an object, push rather than pull it. Use of stronger, larger joints includes hips or elbows to open doors, forearms and palms to carry groceries, and palms rather than fingers to lift, or push, or take weight (see Figure 2). All of these examples use several joint systems to distribute the force.

6. ENSURE CORRECT PATTERNS OF MOVEMENT

Incorrect patterns may be the result of pain, tenosynovitis, deformity, muscle imbalance, or habit. In the hand, the use of the long extensors in the pattern of finger movement should be maintained. Finger flexion should begin at the distal interphalangeal joints (DIP) while maintaining extension at the MCP. When a patient rises from a chair, hip and knee extension should occur together, not sequentially.

7. AVOID STAYING IN ONE POSITION FOR LONG PERIODS

Muscles tire quickly in static holding. Tired muscles cannot support a joint, and the load can go on to the underlying joint capsule and ligaments. Sustained joint compression can lead to damage of articular surfaces. Circulation can be hindered. Activity taking longer than 10 minutes or so can be done seated, but sitting longer than 20-30 minutes without getting up promotes stiffness. A timer is helpful for learning to balance activity and rest. Periodic local rest and joint ROM exercises can be interspersed (Leonard, 1995). Changing positions and tasks can give local rest (Sliwa, personal communication, 1996). Persons sitting at computers should get up and move about regularly, to file, or to make copies.

Individuals with hand involvement who write, use a keyboard, knit, sew, or crochet and who stop the activity several times an hour and move the entire upper extremity through its range of motion report less discomfort during the activity and feel better at the end of the task. If the person has an intrinsic-plus hand, it will be critical for him or her to use intrinsic stretching exercises during these rests.

All the above times can be adjusted for the person's situation. Special attention should be given to helping workers plan how to incorporate rests and stretches into their work routines.

8. AVOID STARTING AN ACTIVITY THAT CANNOT BE STOPPED IMMEDIATELY IF IT PROVES TO BE BEYOND THE PERSON'S ABILITY

The principle here is to prevent the load from going to the joint capsule and ligament if the supporting muscles tire. Modifications might include using a cart on wheels to transport heavy, breakable, or hot items, walking a long distance only if there are seats available along the way, and carrying a package only if there is a place to rest it if it proves to be too heavy.

9. BALANCE REST AND ACTIVITY

Tired muscles provide less protection to damaged joints and allow more force to be put on the joint. The efficient and appropriate use of rest during daily activities is probably the most effective weapon a person with arthritis can use against the demands of the disease. It is also the most difficult to incorporate into daily life (Melvin, 1989). This is discussed further in Fatigue Management.

Persons with a systemic disease like RA need more rest and sleep. Many rheumatologists recommend 10 hours of sleep and another hour of rest during the day. Furst and colleagues (1985) recommended planning a daily 1-hour rest period, and during long periods of activity taking 10-minute rest breaks every 20 minutes. Sliwa proposes that if a person cannot lie down, he or she could sit 15-20 minutes with all body parts supported. Resting with the feet elevated reduces muscle tone and is more restorative to the body (Melvin, personal communication, 1996). "Only trial and error can help sort out the particular level of activity that is appropriate for each individual" (Gerber, 1985, p. 3).

10. REDUCE THE FORCE

Reducing the muscular force needed to perform an activity is a key aspect of protecting joints (see volume 4 of this series: The Hand: Joint Protection). This reduction can be accomplished by using a new method or by using different equipment.

The motions described under most of the principles are not harmful to persons with inflammatory joint disease *unless they involve strong effort.* For example, a light grasp used for eating from a fork or spoon would not require the harmful forces of a tight grip on a knife in food preparation (see Figure 3). Light movements are not painful in the way strong, forceful ones can be. Making handles larger reduces effort, as does using objects that are not slippery or have grip flanges to prevent their slipping through the hands.

Equipment includes functional orthoses, assistive devices, and ordinary household or workshop tools. Functional orthoses can follow the precept of Bennett (1965, p. 1006), who described an ideal orthosis as one that would "permit the essential function but block all faulty planes that might result in functionally significant deformity." Examples of these are a tripoint splint for swan-neck deformity and an orthosis similar to the Quest-Cordery splint for ulnar deviation (1971). The latter is made to fit the deformed position of the digits; its value comes when the hand is used and motion into increased deformity is blocked. Deformity is not always a functional problem; a bigger functional problem is lack of stability of the joints.

Providing assistive devices or orthoses early in the disease process may be important to reduce joint stress and pain. It is helpful to the patient for the therapist to introduce the devices for these purposes and then to point out that they do not represent "giving in" to the disease but are positive actions to avoid pain and reduce stress and damage to the joints. (See chapter 16, Assistive Technology, for the latest devices, resources, and catalogs.)

Work simplification methods also reduce stress on joints. For example, reorganized storage that puts most-used objects near the point of use gets rid of clutter so that the wanted items can be retrieved without lifting others first, and learning how to slide instead of lifting with both hands also reduce effort.

APPLICATION OF JOINT PROTECTION PRINCIPLES TO SPECIFIC JOINT INVOLVEMENT

HANDS WITH INFLAMMATORY JOINT DISEASE

Volume 4 of this series contains expanded descriptions and discussions of JP for the hand including the biomechanical basis for JP of the rheumatoid hand.

The wrists and hands have joint systems of linked bony segments, with power coming from opposing muscle forces that act across each joint in a protagonist-antagonist relationship. The extrinsic muscles exert the primary forces; the intrinsic muscles give the maneuverability and delicate balance to this multiarticular system. The intrinsic muscles also create the counterbalancing constraint forces at the joint surface and surrounding ligamentous structures. In such a system, muscular force is essentially compressive. Landsmeer (1962) showed that a bimuscular, multiarticular system subjected to compressive forces will buckle in a predictable zigzag manner unless it is controlled and stabilized. Swan-neck, boutonnière, and thumb deformities all represent the sequela of this process. When ligaments are elongated by chronic inflammation and tendons shift location, a new equilibrium of force and counterforce is found that will be changed permanently in favor of the direction of the deformity (Smith, Juvinal, Bender, & Pearson, 1966). No conservative treatment can restore the original equilibrium.

MCP SYNOVITIS: VOLAR SUBLUXATION AND ULNAR DRIFT

The causes of MCP volar subluxation and ulnar drift are multiple. The collateral ligaments, normally loose in extension and tight in flexion, become loose on the radial side in flexion and allow the proximal phalanx to sublux volarly and ulnarly. Smith and colleagues (1966) showed that the forces sufficiently powerful to affect the radial collateral ligaments in the index and long fingers were the long finger flexors where they run through the volar tunnel. This tunnel attaches to the accessory collateral ligament which, when it elongates, allows the whole flexor apparatus to displace volarward and ulnarward. The fulcrum of the long flexors shifts from over the metacarpal bone to over the proximal phalanx (see Figure 1). Wise (1975) showed how forces from the long flexors could similarly affect the ring and little fingers.

Hand functions of power grip and palmar, lateral, and tip pinch require MCP flexion. The stronger the grip or pinch, the more force is exerted against the structures of the volar tunnel and the radial collateral ligament. The greater the MCP flexion, the greater the forces exerted against the base of the proximal phalanx. But allowing MCP flexion of not more than 30-35 degrees during grasp and pinch would reduce the "bowstringing" of the flexor tendons and thus would reduce their volar and ulnar pull (Smith et al., 1966). That is the reason why grip and pinch should be avoided during periods of synovitis, and the force of grip and pinch should be reduced as the synovitis remits and leaves an unstable joint (Brewerton & Lettin, 1973; Cordery, 1965; Kay, 1979; Melvin, 1989). Methods to protect MCP ligamentous structures and reduce pain and forces on the joints are listed in Table 2 and Table 3.

SWAN-NECK DEFORMITIES

One of the most disabling rheumatoid deformities is a swan-neck because PIP hyperextension means the finger tips may not be able to reach the thumb and only lateral pinch can be used. Swan-neck deformity has several causes, but the most common is tightness of the intrinsic muscles.

METHODS TO REDUCE PAIN AND FORCES ON THE MCP JOINTS

- Avoid MCP flexion and any forceful activities such as strong grip, strong pinch or external pressure against the collateral ligaments, such as pushing against the fingers laterally or in a volar direction.

- When there is also wrist involvement, maintain wrist ulnar deviation at rest, even if it makes the fingers look more deviated.

- Use the palm and heel of the hand whenever possible. These are the strongest, most stable parts of the hand and the least vulnerable to stress. This practice also serves to encourage use of the finger extensors, since the fingers must actively extend to allow palmar contact (Melvin, 1989).

- Wear an orthosis to reduce MCP flexion in activities (Phillips, 1995; Smith et al., 1966), but only if the PIP joints are not involved as *restricting the MCP joint may cause additional force to be exerted on the PIP joints* (Bell-Krotoski, Breger-Lee, & Beach, 1995; Melvin, 1989).

- Use two hands instead of one when lifting (bilateral prehension) (see Figure 2).

- Use the forearm for carrying, lifting, and pulling. For car doors and handles that are difficult to open, attach a strap loop through the handle to open the door (or drawer) by slipping the forearm or palm of the hand through the loop.

- A cane handle should fit the palm of the hand and not require a strong grip (see Figure 4).

- Enlarged handles, razor-sharp knives, light-weight objects, sliding instead of lifting, and using wheels will all help protect the MCP during activities. Such methods and devices should be presented as "something positive you can do to help your joints," a self-management tool.

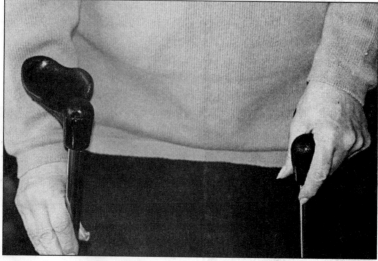

Figure 4. The handles of "arthritis" canes do not require grip by the fingers, and pressure is exerted on a large part of the surface of the palms of the hands.

TURNING JAR LIDS, FAUCETS, AND DOOR KNOBS

Some authors recommend "that movement should be done in a direction opposite to the potential deformity," but this instruction could be very difficult, painful, and frustrating to the patient. Another recommendation is "always turning the fingers toward the thumb side, opening the jar top or door with the right hand and closing it with the left." But these recommendations do not take into account that these actions encourage radial deviation of the wrist, which increases zigzag forces and MCP ulnar drift (Melvin, 1989). These actions require strong finger and thumb flexion to grasp the jar lid or door knob. The arm is used for leverage in this grip and increases the subluxing and deviating forces at the MCP and PIP. *These methods should not be used.* It is much less painful and safer to rely on pressure from the palm of either hand, assisted by devices.

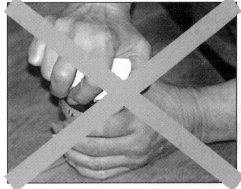

Figure 5a. Opening a jar by hand involves stringly resisted flexion and rotation at the MCPs and PIPs.

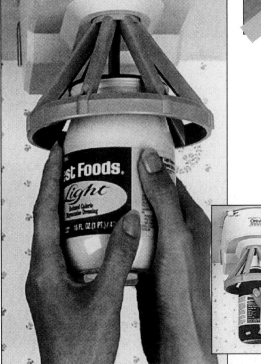

Figure 5b. There are many top openers available. This electric one opens both bottles and jars and allows both hands to support the item and eliminates the need for MCP and PIP flexion (Photo courtesy of North Coast Medical Inc., San Jose, CA).

KNITTING AND CROCHETING

The use of crocheting, knitting, and similar traditional needlecrafts is controversial since they involve prolonged pinch and static holding in an intrinsic-plus position of the hand. These activities are valuable to the patient because they are easily learned, require minimal and available equipment, and produce a useful, desirable product. They can be carried out by persons with severe hand deformities and limited standing tolerance.

In general, the only hand conditions where knitting and crocheting may cause harm are: (1) active MCP synovitis, where MCP volar subluxation and ulnar drift can be ameliorated by wearing an MCP extension or MCP-wrist orthosis, (2) beginning swan-neck deformity, where performing intermittent intrinsic stretching exercises or wearing an orthosis keeping the MCP in extension can give protection against adverse effects, and (3) osteoarthritis of the CMC joint of the thumb, where a CMC stabilization orthosis prevents adverse effects and reduces pain. Padding the lower end of the crochet hook reduces the need for a tight grip; "swallow" knitting needles from Australia allow the yarn to slide more easily; Nordenskiöld (1994) mentions "special tongs" for sewing; limiting time spent reduces the irritation.

The psychological benefit of being productive and making something that is useful, stylish, and valued by others is of great importance to persons with rheumatic disease. This may be of greater importance to the person than whatever amount of hand function might be maintained by not doing the craft. Careful consideration should be given to the psychological benefits of an activity before advising patients about knitting, crocheting, and other beloved hobbies.

Table 4: Knitting and Crocheting. Adapted with permission from Melvin, 1989.

Methods to reduce deforming forces in swan-neck include intrinsic stretching exercises, avoiding pressure that results in PIP hyperextension, use of a tripoint splint during activities to limit hyperextension, and avoiding prolonged intrinsic-plus position with the MCP flexed and PIPs extended, such as holding a book while reading, resting the chin on the dorsum of the hand while resting or watching TV, and craft activities such as knitting and crocheting (see Table 4).

BOUTONNIÈRE OR FLEXION DEFORMITIES

Prevention of boutonnière deformity from becoming a fixed flexion deformity by maintaining passive extension is important: mobility of the PIP and distal interphalangeal (DIP) joints is required for personal hygiene, putting on gloves, and facilitating any surgical outcome (Melvin, 1989).

Measures to reduce forces into flexion at the PIP include avoiding strong grip, performing antideformity exercises, avoiding pinch when the index finger is involved, avoiding keeping the fingers in a flexed position at rest, avoiding extension against resistance (of the involved fingers), and wearing a reverse tripoint splint to restrict PIP flexion.

METHODS FOR REDUCING PAIN AND FORCES ON THE WRIST

- Avoid axial compression at the wrist by avoiding strong use of finger flexors in grip and pinch. Substitute bilateral prehension or use equipment.

- Avoid activities that involve repetitive wrist rotation and flexion, for example, stirring, using a manual screwdriver, or hammering. Substitute power tools and tools with ergonomic handles (Figure 3).

- Use a flexible wrist gauntlet orthosis during the day to prevent circumduction and reduce torque on the wrist (Kjeken, Moller, & Kvien, 1995; Melvin, 1989).

- Avoid lifting and moving heavy objects in a hook grasp, as in carrying a suitcase or a purse. Instead, lighten all loads, substituting another part of the body such as the forearm or shoulder. Use wheels on a suitcase and a rolling table in a work area. Use a fanny pack instead of a purse. Women's purses should weigh less than 3 lbs.

- Avoid using the wrists unnecessarily. Persons with knee involvement must have adequately high seats during chair transfers and must know the correct technique for rising.

- In the kitchen or work place, slide instead of lifting, or use a rolling cart. Keyboard users can consider a wrist bar to provide support during rest breaks, or arm support to reduce stress.

- A cane handle should fit the palm of the hand and not require a strong grip (Figure 4).

Table 5: Methods for Reducing Pain and Forces on the Wrist

THUMB JOINTS

The thumb represents 45% of hand function, and its joints are subject to great forces during activities of daily living. Stabilization orthotics are the most effective way to protect the IP or MCP joints. Avoiding grip and pinch, using lever devices to open car doors, turn the key, or turn a faucet all help reduce forces on the thumb joints. Large diameter or built-up rolling-ball-tipped pens reduce friction on paper and take less pinch when writing. Squeeze bottles cause severe strain on the MCP joint, but their solutions can be transferred to small, easy-to-pour bottles.

After inflammation subsides, protective methods should still be continued. It is particularly important to avoid pressures against the always-vulnerable IP thumb ulnar collateral ligament during pinch or in pushing against objects such as using the lateral side of the thumb in closing a drawer or door.

The CMC joint can be affected by RA, OA, or both. The most troublesome problem occurs when metacarpal motion becomes limited in adduction and the web space becomes narrowed. The patient's grasp activities may unwittingly put force on the MCP ulnar collateral ligament and cause an abduction or lateral-deviation deformity (Swanson, 1995). For this type of problem, handles should be thin and narrow so that the patient can hold them without straining the MCP joint. Pain can be relieved and function improved by an orthosis that stabilizes the CMC and adjacent MCP joint (Melvin, 1989; see chapter on orthotic treatment in Volume 4).

THE WRIST

The axial compressive forces that come from strong grip and pinch, and any repetitive rotational and flexing motions that can exert forces against the vulnerable dorsal and ulnar aspects of the wrist should be avoided. Keeping the wrist straight in activities (see Figure 6b), using only light-weight objects, using other parts of the body and wheels to move, carry, and lift objects will help spare vulnerable structures. Methods for reducing pain and forces in the wrist are listed in Table 5.

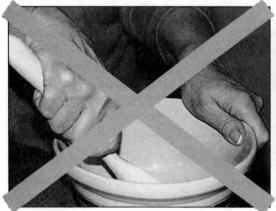 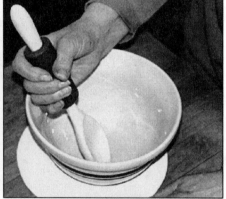

Figure 6a. Holding this small handle requires full MCP flexion and strong grip. The wrist is flexed and deviated and the motion of stirring will involve repetitive wrist rotation.

Figure 6b. The best way to mix is to use an electric mixer. If that is not possible, then padding the spoon handle and turning the hand up reduces stress to MCPs, fingers, and wrist. Note the nonskid mat under the bowl that reduces the effort to hold the bowl stable.

TIMING OF JP EDUCATION

Most patients will absorb joint protection information best during a period of joint involvement because they can see a fairly immediate result from using the techniques for reducing pain. Melvin (personal communication, 1996) considers that people in true, complete remission can probably do whatever they want, but people in so-called drug-induced remission, those who have swelling and no pain because it is masked by medications, and those with fragile hands still need to use JP techniques.

The difficulty lies in judging whether normal use is safe, and whether the residual strength of the joints will be able to withstand the demands that use puts on them. This writer recommends that the decision to continue or discontinue JP techniques for the hands in a true remission be based on an examination of the joints of the hands. Where joint instability is present or shifts in ligamentous structures or tendon location have occurred, care will still be needed to avoid strong grip-and-pinch or lateral pressures against collateral ligaments, etc. (e.g., pushing a drawer shut or lifting a heavy topcoat).

SHOULDERS AND ELBOWS

People primarily reduce stress to the shoulders and elbows by reducing their range of active motion and the weight of what they carry. People with RA of the shoulder or elbow usually have hand involvement and have stopped heavy lifting because of their hands. When there is acute pain or inflammation, joint protection would involve doing activities with as little pain as possible and having someone perform gentle, passive ROM to the shoulder and AROM to the elbow, following a cold modality and conscious relaxation. People in this situation can often benefit from a simple review of how to avoid painful motions such as by donning a jacket with the painful side first and doffing with the least painful side first (Melvin, 1989). When pain and inflammation have subsided, the person's activities should be reviewed to see if activities using unresisted elevation and external rotation can be resumed (for example, keeping a cereal box on a high shelf) as an adjunct to maintaining range. Reachers can reduce strain on the shoulder, but for the RA patient they often create unacceptable forces on the hands and need to be carefully selected.

LOWER EXTREMITIES

Joint protection concepts for the lower extremity involve consideration of the individual joint—hip, knee, and ankle—as well as the combined lower kinetic chain as a unit. Limiting the forces to the entire lower extremity can be done through weight loss, use of assistive devices, and promoting optimal function of the surrounding musculature.

KNEES

When discussing the knee, both the tibiofemoral joint and the patellofemoral joint need to be considered. Force to the knees may be lessened by using seats of an appropriate height: chairs with hip and knee flexion angles at approximately 90 degrees or less will help facilitate proper alignment of the trunk and lower extremities. Excessive knee flexion during sitting may cause increased anterior knee pain secondary to increased forces at the patellofemoral joint (Nordin & Frankel, 1989). Proper alignment of the knees over the feet, moving in a controlled manner, and the avoidance of lower-extremity adduction during transitional movements should be stressed. Rising from sitting to standing will usually be easier if the person slides forward to the edge of the seat before standing and then uses the least-involved lower extremity for push-off or uses a quadriceps facilitation technique prior to rising. A rocking start allows momentum to assist the person in rising. Facilitation of quadriceps strength may be achieved by having the patient (1) do a quad set (isometric contraction of the quadriceps muscle), (2) straighten the knee completely once or twice, or (3) flex and extend the knee two to three times in midrange. The choice of method depends on which causes the least discomfort, since pain inhibits muscle strength.

Other suggestions for reducing forces on the knees include (1) strengthening the knee extensor muscles, (2) avoiding walking on rough, uneven ground, (3) going up steps with the good leg first, descending with the most painful knee first, (4) using knee supports to help keep the knee warm and to serve as a reminder to use the knee in a stable, straight alignment rather than with the body rotated, (5) using ambulation aids if prescribed, and (6) wearing good walking or athletic shoes with a strong heel counter. If biomechanical faults are present in the feet, an internal custom orthosis in the shoe may further decrease stress to the knee by providing improved lower-extremity mechanics during walking (Eng & Pierrynowski, 1993).

HIPS

Reducing the magnitude of the forces on the hip generated by the hip abductor muscles is a focus of hip joint protection. One can reduce myogenic joint forces by using a cane in the hand opposite the involved hip, avoiding single-leg standing on the involved hip by, for example, sitting to put on or take off pants, and carrying loads that are as light as possible. Neumann (1989; Neumann & Hase, 1994) inferred through EMG that the highest forces exerted on the involved hip occurred when the load was carried on the contralateral side. He recommended that if a significant load must be carried and cannot be divided into two and carried on both sides, it should be carried centrally by a backpack on the upper back. If this is not possible, then the load should be carried on the same side as the hip that requires protecting. Neumann goes on to point out that this does not go without a price: the same-side load is a contralateral load experienced on the other hip.

For persons who are overweight, weight reduction can be a valuable method of joint protection. In the case of hip OA, weight loss can decrease the force requirements of the hip muscles. It is estimated that a force equal to 4 times body weight is exerted at the hip joint when the person is bearing weight on one extremity. For every pound one loses, it is estimated that there is a force reduction of 4 pounds of force per square inch per step. Overweight persons should receive dietary counseling and encouragement to participate in a weight-reduction program. For patients with OA of the knees, weight reduction alone can often alleviate symptoms (Templeton, Petty, & Harter, 1978).

Trauma to osteoporotic hips and vertebrae can be reduced if the person controls lowering the body onto the seat. Therapy can be directed toward developing eccentric muscle control of the lower extremity musculature, especially of the quadriceps group. Because of the attachment of the hip muscles to the pelvis, assessment and correction of muscle imbalances of the trunk are also important in management of the hip.

FEET

Joint protection for the feet relies on wearing supportive shoes of proper fit and orthotics as well as maintaining ROM of the feet and ankles. A detailed description of recommended footwear and orthotic options is in appendix A.

A patient who reports that he or she can wear only soft shoes such as slippers should have a medical foot examination to determine if he or she would benefit from shoe adaptations or orthoses.

JOINT PROTECTION FOR THE SPINE

The main objective of neck and back protection is to keep the spine in good alignment during activities. Good alignment consists of trying to maintain the normal curves of the spine—slight lordosis—in the cervical region, slight kyphosis in the thoracic region, and slight lordosis in the lumbar region (Jackson, 1977). The alignment should also be laterally symmetrical. The normal curves allow the spine to function as an effective shock absorber as weight is transmitted through the vertebral bodies. In the presence of neck pain, positions or motions that should be avoided include neck extension (hyperextension), prolonged forward and lateral flexion or rotation, and repetitive motion in any direction (Jackson, 1977).

Education for patients with back pain depends upon the nature of the disorder. Formerly, keeping the back straight and reducing lordosis was the standard recommendation for all back patients. Although reducing the lordotic curve with a posterior pelvic tilt can be an effective and appropriate technique for certain back conditions, decreasing the lordotic curve for some persons may increase pain and is therefore not appropriate (MacKenzie, 1981). The mechanics of the back and its posture and alignment are too complex for a single technique to be appropriate for all patients. The rule of 'keeping the spine straight" as it refers to alignment, however, is still appropriate for most patients. When a person tries to "sit straight," he or she tends to move into a more normal posture, and this encourages the natural curves of the spine. More recently, the concept of the "neutral" back position has been advocated as a desirable position during activities.

Back or neck protection programs with simplistic "rules for all" are not very effective. The most effective programs are based on the findings of a comprehensive musculoskeletal assessment, conducted by a physical therapist, of a person's posture, muscle tone, strength, pain, alignment, ROM, and movement. The physical therapist should determine the postural guidelines for the patient to incorporate and instruct the patient in basic body mechanics. For many patients, learning how to incorporate these measures into daily activities takes practice and experience. This can be done in OT, where there are activities of daily living (ADL) or work capacity stations. The occupational therapist needs to work very closely with the physical therapist.

Posture and alignment, although important, are only two factors that influence neck and back pain. Muscular tension and tightness are also critical and strongly influence spinal pain during functional tasks. For example, a person can drive with good alignment, but with the shoulders and back tight or relaxed, or a person can walk with the pelvis rigid and tight or, conversely, relaxed. Helping people learn to sit, walk, and work with the spine relaxed is a major challenge in back (or neck) treatment (Melvin, 1989).

An effective way to teach patients the desired body mechanics is to instruct them in the principles, present them with the activity, and have them incorporate the principles to accomplish the task. Solutions generated by the person do not have to be taught, but only reinforced. This process simplifies the therapist's job and empowers the patient—a win/win situation (Melvin, 1989).

The effectiveness of spinal protection methods for neck and low-back pain is enhanced when combined with relaxation training and strengthening exercises in physical therapy. Therapists who instruct patients in neck and back protection techniques should be knowledgeable about the patient's specific diagnoses as well as the indications and contraindications for each and the total conservative management of low-back pain. Information on neck and low-back pain is available in numerous resources (Bogduk & Twomey, 1987; Grant, 1994; Grieve, 1988; Hutson, 1990; Macnab & McCulloch, 1990; Saunders, 1985; White & Anderson, 1991).

SPINAL PROTECTION DURING ACTIVITIES OF DAILY LIVING

The following suggestions reflect common techniques for reducing strain on the neck and back. They are presented here only to stimulate ideas on how tasks can be done and are not hard and fast rules.

SITTING

Firm, straight-backed chairs with arms should be used rather than soft, overstuffed chairs. Rocking chairs that support the lower back may be helpful since they allow motions that may help ease back tension. The buttocks and sacrum should be as far back into the chair as possible, so that the backrest will support the back. A pillow to support the lumbar curve may be used if indicated. Sitting for prolonged periods increases compressive loading to the spine, and the person should get up every 20 to 30 minutes to take a stretch break. A timer is useful for remembering this.

SITTING FOR ACTIVITIES

Chair type, desk height, and lighting should facilitate proper posture of the neck, shoulder, and thoracic and lumbar spine. The lumbar spine and pelvis are the base on which the trunk rests, and the chair's position needs to address lumbar position if the cervical region is to achieve good alignment. Changing the position of the femur can change the lumbar curve. For every 3 degrees of femoral motion, the pelvis moves one degree. At approximately 135 degrees thigh-to-torso angle, the lumbar spine is said to be in an anatomically neutral position. By decreasing this angle (bringing the hip into more flexion) more lumbar flexion occurs, and increasing this angle (bringing the hip into more extension) increases lumbar extension (Bohannon, Gajdosic, & LeVeau, 1985;

Keegan, 1953). It is important to realize that everyone may have a slightly different neutral position depending upon the pathology. All patients should avoid a slouched or bent-forward position, which will tend to increase pressure on the intervertebral discs.

The types of activities that a person performs will affect the kind of seating required. A person who performs forward-sitting activities such as reaching, writing, or using a microscope generally has the eyes directed downward and will require a seat and backrest that is inclined forward. A small towel roll placed just posterior to the ischial tuberosities or a wedge-shaped pillow will also help to facilitate a neutral spine position while performing forward-sitting tasks. A person who performs upright-seated tasks such as eating, driving, or using a computer generally has the eyes focused straight ahead and will require a seat and backrest that will help maintain this upright position. A pillow can be used to support the lumbar curve. The third type of seated position is reclined with the eyes oriented upwards. Tasks such as conversing, reading, or relaxing may be performed in a reclined position and require a seat and backrest that are angled backward. The use of a foot prop under the desk or table may provide support in this position (Chaffin & Andersson, 1984).

A desk should be at a height that supports the forearms of the person sitting with the elbows close to the body. If the desk is too low, it become necessary to slouch to support the arms, and the lower the table, the more neck flexion is required to perform desk work. Conversely, if the table is too high, the shoulders will be elevated and cause increased compressive forces in the cervical region.

Prolonged writing should be done on an angle; for example, at a drafting table or on a tilted desk top. The angled work surface reduces the neck flexion necessary for horizontal work (Jackson, 1977). A convenient way to create a small angled work surface is to use a large three-ring binder angled with the rings away from the user, or prop a clipboard up at an angle. A cutting board or drawing board propped against the edge of a table or desk provides a larger working surface.

The person should always face the task directly. For example, when sitting and facing the desk, the person should not reach to pick up the telephone directory by twisting at the waist. He or she should turn the whole body toward the directory and pick it up using the arm muscles, not the back muscles. (Note: People typically lift moderately heavy desk items with their back muscles and need to be taught how to lift using only the arm muscles.) Objects such as telephones, computers, and desk materials should be located close to the body to avoid unnecessary reaching.

Reading. Prolonged reading should be done with the book at eye level on an angle with the desk or table. Bringing the materials up instead of bringing the head down and forward will help to decrease stress to posterior cervical structures. A variety of ergonomic copy holders and inexpensive book racks is available.

Reading slumped in a chair or bed with the neck in full flexion is contraindicated. For the person who cannot tolerate upright sitting for reading, however, the use of a reclining chair with the reading material propped on pillows on the lap may work well. As an alternative, it may be feasible to use a wedge under the head, neck, and back in the supine position with reading material propped on a pillow. A device called an Able Table can support reading material in various positions including sitting and supine.

Bifocal glasses that require hyperextension in order to use the reading portion are not recommended (Johnson & Wolfe, 1972). Bifocals with large lower portions, progressive (blended) lenses, or reading glasses are preferred. Poorly fitting frames may entail frequent repositioning of the head through repetitive cervical movements, which may stress the neck structures and surrounding musculature. All eyeglass users should be encouraged to have the alignment of their frames checked regularly.

Keyboard work. The draft copy should be placed just below eye level to facilitate proper head and neck alignment. A computer screen that is too high will lead to backward bending of the upper cervical spine and may lead to overuse of the suboccipital muscles. A screen that is too low may cause excessive cervical flexion. Placement of the draft copy may need to be altered depending on the type of work. For data entry, place the material from which the person is working straight in front of the visual field with the screen offset to one side to prevent the neck from being held in prolonged rotation to one side. Copy holders that can be attached to the screen are available in office supply stores. When editing typed work that requires looking back and forth from printed material to screen, slightly offset both from the center to help reduce cervical motion. The distance from the visual field will vary depending on the user's vision. A screen that is too far away may cause excessive strain of the suboccipital muscles as the person cranes the neck to see the screen.

Using the telephone. Frequent or prolonged use of a telephone can put severe stress on the neck muscles and cervical joints. The most efficient method for eliminating stress to the neck is the use of a headset, which also leaves the hands free to perform other tasks. A speakerphone is another alternative. Devices that attach to the receiver are not recommended because they require increased shoulder and scapular elevation to hold the receiver between the ear and the shoulder. Holding the receiver to the ear with the hand can be a preferable alternative if a headset or speakerphone are not available.

STANDING AND WALKING

Women and men should wear sturdy, low-heeled shoes. Insoles may provide additional shock absorption (see appendix A). Patients should avoid prolonged standing when possible. Placing one foot up on a low stool or phone book may decrease stress to the lower back. If prolonged standing cannot be avoided, shift weight from one foot to the other; this can be facilitated by standing with the feet on a diagonal. Maintaining good low-back alignment and periodically contracting the abdominal muscles will help increase endurance in standing. Slightly flex the knees while standing and avoid the tendency to lock them in extension. Patients should be sure to avoid standing mainly on one leg with the opposite hip dropped.

Doors should open widely enough to walk through comfortably. Patients in an acute or postacute phase may want to avoid crowded conditions, sports events, and theaters, as these often require turning sideways to walk through such areas. People should at least be conscious of back alignment. The safest solution may be to wear a lumbar corset or cervical collar in these situations.

When walking distances, the person should avoid carrying heavy objects. A "fanny pack" helps keep the load close to the center of gravity and does not add stress to the neck and lower back.

DRIVING

The person should get into the car by sitting on the side of the seat and pivoting into the car, keeping the knees together. To facilitate proper spinal alignment, the seat may need adjusting closer to or farther from the steering wheel. The closer the seat, the more spinal flexion will be encouraged as it will bring the hips and knees into more flexion. If the person is more comfortable in spinal extension, the use of a pillow to support the lumbar curve may be necessary.

Mirrors can be added or adjusted to minimize neck motion. A side mirror on the right side of the car and bubble mirrors attached to both side mirrors can help reduce the need for turning to see blind spots (a task not possible with significant spinal disease, limited ROM, or muscle spasm).

Headrests should be high enough to prevent neck hyperextension. Permanent headrests that are set too far back should be built up with special pads or straps.

For long periods of driving, especially on highways, persons with arthritis can be advised to change the position of the hands on the steering wheel. Instead of holding the hands at 10 o'clock and 2 o'clock, they can change to 4 o'clock and 8 o'clock. This brings the arms in closer to the trunk and shorten the lever arms of the upper extremities.

For severe back problems, a lumbar back support with or without a molded insert may be indicated during distance driving.

Seat belts and shoulder harnesses should always be used to minimize danger in the event of a sudden stop. If prolonged driving exacerbated by associated vibratory forces increases the risk of low back problems, special antivibration pillows are available. Learning conscious-relaxation techniques and periodically assessing and relaxing the shoulders while driving can reduce fatigue and pain associated with driving.

LIFTING AND TRANSPORTING OBJECTS

When lifting items from below waist height (e.g., on a low shelf or on the floor), the object should be faced, and the feet positioned about 12 inches apart with one foot forward; the person then squats down, keeping the spine in neutral (as if doing a deep knee bend). The hands should be placed underneath the object, if possible. Then, keeping the object in close to the body, the person straightens from the hips and knees keeping the spine in neutral. It may be beneficial to tighten the abdominal and buttock muscles to assist with the lift. Lifting with the back by keeping the legs straight and bending at the waist is contraindicated because the mechanical stress to the third to fifth lumbar vertebrae is excessive and approximately 150 percent greater than with the leg-lift method. (Note: The recommended method of lifting with the legs is included in all body mechanics literature; however, a person needs strong quadriceps muscles and good knee joints to carry out this advice. Professional furniture movers and truck drivers with low back problems would have no trouble, but the average person will probably need instruction in strengthening to benefit from this method. Patients often need quite a bit of practice to incorporate this method spontaneously.) Assistance should be sought to lift any items that cannot be lifted in the recommended manner.

Heavy items should not be lifted overhead since this will increase the tendency toward lumbar and cervical hyperextension and increase compressive forces generated in the cervical region. When removing lightweight items from a high shelf, (1) use a step-stool whenever possible, (2) place one foot on a sturdy step to ease low back muscle tension, or (3) place one foot forward toward the object to be reached for, with body weight on the forward foot. As the object is brought down, weight is transferred to the back foot, keeping the back in as neutral a position as possible. The process is reversed for placing an object on the shelf. The feet should not be placed even or parallel when reaching high, as it increases the tendency to arch or hyperextend the spine, especially the thoracic and lumbar regions.

Objects should be carried as close to the body as possible because stress to the spine increases in proportion to the distance of the object from the spine. Avoid carrying heavy objects that require leaning backwards for balance because back hyperextension considerably increases spinal pressure. Objects should be slid instead of lifted whenever possible, and the spine kept in good alignment. Loads should not be unbalanced for carrying. Substitute a nylon carrying bag with shoulder strap for a heavy briefcase or purse, or, better still, use a suitcase on wheels. Newer models can be pushed rather than pulled and allow use of the arm and body in better position.

When pushing an object, keep one foot forward with knees bent, the abdominal muscles tightened to help keep the spine straight, and then use the leg (quadriceps) muscles to move the object.

REST IN BED

Recommended sleeping positions for reducing the lordotic curve are: (1) side-lying with knees and hips flexed (fetal position), or (2) supine with pillows under knees (contraindicated if the knees are involved). If the goal is to maintain or increase the lumbar curve, a lumbar roll or towel roll around the waist may be helpful.

Sleeping in the prone position is contraindicated for patients with neck dysfunction because it maintains the neck in rotation and extension for prolonged periods. Lying prone is not recommended for patients with back dysfunction. If, for some reason, it is essential, a small pillow under the pelvis will reduce the lumbar curve. For persons who have difficulty falling asleep when not in prone because they are used to the contact of the bed against the anterior chest, a body pillow (two to three times longer then a normal pillow) can be used to create a 3/4 prone position. This may improve alignment of the head, neck, and back and allow the patient to sleep more comfortably. When lying in bed, the person should avoid reaching overhead or resting the arms behind the head, since this increases the lordotic curve and spinal pressure.

When rising from a lying position, the person can roll to the side, moving hips and shoulders together to avoid twisting at the trunk, and slide to the edge of the bed. Then, keeping the back straight, the person can use the arms to push up to a sitting position while lowering the feet to the floor.

A firm mattress with a top layer of foam or feathers and firm box springs should be used. Persons are encouraged to try a variety of mattresses before buying one. A bed board (3/4-inch plywood) placed between the box springs and mattress should be a last resort, when it is not possible to purchase a firm bed. The value of a waterbed for neck or back pain is uncertain and appears to depend on the individual. The supportive effect depends on how much it is filled. An air-filled or padded bumper facilitates transfer in and out of bed.

Electric blankets or down comforters are often helpful since they provide consistent warmth and are lightweight and easy to manage. Because of the possible effects of electromagnetic radiation, the use of electric blankets is now discouraged except to warm the bed prior to getting in. An electric blanket should be turned off before going to sleep.

A variety of fillings exists for pillows. Down, feathers, and some synthetic fillings conform well, but foam rubber tends to be unyielding. Various types of air and foam pillows are also now available; one is by Tempurpedic and has had good success with a wide variety of patients with cervical dysfunction.

The type of pillow one uses is important and will vary depending upon the position assumed. In supine, the thickness or number of pillows used will depend on the amount of thoracic kyphosis. If the person has a flat or normal thoracic kyphosis, he or she will usually benefit from one thin to medium-size pillow. Sleeping on too many pillows will result in excessive neck flexion. With an increased kyphosis, two pillows may be necessary to support the head and prevent cervical hyperextension. In side-lying, the thickness of the pillow will be related to the "empty space" between the head and the shoulder. People with very wide shoulders will require thicker pillows. If the head is not properly supported then the person will tend to be in cervical lateral flexion for a prolonged period. The Cervipillo®, a round tubular pillow designed for cervical pain, helps maintain optimal neck alignment in supine and side-lying by conforming to the cervical contours (Jackson, 1977). For more acute patients, sleeping with a cervical collar or a towel roll safety-pinned around the neck may provide better support. It is support to the neck that is needed, not to the head.

Persons with respiratory difficulties or gastrointestinal reflux who need head elevation should raise the head of the bed 4 to 8 inches on blocks, since thick multiple pillows will cause excessive neck flexion.

SEXUAL POSITIONING

The recommended positions are those that allow hip and knee flexion (e.g., the lower position in the traditional male-superior position or various side-lying positions). Many, if not most, patients are able to alter their position to accommodate back pain without any advice. However, many patients use only the traditional position and may need to hear advice from an authoritative medical person to consider alternative methods (Grieve, 1988; Hebert, 1992). Patient education booklets are available for patients (Arthritis Foundation; Herbert, 1994; see Resources).

SELF-CARE

In general, commonly used items should be placed within easy reach. Reaching high or low requires end ranges of spinal extension or flexion.

Dressing. Lower-extremity dressing (including shoes) should be done from a sitting position, bending the knees one at a time instead of the back. If dressing in this manner is not possible, devices such as a long-handled shoe horn, dressing stick, and stocking aid are helpful. For more acute patients, lower-extremity dressing in the supine position may be a more comfortable alternative, as the back is completely supported. Donning and doffing shoes can be made easier by encouraging the use of slip-ons or elastic shoe laces.

Comfortable garments with front openings should be used to minimize the need for twisting during upper-extremity dressing. Putting on pullover garments may require cervical hyperextension and is best avoided.

Hair care. Washing the hair over a sink will create excessive neck flexion and should be avoided. The hair should be shampooed in the shower, where proper neck and back alignment can be maintained. The person should be instructed to position him or herself so that hyperextension is not required, especially when rinsing.

Bathing. Whether bathing or showering, a cloth back-scrubber (one pulled from side to side) for back washing is better than a long-handled brush. A long-handled back-brush, however, is helpful for lower extremity washing.

Facial hygiene. Keep the neck in good alignment when using a washcloth on the face. The neck can be put into hyperextension by leaning over a basin to splash water into the face or brush the teeth. If bending over the sink is necessary, it should be done by bending at the hips and knees—not at the waist—and maintaining a neutral back position and a slight chin tuck. For men, an electric shaver requires less hyperextension than a safety razor. Shaving can also be done in the shower.

Drinking. Drinking from bottles, small glasses, or cans for which the head must be tipped back should be avoided. Wide-mouth glasses and cups or straws are recommended.

HOUSE AND YARD CARE

Light and heavier tasks can be alternated and interspersed with short rest breaks to avoid fatigue (see section on fatigue management and energy conservation). Unnecessary motions and tasks should be eliminated. Equipment and supplies should be located above the floor, and adaptive equipment such as long handles and ergonomically designed tools reduce the need for bending over.

Mopping, vacuuming, sweeping, and raking. When using long-handled equipment, the material or area being cleaned should be faced. The work should be done in front, not to the side, to minimize twisting. Keeping the knees slightly bent while working also helps reduce the tendency to twist. The feet should be kept moving. The tendency is to move the trunk and keep the feet fixed, but if the tool is held close to the body, then the lever arm is reduced and the stress to the back is decreased.

Washing the car, walls, or windows. For areas above head level, keep one foot on a stepstool or use a stepladder. Keep the feet at different levels and position the ladder as closely as possible. For the lower area, kneel (as described for lifting) or squat, and keep the back straight. Place the water bucket and cleaning materials on a chair or stool to avoid bending.

Bed-making. Raising the bed 3 to 4 inches on blocks will help minimize bending. If this is not sufficient or possible, an alternate method is to make the bed while kneeling. The bed can be moved away from the wall or be put on casters for easy moving. Straightening the covers while in bed before arising will minimize this daily chore. A down comforter can reduce the weight of covers.

Cleaning the bathtub. After bathing in the tub, putting a strong detergent into the water can reduce or prevent bathtub ring and reduce the need for scrubbing. An extended-handle brush can be used for cleaning.

Washing and drying clothes. Front-loading washers and dryers are preferred over top-loading models because they allow loading from a kneeling or squatting position, or from a low stool. The top-loader requires bending over the top to remove the load. If only a top-loader is available, one can use a "golfer's bend" (Melnick et al., 1989) where one leg is extended behind the body to help maintain the lumbar spine's neutral position. Washing smaller loads of laundry more frequently means there will be smaller loads to transfer. Lower the clothesline to shoulder height and elevate the wash basket with a chair or table.

Infant and Child Care

Always use the arm or leg muscles rather than the back muscles when lifting an infant. To avoid bending, have small children stand on a chair or step-stool for dressing or facial hygiene. Kneel while washing a child in the tub. When transferring a child in and out of the car, try to get in as close as possible. Swivel car seats for infants and children eliminate the need for twisting. Consider the weight of equipment such as strollers and carriers before purchasing.

INSTRUCTION IN NECK PROTECTION

A mirror is an excellent teaching tool for training a person to achieve and maintain proper lateral neck alignment. Use a three-way mirror to observe anterior-posterior alignment. This is particularly effective because there are no visual body clues regarding neck position when the head is in proper postural alignment (Melvin, 1989). People who have developed poor postural habits will require retraining to learn where the correct head-and-neck position is.

A soft neck collar can be excellent for instructing people in neck protection techniques because it serves as a reminder of proper cervical position. This technique is effective for those persons who do not have fixed postural deformities and have the ability to correct their alignment. The collar can be worn while practicing activities in a correct manner. Once a person has learned the proper way to position the neck, the collar should be discontinued and used only during prolonged activities that place stress on the neck or that the person finds too difficult to do without support. Using a collar only as a teaching aid versus having the patient wear it all the time needs to be cleared with the referring physician. As an alternative, use a towel roll fastened with a safety pin or Velcro®.

In patients with cervical involvement, it is essential to consider not only the posture of the neck but also the posture of the shoulders, thoracic and lumbar spine, and pelvis. Another helpful teaching tool may be the use of an upper-back support. These supports serve as postural reminders for the person who tends to maintain the shoulders in an internally rotated position with the thoracic spine in flexion.

Educating a person to move the entire trunk properly may also help to lessen stress to the neck. For example, in the case of a person with limited cervical rotation who is having difficulty turning the head to back a car out of a driveway, he or she could be instructed to shift weight through the pelvis and use the available ROM in the lumbar and thoracic regions to see what is behind (using car mirrors may be preferable).

For a patient with cervical subluxation, a soft or semirigid (Plastazote®) collar should be used when indicated, especially during activities with a high risk of neck injury such as being a passenger in a car. (For patients with limited hand or shoulder involvement, it is helpful if the collar can be adapted with a side opening.) The type of collar used should be discussed with the referring physician.

FATIGUE MANAGEMENT AND ENERGY CONSERVATION

Fatigue is one of the most disabling aspects of rheumatic disease. McCarty (1993) noted that 80% of patients with RA complained of fatigue. Fatigue peaked 4 to 5 hours after arising with the interval varying inversely with the disease activity. Of patients with SLE, 80-100% complain of fatigue (Schur, 1993). Calin, Edwards, and Kennedy (1993) reported that fatigue was the most important symptom for more than 50% of patients with ankylosing spondylitis. The American College of Rheumatology Multicenter Criteria Committee for Fibromyalgia found 80% of these patients reported fatigue (Wolfe, Smythe, Yunus, et al., 1990).

In a descriptive, exploratory study of fatigue in 20 patients with RA (Tack, 1990), the comment of one participant was, "I would rather do an activity with pain than be wiped out with fatigue. With the pain, I would cook the dinner and just find a different way to do it. With the fatigue, I couldn't even attempt it. I don't have any control" (p. 67).

Fatigue has been described as the enduring subjective sensation of generalized tiredness or exhaustion (Belza, 1995a). To healthy people, rest brings relief; not so for the person with a chronic illness such as arthritis. The cause of fatigue may not be readily apparent. A good night's sleep alone may not completely relieve the fatigue, and the fatigue condition may not be transient (Tack, 1990).

Fatigue can have a muscle component or be more generalized. The generalized fatigue called exhaustion is multidimensional, may be of central-nervous-system origin, and may consist of emotional, behavioral, and cognitive components (Goldenberg, 1995). Fatigue in the inflammatory rheumatic diseases generally refers to the more generalized form. Fatigue severity is associated with joint pain, poorer overall mood, depression (Tack, 1990), fragmented sleep, and reduced functional abilities (Crosby, 1991). Inefficient joint movement resulting from swelling in the joint can use more energy than normal motion, as can the psychological stress of a fluctuating disease that does not allow the person to predict from day to day the level of functional capacity or pain that will be present (Gerber, 1985). Crosby considered that reducing pain through medication, rest, and splinting would perhaps improve the quality of sleep, enhance functional abilities, and reduce the level of fatigue.

Melvin (1989) determines a person's energy pattern using the following interview questions: Pattern or time of peak and low energy? Time of day fatigue occurs? Duration of fatigue? How does the person handle the fatigue? (What does he or she do to improve endurance or reduce fatigue? Takes naps or pushes through the day?) What factors besides illness contribute to the person's fatigue or endurance level? Melvin uses these data for planning education related to energy conservation, exercise, rest, relaxation techniques, improving sleep patterns, and psychological support for reducing depression.

Tack (1990) considered those activities and thoughts that generated energy for the individual as "energy enhancers." These included social resources (family, friends, coworkers), cognitive processes (distraction, energy audits, renormalization), and behavioral responses (taking time out and organizing one's environment to reduce walking, standing, reaching).

The cognitive process of "distraction" allows the person to ignore temporarily the fatigue. Work and pleasurable leisure activities are important distracters because they can improve mood and therefore energy. "Energy audits" take stock of how much energy one has and what activities are still to be done in an upcoming time. Energy is rationed based on a fatigue assessment similar to the way a dieter counts calories. "Renormalization" is readjusting to reduced activities (Weiner, 1975). Tack (1990) quoted one of her subjects as saying, "Having limited energy has made me look at what is really important in my life."

Organizing one's environment, taking time out (resting), and pacing activities are some of the steps a person can use to moderate fatigue. Recommending the alternation of heavy and light tasks is useful. For example, keyboard use can be broken up by filing or copying, and home vacuuming broken up by dusting.

Finding the balance of rest and activity is a fundamental aspect of energy conservation and fatigue management. The most effective method to increase functional endurance is to rest before becoming tired (Melvin, 1989). Taking a 5-10 minute rest during activities is difficult but can significantly increase overall functional endurance. The concept of resting for 10 minutes in the middle of vacuuming is totally foreign for the majority of homemakers. This practice implies lengthening the total time spent doing housework, and the desire to get housework over with is usually strong. Resting is also effective during activities such as shop work, gardening, yard work, or shopping; sitting for only a few minutes *before* one becomes tired will greatly expand the total endurance for the activity. Working to fatigue before stopping makes it harder to resume the task. Rest breaks during work not only increase functional endurance but also allow more energy for activities the person enjoys.

Resting before one becomes tired or exhausted is so effective that it should be the number-one priority in energy-conservation instruction. Once a person employs this practice, the benefits are usually self evident. With encouragement and self-discipline, patient and therapist can use this process to advantage (Melvin, 1989). This was shown in the 6-week course of energy conservation and joint protection training for patients with RA (Furst et. al., 1987) in which participants took a 10-minute rest after each 20 minute segment of a prolonged task. The 10 minutes of rest could include reading, watching TV, relaxation tapes, etc. As a result, 50% of these persons increased the amount of time they were active, compared with 11% of controls (Gerber et al., 1987).

Fatigue secondary to chronic illness is often progressive and of long-standing duration. Packer, Sauriol, and Brower (1994) were encouraged that preliminary results of their course of energy conservation for patients with postpolio syndrome, chronic-fatigue syndrome, and other conditions found positive trends in decreasing fatigue severity and impact in only 6 weeks. They proposed energy management as a positive concept that implied choice, a sense of control, and positive participation in activity. Energy management has two main concepts: banking energy (saving energy by using efficient body mechanics, rearranging work areas, using technology, simplifying, and delegating activities) and budgeting energy (deciding on which activities to spend the energy). Three steps are involved in planning energy expenditure: (1) Examine priorities, (2) examine standards, and (3) make choices and decisions about activities. The goal is to spend energy on what is most important. Furst and colleagues (1985) recommend specific steps for accomplishing activities that cause pain and fatigue (see Table 6).

The *Energy Conservation and Joint Protection Workbook* of Furst and colleagues (1985) and the *Managing Fatigue Manual* by Packer, Brink, and Sauriol (1995) provide techniques for combating fatigue in people with limited energy. They do not address increasing energy for patients with RA through endurance training that involves repeated exercise of large muscle groups of sufficient intensity to evoke a moderate cardiovascular

HOW TO ACCOMPLISH ACTIVITIES THAT CAUSE PAIN AND FATIGUE

1. Take rest breaks during the activity.
2. Analyze the activity:
   - time of day the activity is done
   - body position during the activity
   - height of work surfaces
   - location of supplies and equipment
3. Break the activity down into parts.
4. Use adaptive equipment.
5. Consider eliminating the activity.
6. Have someone else do the activity.
7. Plan your regular activities for the coming week.
   a. Divide jobs into heavy and light.
   b. Balance light and heavy activities and rest periods.
   c. Consider which jobs can be changed and which are fixed.
   d. Consider which jobs can be done by others.
   e. Analyze and change or eliminate jobs.
   f. Plan fewer activities for days when evening activities are planned.
8. Planning your time helps others plan their time.

Table 6: How to Accomplish Activities That Cause Pain and Fatigue (Furst, 1985)

response (Belza, 1995b); nor do they address the influence that speed has on energy. Fatigue can strike suddenly in anyone if he or she tries to do things too quickly. Therefore, don't rush: take your time.

JOINT PROTECTION FOR OSTEOARTHRITIS

Osteoarthritis affects primarily articular cartilage and subchondral bone. The joints may show an inflammatory response, but there is no systemic disease as in RA. Osteoarthritis does not have the proliferating synovium that in RA can elongate and destroy joint capsules, ligaments, and tendons.

Bland (1997b) prefers to consider OA an active process by which the body attempts to repair itself following injury, that joints are complex organs, and that their successful function is not simply the consequence of a single tissue or structure. All the tissues around a joint are involved. For example, healthy knee joints have a negative or subatmospheric pressure creating a suction force. Bland (1997a) suggests that this suction plays a part in stabilizing joints by drawing the articulating surfaces into the best possible fit as they move through ROM. This guidance is impaired and increased strain put on ligament and cartilage if the joint develops an effusion and thus develops a positive pressure.

It does not take a large effusion to have a profound effect upon joint function. For example, 20 ml of extra fluid are sufficient to cause a reflex inhibition of the action of quadriceps vastus medialis (Spencer, Hayes, & Alexander, 1984). Control of joint effusion is an essential part of management.

Healthy joints cannot wear out; the lubrication is so efficient that the friction in them is about that of rubbing ice against ice. But unguided motion resulting from ligamentous laxity and abnormalities of joint shape results in tensile (pulling) forces on articular cartilage, which is vulnerable to damage in this way. Under load, the leading and following edges of the bearing surfaces will dig into the cartilage in what is known as "plowing." Functional orthoses may be used to give stability to the rheumatoid arthritic joint and block movement toward increased deformity, but functional orthoses for the hand should never reposition the joints to correct the deformity (Brewerton, 1973; Quest & Cordery, 1971). A different and dangerous pattern of "plowing" could result.

Articular cartilage is strong in compression. It transmits loads to the underlying subchondral bone, and both act as shock absorbers. However, the cartilage is too thin to protect against repetitive impact loading, which produces the most destructive effects on cartilage. Major factors that attenuate forces delivered to the joint are joint motion together with the associated lengthening of muscles under tension, and deformation of subchondral bone (Brandt & Mankin, 1993). Bland (1997a) points out in volume 2 of this series that the principal protection to ordinary joints is through neuromuscular mechanisms and normally functioning proprioceptors. Since the reaction time to prepare the neuromuscular apparatus reflexively for an impact load is about 75 milliseconds, unexpected falls of only about one inch do not allow sufficient time to activate these protective reflexes. We have all experienced the spine-shaking jar that comes with stepping off what we thought was a last step when it was not. The load goes to articular cartilage, subchondral bone, and ligaments, and can result in injury even to a healthy person. McCloy (1982) recommends that activities involving a faster reaction time than the neuromuscular system is capable of, such as tennis and jogging, should be discouraged for persons with OA.

Factors that lead to muscle fatigue would tend to impair this shock-absorbing mechanism (Brandt & Mankin, 1993), as would muscle weakness and atrophy. Bland (1997b) recommends that patients be educated in joint physiology, including the role of the proprioceptors.

Most of the force across a joint is the major product of muscular contraction and not of weight bearing. Joints of the upper extremity are therefore probably subjected to stress (force per unit area) similar to those of the lower extremity joints (Radin, 1987). Brandt (1993) considers it important that every patient with OA have an analysis of his or her vocational and avocational use of the involved joint to find activities that result in excessive loading of the joint and recommend measures that will avoid or ameliorate them. Bland (1997b) proposes that underuse of joints could be harmful because the joint remodeling that occurs in response to stress is not operating properly, and so loss of ROM and damage to the cartilage occur.

OA does not progress inexorably (Brandt, 1993); a survey of 682 elderly people showed that prevalence and severity of symptoms suggestive of OA of the knee increased with age but remained constant from the seventh through the ninth decades.

Brandt (1993) states that "measures that protect the involved joint from mechanical damage, instructing the patient in the use of assistive devices; in patterns of joint use that avoid excessive loading of the articular cartilage; strengthening the supporting muscles to increase joint stability are important in diminishing pain and discomfort. . . . Although no evidence is available to indicate such measures are prophylatic, it is logical to consider that they may retard or prevent progression of the disease by preventing further cartilage damage" (p. 1385).

JOINT PROTECTION WITH OSTEOARTHRITIS: RATIONALE AND TREATMENT IMPLICATIONS

At first consideration, joint-protection principles designed to reduce loading on the fragile capsules, ligaments, and tendons of joints with RA might seem unpromising in reducing loading on articular cartilage and subchondral bone in osteoarthritis. But joint protection principles are appropriate for OA, although they are based on a different rationale. For OA, protection is directed to strengthening the muscular support and shock absorption for a joint, reducing total load on the joint with different techniques or devices, managing inflammation, avoiding pain (which inhibits muscle strength and function), and getting physically fit to reduce muscle tiredness and fatigue.

(1) INCREASE MUSCLE STRENGTH AND FITNESS

Increasing muscle strength is thought to protect a joint by reducing load and providing a more efficient shock absorber (Schnitzer, 1993). Strengthening the supporting muscles increases joint stability and reduces or eliminates pain (Brandt, 1993). Joint stability reduces the risk of "plowing" the articular cartilage. Improving muscle strength is also important for maintaining ROM. Muscle strengthening is now frequently addressed through a fitness or aquatics exercise program.

Patients with OA have poor endurance due in part to pain and inactivity, and they are generally overweight. Aerobic exercise has been shown to be beneficial and safe (Minor, Hewelt, Webel, Anderson, & Kay, 1989). It may even be prophylactic. Individuals who maintained a regular weight-bearing exercise program were shown to exhibit less osteophyte formation at the hip (Michel, Fries, Bloch, Lane, & Jones, 1992). Bland (1997b) considers that educating the older population in maintaining optimum overall fitness is probably the greatest deterrent to the development of osteoarthritis.

(2) MAINTAIN JOINT RANGE OF MOTION

Maintaining as full a ROM as possible enables the joint to distribute the load over the largest area. Joint position is critical for optimal function of muscles, and normal

ROM with normal loading (Palmoski, Colyer, & Brandt, 1980) maintains healthy cartilage and joint mobility through lubrication of the joint (Bland, 1997a; Maehlums, 1994).
It enables the joint to work at a biomechanical advantage and therefore with the greatest
efficiency. Change of ROM of one joint will cause loads to be transmitted (unduly) to
another.

(3) REDUCE EXCESSIVE LOADING ON JOINTS

Although cartilage needs intermittent compression for its health, activities that cause
excessive loading of involved joints should be avoided wherever possible (Brandt, 1993).
To lower the overall force across a joint, one can use the muscles more efficiently so they
do not have to contract as strongly to have the same effect (Radin, Paul, & Rose, 1975).
The load being carried on an involved joint can be reduced by using and carrying lighter-
weight objects and equipment, using assistive devices and ambulation aids (Neuman &
Hase, 1994), and by eliminating activities such as stair climbing and single-leg standing
(e.g., to get in and out of a tub). Swimming and biking are better sports than tennis or
jogging. Peak dynamic load can be attenuated by adding shock absorbers (Radin, 1987).
Thick rubber mats to stand on have helped ticket agents with OA of the lumbar spine;
viscoelastic shoe inserts have reduced pain in the OA knee; and better shock absorbers
have reduced vibration for truck and bus drivers.

(4) AVOID PAIN IN ACTIVITIES

Pain plays a different role in OA compared to RA. In OA the major structure to be
protected is the articular cartilage, which has no nerve supply and is, therefore, insensitive
to pain. Pain with OA has little value as a warning signal (compared with RA). When pain
occurs it is related to inflammation, weight-bearing on thin cartilage, or pressure from
osteophytes. Inflammation can increase osteophytosis. Pain can lead to protective muscle
splinting, which will restrict joint ROM. Pain during use of an involved joint causes
uncoordinated function, which can lead to undesirable joint loading. Any activity or posture that causes pain should be avoided. Muscle strengthening, stabilizing orthoses, assistive devices, and modification of activities can reduce pain.

(5) BALANCE ACTIVITY AND REST

Persons with OA do not have a systemic disease to create exhaustion as do those
with inflammatory joint diseases. The person with OA may be biomechanically inefficient, however, and expend more energy than a person without OA on everyday activities
such as walking (Schnitzer, 1993). He or she may also be physically deconditioned.

Brandt (1993) recommends rest periods of 30 to 60 minutes in the morning and
afternoon to diminish discomfort in lower extremity joints and the lumbar spine. Several
shorter periods are more desirable. Women in a group workshop for OA of the hands
appreciated the "legitimization of rest periods, not so easy in our demanding culture with
norms of efficacy and production" (Schreuer, Palmon, & Nahir, 1994).

Some persons with OA consider that they can prevent stiffness by using their joints continuously. This should be discouraged, as it can contribute to inflammation and pain (Brandt, 1993). Instead, the person can have demonstrated the advantages of substituting ROM carried out intermittently.

Tired muscles cannot take control of the loading of the joint or act properly as shock absorbers. They cannot act fully to protect articular cartilage. Increasing physical fitness and muscle strength and taking intermittent rest periods are helpful.

(6) AVOID STAYING IN ONE POSITION FOR LONG PERIODS

People with OA are prone to "gelling," stiffness and discomfort that occur after periods of inactivity. Instructing the patient to put the involved limb through its ROM every 15 to 20 minutes may minimize stiffness and facilitate muscle function (Brandt, 1993). In addition, muscles tire quickly in static holding and are less effective in supporting the joint.

THE AMERICANS WITH DISABILITIES ACT (ADA)

The ADA requires employers to make "reasonable accommodations" to help persons perform the "essential elements" of their jobs. In the office, ergonomic computer equipment, ergonomic chairs, telephone headsets, and large-button phones and calculators are all comparatively inexpensive and, therefore, can be considered reasonable. A carpenter or other tradesperson can ask for ergonomic tools; the worker who must stand can ask for a cushioned mat to stand on or a step on which to rest feet. Changing door knobs from the round type to levers would assist everybody.

Specific ADA requirements are being phased in slowly and, for the individual, are still in the process of definition. Publications and information can be obtained by calling the Equal Employment Opportunity Commission (EEOC) at (800) 669-3362. The location of the nearest EEOC office can be found by calling (800) 669-4000.

QUESTIONS FOR RESEARCH INTO JOINT PROTECTION AND ENERGY CONSERVATION

The most pressing aspect of joint-protection research is to identify whether or not it has effectiveness in preserving joint function. Although demonstrating effectiveness is exceedingly difficult, further descriptive studies would be helpful. For example, the broad classification of hand use in OA (Lane et al., 1989) could be refined, and the preliminary activity analysis of hand use in housework by women with RA (Fitinghoff, Söderback, & Nordeman, 1994), an excellent beginning, could be expanded. Analysis and categorization of "hand use" would be a step on the way to seeing if patterns of hand use were related to the development of rheumatoid deformity (Feinberg & Trombley, 1995; Hasselkus, 1981; Palmer & Simons,1989).

Each deformity needs to be analyzed more precisely and its stages identified. With the development of new imaging techniques, will it be possible to measure the subtle shifts of tendons and ligamentous structures in early RA? Can methods of measurement of the various deformities be developed to provide objective and sensitive methods of assessing progression that are applicable during functional use? This is where the collaboration of the bioengineers would be most helpful if they can be encouraged to become involved. Another important area to explore with bioengineers is whether or not the joint-protection methods proposed for reducing the forces on joints during activities actually do reduce them.

Reports of reduction in pain after joint-protection instruction have been mainly anecdotal or observed as part of other studies. Does the behavioral change last when pain is reduced but protection needs to be continued for the then-unstable joints?

The pilot studies in energy conservation and fatigue management were relatively short-term with small numbers of participants. Will the results be confirmed in larger, longer-term studies? Were the instruments used to detect change sufficiently sensitive? What are the differences in approach or results between such conditions as RA, fibromyalgia, and other diagnoses? For patients who are in such programs but do not change behavior, what factors prevent them from adopting new habits?

Many of the attempts to change behavior by making a change in knowledge (traditional hand-outs, discussion) have been largely unsuccessful. Using cognitive, behavioral, and learning theories to develop teaching programs has been effective in arthritis patient education (see chapter 2, Patient Education, and chapter 3, Adherence). Only a few education programs for joint protection have used such theories, and more work needs to be done.

Palmer and Simons (1991) pointed out the mounting evidence for the importance of psychological factors in disease progression. If the ultimate goal is to reduce disability, they asked, should therapists, instead of teaching joint protection, be adopting a more psychodynamic approach? Leonard (1995) considers that living comfortably with a chronic condition requires lifelong commitment to protective methods.

But are these two differing views mutually exclusive? How is this question and all others to be answered? By research and by clinicians who, in their everyday work, are close to people with rheumatic disease. Only by research can anecdote and opinion be changed into fact and action, and—in this era of managed care—only by research into outcomes can the use of therapists' time be validated.

REFERENCES

Agnew, P. J. (1987). Joint protection in arthritis: Fact or fiction. *British Journal of Occupational Therapy, 50*, 227-230.

Bell-Krotoski, J. A., Breger-Lee, D., & Beach, R. B. (1995). Biomechanics and evaluation of the hand. In Hunter, Mackin, Callahan (Eds.), *Rehabilitation of the hand*, Vol 1 (4th ed.). St. Louis, MO: Mosby.

Belza, B. (1995a). Comparison of self-reported fatigue in rheumatoid arthritis and controls. *Journal of Rheumatology, 22*, 639-643.

Belza, B. (1995b). Fatigue modulation program. Presented at Association of Rheumatology Health Professionals, San Francisco, CA.

Bennett, R. L. (1965). Orthotic devices to prevent deformities in rheumatoid arthritis. *Arthritis and Rheumatism, 8*, 1006-1018.

Bland, J. H. (in press-a). Pathophysiology of cartilage and joint structures in the adult rheumatic diseases. In J. Melvin & G. M. Jensen (Eds.), *Rheumatologic rehabilitation*, Vol. 2. Bethesda, MD: American Occupational Therapy Association.

Bland, J. H. (in press-b). Osteoarthritis. In J. Melvin & G. M. Jensen (Eds.), *Rheumatologic rehabilitation*, Vol. 2. Bethesda, MD: American Occupational Therapy Association.

Bogduk, N., & Twomey, L. (1987). *Clinical anatomy of the lumbar spine.* New York: Churchill Livingstone.

Bohannan, R. J., Gajdosic, R., & LeVeau, B. (1985). Relationship of pelvic and thigh motion during unilateral and bilateral hip flexion. *Physical Therapy 65*, 1501-1504.

Brandt, K. D. (1993). Management of osteoarthritis. In W. N. Kelly, E. D. Harris, S. Ruddy, & C. B. Sledge, (Eds.), *Textbook of rheumatology* (4th ed.). Philadelphia, PA: Saunders.

Brandt, K. D., & Mankin, H. J. (1993). Pathogenesis of osteoarthritis. In W. N. Kelley, E. D. Harris, S. Ruddy, & C. B. Sledge (Eds.), *Textbook of rheumatology* (4th ed.). Philadelphia, PA: Saunders.

Brewerton, D. A., & Lettin, A. W. F. (1973). The rheumatoid hand and its management. In C. B. Wynn Parry, *Rehabilitation of the hand* (3rd ed.). London: Butterworth.

Buckland-Wright, J. C., Macfarlane, D. G., & Lynch, J. A. (1991). Osteophytes in the osteoarthritic hand: their incidence, size, distribution and progression. *Annals of the Rheumatic Diseases, 50*, 627-630.

Calin, A., Edwards, L., & Kennedy, L. G. (1993). Fatigue in ankylosing spondylitis: Why is it ignored? *Journal of Rheumatology, 20*, 991-995.

Castillo, B. A., El Sallab, R. A., & Scott, J. T. (1965). Physical activity, cystic erosions and osteoporosis in RA. *Annals of Rheumatic Disease, 24*, 522-527.

Chaffin, D. B., & Andersson, G. (1984). *Occupational biomechanics.* New York: Wiley.

Chamberlain, M. A. (1994). Strategies to prevent disability and lessen its impact. In J. H. Kippel & P. A. Dieppe (Eds.), *Rheumatology*. St. Louis, MO: Mosby.

Chamberlain, M. A., Ellis, M., & Hughes, D. (1984). Joint protection. *Clinics in Rheumatic Diseases, 10*, 727-742.

Cordery, J. C. (1962). The conservation of physical resources as applied to the activities of patients with arthritis and connective tissue diseases. *Study course III. Third International Congress, World Federation of Occupational Therapists.* Dubuque, IA: William C. Brown.

Cordery, J. C. (1965). Joint protection: A responsibility of the occupational therapist. *American Journal of Occupational Therapy, 19*, 285-294.

Crosby, L. J. (1991). Factors which contribute to fatigue associated with rheumatoid arthritis. *Journal of Advanced Nursing, 16*, 974-981.

Eng, J., & Pierrynowski, M. (1993). Evaluation of soft foot orthotics in the treatment of patellofemoral pain syndrome. *Physical Therapy, 73*, 62-70.

Feinberg, J. A., & Trombley, C. A. (1995). *Arthritis: Occupational therapy for physical dysfunction* (4th ed.). Baltimore, MD: Williams and Wilkins.

Fitinghoff, H., Söderback, I., & Nordeman, R. (1994). An activity analysis of hand grips used in housework by female rheumatoid arthritics. *Work, 4,* 128-136.

Furst, G. P., Gerber, K. H., & Smith, L. B. (1985). *Rehabilitation through learning: Energy conservation and joint protection. A workbook for persons with rheumatoid arthritis.* Washington, DC: United States Department of Health and Human Services.

Furst, G. P., Gerber, L. H., Smith, C. C., Fisher, S., & Shulman, B. (1987). A program for improving energy conservation behaviors in adults with rheumatoid arthritis. *American Journal of Occupational Therapy, 41,* 102-111.

Gerber, L. H. (1985). *Introduction: Rehabilitation through learning. Energy conservation and joint protection. A workbook for persons with rheumatoid arthritis.* United States Department of Health and Human Services, Public Health Service, National Institutes of Health.

Gerber, L. H., Furst, G.P., Smith, C., Shulman, B., Liang, M., Cullen, K., Stevens, M. B., & Gilbert, N. (1987). Patient education program to teach energy conservation behaviors to patients with rheumatoid arthritis: A pilot study. *Archives of Physical Medicine and Rehabilitation, 68,* 422-445.

Goldenberg, D. L. (1995). Fatigue in rheumatic disease. *Bulletin of Rheumatologic Diseases, 44,* 1.

Grant, R. (Ed.). (1994). *Physical therapy of the cervical and thoracic spine* (2nd ed.). New York: Churchill Livingstone.

Grieve, G. (1988). *Common vertebral joint problems* New York: Churchill Livingston.

Hammond, A. (1994a). Joint protection behavior in patients with rheumatoid arthritis following an education program. *Arthritis Care and Research, 7,* 5-9.

Hammond, A. (1994b). Helping rheumatoid arthritis patients adopt joint protection behaviors. *Arthritis Care and Research, 7,* abstract S9.

Hammond, A. (1994c). The Joint Protection Behavior Assessment. *Arthritis Care and Research, 7,* abstract, S15.

Hasselkus, B. R., Kshepakaran, K. R., & Safrit, M. J. (1981). Handedness and hand joint changes in rheumatoid arthritis. *American Journal of Occupational Therapy, 35,* 705-710.

Hebert, L. (1992). *Sex and back pain* [library ed.]. Minneapolis, MN: Orthopedic Physical Therapy Products.

Hertling, D., & Kessler, R. M. (1996). *Arthrology: Management of common musculoskeletal disorders* (3rd ed.). Philadelphia, PA: Lippincott.

Hutson, M. (1990). *Back pain: Recognition and management.* London: Butterworth Heinemann.

Jackson, R. (1977). *The cervical syndrome* (4th ed.). Springfield, MO: Charles C. Thomas.

Johnson, E. W., & Wolfe, C. V. (1972). Biofocal spectacles in the etiology of cervical radiculopathy. *Archives of Physical Medicine and Rehabilitation, 53,* 210.

Kay, A. G. L. (1979). Management of the rheumatoid hand. *Rheumatology Rehabilitation, 18* (Suppl. 1), 76-81.

Keegan, J. (1953). Alterations of the lumbar curve related to posture and seating. *Journal of Bone and Joint Surgery, 35,* 598-603.

Kjeken, I., Moller, G., & Kvien, T. K. (1995). Use of commercially produced elastic wrist orthoses in chronic arthritis: a controlled study. *Arthritis Care and Research, 8,* 108-113.

Landsmeer, J. M. F. (1962). Power grip and precision handling. *Annals of the Rheumatic Diseases, 21,* 164.

Lane, N. E., Bloch, D. A., Jones, H. H., Simpson, V., & Fries, J. F. (1989). Osteoarthritis in the hand: A comparison of handedness and hand use. *Journal of Rheumatology, 16,* 5.

Leonard, J. B. (1995). Joint protection for inflammatory disorders. In J. M. Hunter, E. J. Mackin, & A. D. Callahan (Eds.), *Rehabilitation of the hand: Surgery and therapy* (4th ed.). St. Louis, MO: Mosby.

Mackenzie, R. A. (1981). *The lumbar spine: Mechanical diagnosis and therapy.* Waikanae, New Zealand: Apinnal Publications.

Macnab, I., & McCulloch, J. (1990). *Backache.* Baltimore, MD: Williams and Wilkins.

Maehlums, S. (1994). Strategies to improve strength and stamina. In J. H. Klippel & P. A. Dieppe, *Rheumatology.* St. Louis, MO: Mosby.

McCarty, D. J. (1993). Clinical picture of rheumatoid arthritis. In D. J. McCarty & W. J. Koopman (Eds.), *Arthritis and allied conditions.* Philadelphia, PA: Lea and Ferbiger.

McCloy, L. (1982). The biomechanical basis for joint protection in osteoarthritis. *Canadian Journal of Occupational Therapy, 49*(3), 85-87.

Melnik, M., Saunders, R., & Saunders, H. (1989). *Self-help manual: Managing back pain.* Minnesota: Educational Opportunities.

Melvin, J. (1989). *Rheumatic disease in the adult and child: Occupational therapy and rehabilitation* (3rd ed.). Philadelphia, PA: F. A. Davis.

Melvin, J. (1995). Orthotic treatment of the hand: What's new? *Bulletin of Rheumatic Diseases, 44*(4).

Michel, B. A., Fries, J. F., Block, D. A., Lane, N. E., & Jones, H. H. (1992). Osteophytosis of the knee: Association with changes in weight bearing exercise. *Clinical Rheumatology, 11,* 235-238.

Minor, M. A., Hewett, J. E., Webel, R. R., Anderson, S. K., & Kay, D. R. (1989). Efficacy of physical conditioning exercise in patients with rheumatoid arthritis and osteoarthritis. *Arthritis and Rheumatism, 32:* 1396-1405.

Mody, G. M., Meyers, O. L., & Reinach, S. G. (1989). Handedness and deformities: Radiographic changes and function of the hand in rheumatoid arthritis. *Annals of Rheumatic Diseases, 48,* 104-107.

Moskowitz, R. W. (1979). Osteoarthritis. In D. J. McCarty, & W. J. Koopman (Eds.), *Arthritis and allied conditions.* Philadelphia, PA: Lea and Febiger.

Neumann, D. A. (1989). Biomechanical analysis of selected principles of hip joint protection. *Arthritis Care and Res, 2,* 146-155.

Neumann, D. A., & Hase, A. D. (1994). An electromyographic analysis of the hip abductors during load carriage: Implications for hip joint protection. *Journal of Orthopedic and Sports Physical Therapy, 19,* 296-304.

Nordenskiöld, U. (1994). Evaluation of assistive devices after a course in joint protection. *International Journal of Technology Assessment in Health Care, 10*(2), 283-304.

Nordin, M., & Frankel, V. (1989). *Basic biomechanics of the musculoskeletal system* (2nd ed.). Philadelphia, PA: Lea & Febiger.

Packer, T. L., Sauriol, A., & Brouwer, B. (1994). Fatigue secondary to chronic illness: Postpolio syndrome, chronic fatigue syndrome and multiple sclerosis. *Archives of Physical Medicine and Rehabilitation, 75,* 1122-1126.

Packer, T. L, Brink, N., & Sauriol, A. (1995). *Managing Fatigue: A six-week course for energy conservation.* Catalogue. Therapy Skill Builders.

Palmer, P., & Simons, J. (1991). Joint protection: A critical review. *British Journal of Occupational Therapy, 54*(12) 453-458.

Palmoski, M., Colyer, R. A., & Brandt, K. D. (1980). Joint motion in the absence of normal loading does not maintain normal articular cartilage. *Arthrits and Rheumatism, 23,* 325-334.

Pedretti, L. W., & Zoltan, B. (1990). Treatment applications: Rheumatoid arthritis. *Occupational therapy practice skills for physical dysfunction* (3rd. ed., pp. 468-71). St. Louis, MO: Mosby.

Phillips, C. A. (1995). Therapist's management of patients with rheumatoid arthritis. In J. M. Hunter, E. J. Mackin, & A. Callahan (Eds.), *Rehabilitation of the hand: Surgery and therapy.* St. Louis, MO: Mosby.

Poole, J. L. (1995). Learning. In C. A. Trombley, *Occupational therapy for physical dysfunction* (4th ed.). Baltimore, MD: Williams & Williams.

Quest, I., & Cordery, J. C. (1971). A functional ulnar deviation cuff for the rheumatoid deformity. *American Journal of Occupational Therapy, 25*(1), 1-7.

Radin, E. L. (1987). Osteoarthritis: What is known about prevention. *Clinical Orthopedics and Related Research, 222,* 60-65.

Radin, E. L., Paul, I. L., & Rose, R. M. (1972, March). Role of mechanical factors in pathogenesis of primary osteoarthritis. *The Lancet,* 519-522.

Radin, E. L., Paul, I. L., & Rose, R. M. (1975). The mechanical aspects of osteoarthrosis. *Bulletin on the Rheumatic Diseases, 26,* 862-865.

Saunders, H. D. (1985). *Evaluation and treatment of musculoskeletal disorders.* Minneapolis, MN: Viking.

Schnitzer, T. J. (1993). Management of osteoarthritis. In D. J. McCarty & W. J. Koopman (Eds.), *Arthritis and allied conditions* (12th ed.). Philadelphia, PA: Lea & Febiger.

Schur, P. (1993). Clinical features of SLE. In W. Kelly, E. Harris, S. Ruddy, & C. Sledge (Eds.), *Textbook of rheumatology.* Philadelphia, PA: W. B. Saunders.

Schreuer, N., Palmon, O., & Nahir, A. M. (1994). An occupational therapy group workshop for patients with osteoarthritis of the hands. *Work 4,* 147-150.

Shumway-Cook, A., & Wollacott, M. H. (1995). *Motor Control: Theory and practical applications.* Baltimore, MD: William and Wilkins.

Sliwa, J. L. (1983). Teaching approach. Joint protection and energy conservation: Re-examining the biomechanics, the principles for specific connective tissue diseases, and the teaching approach. Workshop meeting of the Arthritis Health Professional Section Workshop, San Antonio.

Sliwa, J. L. (1986). Occupational therapy management. In G. Erlich, *Rehabilitation management of rheumatic conditions* (2nd ed.). Baltimore, MD: Williams and Wilkins.

Smith, E. M., Juvinal, R. C., Bender, L. F., & Pearson, J. R. (1964). Role of the finger flexors in rheumatoid deformities of the metacarpophalangeal joints. *Arthrits and Rheumatism, 7,* 467-480.

Smith, E. M., Juvinal, R. C., Bender, L. F., & Pearson, J. R. (1966). Flexor forces and rheumatoid metacarpophalangeal deformity. *Journal of the American Medical Association, 198,* 2.

Spencer, J. D., Hayes, K. C., & Alexander, I. J. (1984). Knee joint effusion and quadriceps reflex inhibition in man. *Archives of Physical Medicine and Rehabilitation, 65,* 171-177.

Tack, B. B. (1990). Fatigue in rheumatoid arthritis: Conditions, strategies and consequences. *Arthritis Care and Research, 3,* 2.

Templeton, C. L., Petty, B. J., & Harter, J. L. (1978). Weight control group approach for arthritis clients. *Journal of Nutrition Education, 10,* 1.

Weiner, C. (1975). The burden of rheumatoid arthritis: Tolerating the uncertainty. *Social Science Medicine, 9,* 97-104.

White, A., & Anderson, R. (1991). *Conservative care of low back pain.* Baltimore, MD: Williams and Wilkins.

Wolfe, F., Smythe, H. A., Yunus, M. B., et al. (1990). The American College of Rheumatology criteria for the classification of fibromyalgia: Report of the Multicenter Criteria Committee. *Arthritis and Rheumatism, 33,* 160-172.

BIBLIOGRAPHY

Arthritis Foundation Booklets: A single copy is free to patients and professionals. *Managing Your Arthritis: Using your joints wisely. Managing Your Fatigue. Managing Your Pain. Managing Your Stress. Living and Loving: Information about sexuality and intimacy.* The Arthritis Foundation, P. O. Box 19000, Atlanta, GA 30326; 1-800-283-7800 or the local chapter.

Brattstrom, M. (1987). *Joint protection and rehabilitation in chronic rheumatic disorders* (2nd ed.). Rockville, MD: Aspen.

Covey, Stephen R. (1990). *The seven habits of highly effective people. Powerful lessons in personal change.* New York: Simon & Schuster.

Furst, G. P., Gerber, K. H., & Smith, L. B. (1985). *Rehabilitation through learning: Energy conservation and joint protection. A workbook for persons with rheumatoid arthritis (1985). Instructor's Guide.* United States Department of Health and Human Services. Available from the Department of Rehabilitation, National Institutes of Health, Building 10, Room 6S-235, 10 Center Drive MSC 1604, Bethesda, MD 20892-1604.

Hebert, L. (1994). *Sex and back pain* (2nd ed., patient booklet). Available through Orthopedc Physical Therapy Products (OPTP), PO Box 47009, Minneapolis, MN 55447-009.

Jacobs, K., & Bettencourt, C. M. (Eds). (1995). *Ergonomics for therapists.* Boston: Butterworth-Heinemann.

Melvin, J. L. (1995). *Rheumatoid arthritis: Caring for your hands* and *Osteoarthritis: Caring for your hands.* American Occupational Therapy Association, 4720 Montgomery Lane, Bethesda, MD 20824; Phone: 1-800-SAY-AOTA.

Packer, T. L, Brink, N., & Sauriol, A. (1995). *Managing fatigue: A 6-week course for energy conservation.* Catalogue No. 4368. Tucson, AZ: Therapy Skill Builders, PO Box 42050 85733; (800) 763-2306.

Pirie, A., & Herman, H. (1995). *How to raise children without breaking your back.* West Summerville, MA: IBIS Publications.

Snijders, C. (1987). Biomechanics of footwear. *Clinics in Podiatric Medicine and Footwear, 4,* 629-643.

Swanson, A. (1995). Pathomechanics of deformities of the hand and wrist. In J. M. Hunter, E. J. Mackin, & A. D. Callahan (Eds.), *Rehabilitation of the hand: Surgery and therapy* (4th ed.). St. Louis, MO: Mosby.

Thornton, B. (1996). Hand therapy for clients with arthritis. In L. F. Collins, *OT practice, 1*(4), 1996.

Volowitz, E. (1988). Furniture prescription for the conservative management of low back pain. *Topics in Acute Care Trauma Rehabilitation, 2,* 8-32.

Winston, S. (1995). *Stephanie Winston's best organizing tips.* New York: Simon & Schuster.

Wise, K. S. (1975). The anatomy of the metacarpophalangeal joints with observations the aetiology of ulnar drift.

SUPPLIERS

1. Arthritis Cane
   Union City/Bio-dynamic Technologies, Inc. (800) 879-2276.

2. Silver Ring Splint Company
   PO Box 2856, Charlottesville, VA 22902. (804) 971-4052.

3. Sammons-Preston
   (800)-323-5547.
   Distributes the Cervipillo®.

4. Back Designs
   Berkeley, CA (510) 849-1923.
   This company makes a variety of back supports including auto head rests.

5. The Saunders Group
   (800) 456-1289.
   This company makes a variety of back supports.

6. Tempurpedic Swedish Neck Pillow
   Lexington, KY. (800) 878-8889.

7. Rugg Manufacturing
   PO Box 507
   105 Newton Street
   Greenfield, MA 10302
   (800) 633-8772.
   This company offers ergonomic tools.

8. First Step Catalog
   This company offers baby equipment including a swivel car seat. 1 (800) LITTLE 1.

9. Bardeck Yarns
   Bardeck, Nova Scotia, Canada. (902) 707-5512.

13

THERMAL AGENTS FOR INFLAMMATORY ARTHRITIS

Sue Schuerman, MBA, GCS, PT

INTRODUCTION

A number of physical agents can assist in treating the musculoskeletal manifestations of inflammatory arthritis. Teaching the patient to apply home agents appropriately enhances his or her sense of self-worth and self-efficacy (Minor & Sanford, 1993). It also allows the patient to treat exacerbations early. Finally, application of physical agents at home as part of the total self-management program for arthritis will assist the patient in exercising and working more comfortably. Maintaining normal activities helps prevent further impairment, loss of function, and disability (Kirby, 1993).

This chapter will review the clinical and home use of heat and cold agents listed in Table 1 in the treatment of the musculoskeletal manifestations of rheumatoid arthritis (RA). The chapter will emphasize the treatment of inflammation and associated symptoms, discuss applications for each agent, and review the literature of the use of that agent in inflammatory arthritis. A summary of thermal agents, their purposes, contraindications, precautions, and application procedure is provided in table format. Although inflammation is usually associated with RA, it may also occur in osteoarthritis. This is particularly true after overuse or trauma, or during exacerbation of the disease (Sotosky & Michlovitz, 1996).

THERAPEUTIC USE OF COLD

Cold has long been used to decrease pain and symptoms associated with acute inflammation. Physiologically, cold has been shown to (1) raise the pain threshold, (2) decrease the release of vasoactive agents that catalyze the inflammatory response, and (3) reduce swelling by decreasing the activity of vasoactive agents to reduce outward fluid filtration (Von Nieda & Michlovitz, 1996). In RA, the primary treatment goal is to reduce the inflammatory response, usually manifested as pain, swelling, heat, redness, and loss of function in the joint during an acute exacerbation. Cold is also used in the subacute period to reduce any increased inflammation that might develop after range of motion exercises or daily activities. Cold is the treatment of choice when swelling is the primary problem limiting joint or tendon motion, as for example in tenosynovitis of the hands or feet, or for swollen joints that may not be painful because the pain is masked by medication, especially corticosteroids. Cold is contraindicated for treatment of inflammation associated with systemic lupus erethymatosus (SLE) and mixed connective-tissue disease when Raynaud's phenomenon is present or if concomitant conditions such as diabetes compromise sensation.

Methods of application include cold packs, ice massage, cold immersion baths, and contrast baths. Contrast baths combine cold and heat in alternation to decrease inflammation in hands and feet when cold alone has been unsuccessful. (Although this method has proven effective in the clinic, there has not been any research on the effectiveness of contrast baths.) Table 1 summarizes the purposes, contraindications, precautions, and techniques for use of these cold modalities.

Research on Cold Modalities and Arthritis

In applying ice massage to the ring PIP joint in 15 patients with RA, researchers Curkovic, Vitulic, Babic-Naglic, and Durvigl (1993) showed a pain threshold increase compared to baseline with a single 1-3 minute application, and the increase was maintained at 10 and 30 minutes posttreatment. Utsinger, Bonner, and Hogan (1982) compared cryotherapy (cold packs placed circumferentially around the knee for 20 minutes twice per day for 1 week) and thermotherapy (hot packs placed circumferentially around the knee for 20 minutes, three times per day, for 1 week) on 100 patients with RA and knee pain. They treated the same knee for 1 week with cryotherapy, 1 week for evaluation only, 1 week with thermotherapy, and 1 week with cryotherapy. They assessed knee ROM, strength, circumference, timed functional tests, sleep duration, and visual analogue pain scales on all patients. Fifty patients improved in one to five of these parameters, and 32 patients improved in three to five parameters. Although cold is anecdotally said to be tolerated poorly by patients with RA, a study by Kirk and Kersley (1968) found that 12 out of 14 subjects preferred cold. In the study of Utsinger and colleagues described above, 50% of their patients preferred heat, 32% preferred cold, and 18% had no preference. They reported that the 32% who preferred cold generally demonstrated more intense inflammation in the treated knee.

Cold is also anecdotally associated with increases in patient-reported joint stiffness. However, Pegg, Littler, & Littler (1969), Utsinger et al. (1982), and Kirk and Kersley (1968) have shown patient-reported stiffness in chronically inflamed joints with RA to be decreased with cold. This is typically true when the stiffness is associated with swelling. All of the studies relied on self-report of stiffness change except Kirk and Kersley, who used ROM as a measure of stiffness and did not find a significant change with this measure. Further study is needed to quantify stiffness changes. The specific impact of ice on stiffness associated with swelling is needed as ice would be more likely to decrease stiffness and improve ROM in the presence of swelling.

THERAPEUTIC USE OF COLD

COLD AGENT	ADVANTAGES AND LIMITATIONS	PROCEDURE	CONTRAINDICATIONS AND PRECAUTIONS
COLD PACKS (NONRIGID), COMMERCIAL PACKAGES OF SMALL FROZEN VEGETABLES	Easily contoured. Various sizes and shapes. Conform to almost any body part.	Store in freezer for a minimum of 2 hours. Use thin, moist cloth over skin to enhance cold transfer and protect skin. Compress gently for good surface contact. Apply 15-20 minutes. Wait at least 1 hour before reapplying.	Cold intolerance. Cold insensitivity. Vasospastic disorders. Over areas of poor circulation (arterial, venous, or neuropathic). Hypertensive patients if large area involved.
ICE MASSAGE	Small areas.	Freeze water in small paper cup (may use tongue depressors or popsicle sticks for handles). Peel back cup as ice is used. Gently apply over postcard-size area for 5-8 minutes. Patient will note cold, burning, aching, and numbness. Stop when no light-touch sensation is present.	Same as above.
IMMERSION BATHS	Distal extremities. Surround part for complete contact. Very effective method of cold transfer. Good for finger, wrist.	Container of water at 55-65 degrees Fahrenheit. Immerse to tolerance (shorter times in colder water, typically 1-2 minutes).	Same as above.
CONTRAST BATHS	Distal extremities.	Container of water 55-65 degrees Fahrenheit, and another 100-104 degrees. Alternate warm and cold at a 3:1 or 4:1 ratio for 30 minutes. End in cold if swelling and inflammation are main problems.	Same as above.

Table 1: Therapeutic Use of Cold

THERAPEUTIC USE OF SUPERFICIAL HEAT

Heat can have a variety of physiological effects at the local level, depending on the method of application and how vigorously it is applied. These effects include (1) increased pain threshold, (2) relaxation, (3) increased blood flow to an area to assist in removing metabolites that prolong the inflammatory response, and (4) altering the viscoelastic properties of connective tissue, decreasing stiffness, and facilitating stretching and movement (Rennie & Michlovitz, 1996).

In RA, heat is the treatment of choice when stiffness and aching, as opposed to swelling, are the primary problems. Heat is appropriate to reduce discomfort and facilitate movement in the chronic period and possibly in the subacute period as well, especially if cold is ineffective. However, heat has been consistently shown to increase inflammation and swelling by increasing blood flow, and patients should not apply heat during the acute or early subacute periods following an exacerbation. They should be advised to be alert for the signs of inflammation at any time heat is applied and switch to cold if any swelling or increased pain occurs. Research by Weinberger, Fadilah, Lev, and Pinkhas (1989) indicates that even superficial heating agents such as hot packs were able to increase intra-articular temperature to 35-36 degrees Celsius in patients with knee effusions. (Four of their patients had RA and one had osteoarthritis.) Sotosky & Michlovitz (1996) discuss the possibility that further increases in intra-articular temperature from heating agents (superficial or deep) might increase joint enzyme activity and thus facilitate joint destruction. Until more research is done, it is prudent to recommend only cold applications for the acutely inflamed joint. If using heat, the need to reduce stiffness in the subacute period should significantly outweigh the risk of increasing enzyme activity and inflammation at that time.

In the subacute or chronic-active stages of RA or SLE, stiffness and aching are often responsive to the warmth provided by gloves or cloth elbow, knee, or ankle sleeves. The heat source does not have to be as strong as a hot pack or heating pad.

Many superficial heating agents are available for home use. The clinician must recommend these devices with consideration of the great care that must be used to prevent skin damage or burning in the application of any heating device. Commercially available hydrocollator packs are *not* recommended for home use. Only dedicated paraffin baths designed for home use should be used. Waterproof electric heating pads allow placing a moist, warm towel near the skin to provide moist heat. Small packs that may be heated in the microwave oven are available but must be handled carefully. The clinician must provide clear and concise instructions and ideally should require the patient to demonstrate correct technique in the clinical setting prior to the home use. The purposes, contraindications, precautions, and procedures for the application of superficial heating devices discussed in this section are located in Table 2. Infrared heating is rarely used in the U.S. and is therefore not included.

THERAPEUTIC USE OF SUPERFICIAL HEAT

HEAT AGENT	ADVANTAGES AND LIMITATIONS	PROCEDURE	CONTRAINDICATIONS AND PRECAUTIONS
HOT PACKS, HEATING PADS	Many shapes and sizes available. Can apply to many body parts.	Commercial packs are kept in water at 160 degrees Fahrenheit and must be padded with minimum of six-eight layers of toweling. Do not lie on pack. Apply for 20 minutes. Follow specific instructions for heating pads and over-the- counter products. Aim for only mild to moderate warmth. Monitor skin every 5 minutes to watch for red and white blotches (mottling), which indicate overheating.	Patient must have normal light touch and temperature sensation. Do not apply over areas of decreased circulation. Do not apply over areas prone to bleeding or on patients with bleeding disorders such as hemophilia. Do not apply over malignancies.
PARAFFIN	Use for application to distal extremities. Use only commercial units.	Unit should be kept at 118-130 degrees Fahrenheit. Dip part eight-ten times. Wrap part in plastic. Wrap in towel and fasten towel with rubber bands. Elevate part if any risk of swelling. Remove all jewelry. Clean the part first. Treat 20 minutes.	Same as above.
FLUIDOTHERAPY®	Primarily used on extremities. Forced convection dry heat with adjustable agitation and adjustable temperature between 102 and 118 degrees Fahrenheit. Part can easily move allowing ROM during heat treatment.	Set temperature lower in range if risk of swelling. Encourage ROM during treatment. Treat 20 minutes.	Same as above.
INFRARED	Radiant energy through air so nothing touches part. Selected if patient is sensitive to weight. Rarely used	Energy is set in device so dosage is controlled by moving source closer to or further from body part. High-energy source so patient must be closely monitored. Treat as tolerated up to 20 minutes.	Same as above.

Table 2: Therapeutic Use of Superficial Heat

RESEARCH ON USE OF SUPERFICIAL HEAT

Several studies have documented the effectiveness of superficial heat for raising the pain threshold, decreasing self-reported pain, and improving self-reported well-being in patients with chronic inflammation associated with RA (Curkovic et al., 1993; Kirk & Kersley, 1968; Mainardi, Walter, Spiegel, Goldkamp, & Harris, 1979). Gains in ROM or decreases in stiffness were observed by Dellhag, Wollersjo, & Bjelle (1992) and Kirk & Kersley (1968).

Mainardi and colleagues (1979) were interested in proving or disproving the long-term effects of the use of electric mittens on the RA disease process, as these devices were in common use in the northeast. They followed 17 volunteers with RA over 2 years and treated one hand daily with an electric mitten. Their study documented that this type of heat treatment is neither beneficial nor destructive for the RA hand. No changes in range of motion (ROM), stiffness, or joint swelling in the treated hand compared to the nontreated hand were observed over the 2 years. (At the time of this study, cold modalities were not being used for RA, and clinicians were not aware of the negative effects of heat on inflammation.)

THERAPEUTIC USE OF DEEP HEAT

Deep-heating agents are able to cause tissue temperature elevation at depths of 3 cm or more. The heat energy needs to be delivered to the deeper tissues without overheating superficial tissues (McDiarmid, Ziskin, & Michlovitz, 1996). Ultrasound (US), continuous short-wave diathermy (CSWD), and microwave diathermy (MWD) are the common deep-heat methods used today. Ultrasound is used much more frequently than diathermy in the United States, and microwave diathermy is used very rarely. In the treatment of the patient with RA, US is indicated only if the patient has decreased soft-tissue extensibility that limits necessary joint range of motion. These tissues, usually tendinous in nature, are quite deep below the surface. Continuous US might be applied to heat tissues with high collagen content that limit the range. Evidence of any acute inflammation precludes the use of US, and evidence of the development of any signs of inflammation limits further treatment.

The physiological effects of deep heat are the same as those for superficial heat when applied to target tissues. As with superficial agents, the clinician must use extreme caution not to apply these devices to patients during acute periods with joint inflammation. In applying deep heat during the subacute and chronic periods, the clinician must be sure that there is no increase in the inflammatory response. Use of these agents is largely confined to the clinical setting, although portable ultrasound units are available for use by home therapists. Since the ultimate goal of therapy for chronic illness is to teach the patient self-management, clinic-based or therapist-applied modalities should be kept to a minimum (Moncur & Shields, 1987).

As noted earlier, superficial heating agents such as hot packs have also been shown to increase peri- and intraarticular temperature in patients with chronic rheumatoid conditions (Weinberger et al., 1989). As a result, a superficial heating agent used appropriately at home might provide effective heating of a periarticular tendon. In such a case, the therapist would provide the patient with appropriate instruction in the treatment and in the posttreatment stretching exercises. Some diathermy (radio frequency radiation) devices and most newer ultrasound devices allow the use of a pulsed setting. For these settings, "off" time is usually much longer than "on" time to allow any heat built up to be dissipated. Some of the pulsed radio frequency radiation devices (PRFR) have adequate power to produce heat, but others do not. In both US and PRFR, the nonthermal effects of the devices are desired. In US these effects include acoustical streaming or fluid movement along cell membranes. This movement may be associated with changes in cellular activity and ion fluxes (McDiarmid et al., 1996). Some therapists believe that these nonthermal effects might speed the resolution of the inflammatory process. However, the timing for effective application is not yet clear in the research, and at this time no definitive research has been done on patients with RA. The reader is referred to the chapter on US by McDiarmid, Ziskin, and Michlovitz (1996) for a more complete discussion of the nonthermal effects of ultrasound. Nonthermal effects of PRFR devices will not be discussed in this chapter, as their relationship to the treatment of inflammation associated with RA is not yet established in rheumatologic literature. The reader is referred to the chapter on diathermy and PRFR devices by Kloth and Ziskin (1996) in Michlovitz (1996) for more information on the nonthermal effects of PRFR devices.

PHONOPHORESIS

Phonophoresis is the use of ultrasound (US) to facilitate the transfer of molecules of medication through the skin to underlying tissues (McDiarmid et al., 1996). Anti-inflammatory agents such as 1%, 5%, or 10% hydrocortisone are usually used. Phonophoresis is used on some symptoms associated with acute inflammation in RA. Unfortunately, US is not transmitted well through many of the anti-inflammatory agents used, and the effectiveness of the treatment is uncertain (Cameron & Monroe, 1992). The recommended procedure is to rub the drug completely into the skin in the painful area with a gloved hand, apply the US transmission gel over the area, and begin the ultrasound treatment (McDiarmid et al.). Dosage control and analysis of depth of penetration are also challenging in phonophoresis.

The purposes, precautions, contraindications, and procedures for application of deep heating devices are in Table 3. Diathermy is not appropriate for the treatment of RA and is therefore not included in this table.

RESEARCH ON USE OF DEEP-HEATING DEVICES FOR ARTHRITIS

There is very little research on deep-heat modalities for arthritis, primarily because they are contraindicated for joint inflammation. Bromley, Unsworth, and Haslock (1994) applied pulsed US to 13 patients treated with paraffin and to 11 untreated patients all with acute rheumatoid involvement of the MCP joints, twice a week for 6 weeks, but

THERAPEUTIC USE OF DEEP HEAT

HEATING AGENT	ADVANTAGES AND LIMITATIONS	PROCEDURE	CONTRAINDICATIONS AND PRECAUTIONS
ULTRASOUND, CONTINUOUS US (More research is needed to establish role of pulsed US in RA.)	Decrease pain, increase connective-tissue extensibility.	Frequency of 1 MHz for deeper target tissues, 3 MHz for superficial target tissues. Intensity adjusted between 1 and 2 W/cm^2 depending on heating dosage desired. Decrease intensity over bony areas. Apply for about 5 minutes over postcard-size area. Use adequate US conductive gel between US transducer and skin.	Demand-type cardiac pacemaker. Over pregnant uterus. Over eye or testes. Over malignancies. Where sensation decreased to touch or temperature. Where circulation decreased or potential for thrombophlebitis. Over open epiphyseal growth plates or fracture sites. US head must be kept moving at all times.
PHONOPHORESIS (More research needed to establish safety in use during acute inflammation in RA.)	Decrease inflammation.	Use only pulsed US versus continuous in RA. More research needed but intensity should be limited to 0.5 to 1.0 W/cm^2. Use only technique where medication completely rubbed in to target site, then apply US gel and follow all above procedures.	As above. Allergies to medications.
CONTINUOUS SHORT-WAVE DIATHERMY (More research needed to establish whether pulsed radio-frequency radiation devices have a role in the treatment of RA.)		Follow specific instructions for each device. Usual application time is 20 minutes.	Any internal or externally worn metallic object or electromedical device. Within 15 feet of an individual with a demand-type pacemaker. Over high fluid volume areas such as the eyes, testes, hemorrhages, perspiration, and wound dressings. Over malignancies. Where sensation reduced to touch or temperature. Near pregnant uterus. Over open ephiphyseal plates. Near synthetic materials in the treatment area.

they could not demonstrate a positive change compared to groups receiving the paraffin alone, active ROM alone, and a control group. Unfortunately there was no comparison to the use of cold modalities, which are the treatments recommended for acute inflammation. This study is limited by its small sample size.

Continuous US (used for heating or thermal effects) has been compared to other modalities in several studies. However, very few studies with reasonable clinical treatment parameters include subjects with RA. At this time too little literature exists to support or rule out the use of continuous US in reducing joint stiffness in RA. Further isolated study with good control and placebo groups is needed.

Short-wave diathermy (SWD) is not indicated for acute joint inflammation, which is the primary reason most people with inflammatory arthritis are referred to PT. If a patient was referred with chronic arthritis or OA for range of motion problems due to decreased soft-tissue extensibility, it would be preferable to use a device such as US, which could better target specific structures, than to use SWD, which would heat the entire joint. No studies were found that reported significant improvement in patients with RA after SWD.

Phonophoresis specifically for arthritis has been evaluated in only one study. Griffin, Echternach, Price, and Touchstone (1967) compared the results of ultrasound with 10% hydrocortisone ointment and ultrasound with a placebo cream on patients with osteoarthritis and RA. Ultrasound intensity was 1.5 W/cm^2, application time was 5 minutes, and frequency was once per week. Sixty-eight percent of patients in the experimental group reported improved range of motion and decreased pain versus only 25% in the placebo group. However, the hydrocortisone was also used as the transmission gel in the experimental group. Cameron and Monroe (1992) showed that hydrocortisone is a poor transmission agent for ultrasound, and this study needs to be repeated with a different transmission technique to assure valid results. A discussion of the literature to date in McDiarmid and colleagues (1996) indicates that more study is needed to assure that the phonophoresis can do more than ultrasound alone and more than topical application of the medication alone.

SELECTION OF MODALITIES: CLINICAL REASONING

In the treatment of arthritis, the amount of inflammatory activity in the involved structures guides the clinician in selecting the appropriate physical agent (Hayes, 1993). There are several questions useful to the clinician in deciding on the best modality.

1. Is the joint inflammation acute or chronic?

2. Is there limited joint motion or function?

3. If so, is that limitation a result of pain, swelling, or stiffness?

4. Is the joint involvement local or systemic?

5. Where should the treatment be provided? (clinic, home, both?)

6. How often does it need to be done, e.g. daily, three times a week?

7. Are there any precautions or contraindications for the selected agent in the patient?

8. If home use is indicated, has adequate instruction been provided to the patient so that the agent can be used safely and effectively?

9. A final question should be asked. Has the patient's preference been considered? Patients who have tried thermal agents will have opinions about their effectiveness. These will need to be included in the treatment plan. All of the above factors will affect the choice of treatment modality and the manner in which it is applied for the specific condition. Read the following case and ask the questions in the section above as you read it.

Patient: Mary Smith; 79 y.o.; retired; lives alone; was independent in self-care and community prior to exacerbation of her RA 1 week ago.

Referral: Treatment of recent exacerbation of RA with inflammation of left knee. Patient has pain with inability to ambulate on a level surface without a walker and cannot negotiate stairs.

Evaluation: P & AROM are decreased and painful. Significant pain was reported moving from sitting to standing and with weight bearing. Redness, swelling, tenderness, and warmth are noted about the left knee.

The patient described above has the cardinal signs of acute inflammation including redness, swelling, tenderness, warmth, and pain about the left knee. The initial treatment goal is to reduce inflammation in order to decrease pain and facilitate movement and function. Cold agents such as a cold pack or ice massage are most indicated and could reduce both pain and inflammation. As the signs of inflammation were noted about the entire knee, cold packs would probably be more effective and efficient in providing relief than ice massage, which is more effective over a small, painful area. The patient should be instructed in the home use of cold packs.

As the swelling, redness, and warmth decrease, the patient's joint inflammation will be described as subacute. She will likely report less pain with movement at this time. Stiffness usually persists for a longer period due to mild residual swelling and lack of motion during the acute period. In this subacute period, cold has been shown in most studies to be appropriate for both pain and stiffness.

Superficial heat may be indicated now as it will assist in decreasing pain and stiffness as well. Hot packs in the clinic or a heating pad at home would probably be the most effective and efficient application of superficial heat for the knee. The patient should be instructed on proper use of a heating pad at home. Deep heat such as ultrasound or diathermy is probably not indicated in either the acute or subacute stages for a patient with RA due to the potential for increasing the inflammatory response and destructive joint-enzyme activity. Patients must be instructed not to increase their activity during the acute phase when treatment has reduced the associated discomfort. Increased activity could cause further joint destruction. For acute inflammation the use of modalities should be combined with instruction in joint-protection techniques for the lower extremities (see chapter 12).

SUMMARY

Investigations on the use of cold in this chapter strongly support its role in reducing inflammation. This is particularly true in the period during and immediately following an acute exacerbation of RA. Superficial heat is also strongly supported in reducing discomfort, increasing well-being, and reducing stiffness in the subacute and chronic periods as long as it does not increase the inflammatory response. Deep-heating agents including continuous ultrasound and diathermy should not be used in the presence of inflammation. This limitation and the fact that they are clinic-based and do not encourage self-management greatly limit their usefulness in the treatment of rheumatic diseases. Superficial heat and cold agents can be applied safely and effectively at home as needed. This will encourage self-management and result in improved well-being and function. Clinicians must emphasize appropriate home interventions and provide clear instruction for their safe and effective use.

REFERENCES

Bromley, J., Unsworth, A., & Haslock, I. (1994). Changes in stiffness following short-and long-term application of standard physiotherapeutic techniques. *British Journal of Rheumatology, 33*(6), 555-561.

Cameron, M. H., & Monroe, L. G. (1992). Relative transmission of ultrasound by media customarily used for phonophoresis. *Physical Therapy, 72,* 142-148.

Curkovic, B., Vitulic, V., Babic-Naglic, D., & Durvigl, T. (1993). The influence of heat and cold on the pain threshold in rheumatoid arthritis. *Zeitschrift fur Rheumatologie, 54*(5), 289-291.

Griffin, J. E., Echternach, M. S., Price, R. E., & Touchstone, J. C. (1967). Patients treated with ultrasonic driven cortisone and with ultrasound alone. *Physical Therapy, 47,* 594.

Hayes, K. W. (1993). Heat and cold in the management of rheumatoid arthritis. *Arthritis Care and Research, 6*(3), 156-166.

Kirby, R. L. (1993). Impairment, disability, and handicap. In J. A. De Lisa, B. M. Gans, D. M. Currie, L. H. Gerber, J. A. Leonard, Jr., M. C. McPhee, & W. S. Pease (Eds.). *Rehabilitation medicine: Principles and practice* (2nd ed., pp. 40-42). Philadelphia, PA: J. B. Lippincott.

Kirk, J. A., & Kersley, G. D. (1968). Heat and cold in the physical treatment of rheumatoid arthritis of the knee: A controlled clinical trial. *Annals of Physical Medicine, 9,* 270-274.

Kloth, L. C., & Ziskin, M. C. (1996). Diathermy and pulsed radiofrequency radiation. In S. L. Michlovitz (Ed.), *Thermal agents in rehabilitation* (3rd ed., pp. 213-254). Philadelphia, PA: J. B. Lippincott.

Mainardi, C., Walter, J. M., Spiegel, P. K., Goldkamp, O. G., & Harris, E. D. (1979). Rheumatoid arthritis: Failure of daily heat therapy to affect its progression. *Archives of Physical Medicine and Rehabilitation, 60,* 390-392.

McDiarmid, T., Ziskin, M. C., & Michlovitz, S. L (1996). Therapeutic ultrasound. In S. L. Michlovitz (Ed.), *Thermal agents in rehabilitation* (3rd ed., pp. 168-212). Philadelphia, PA: J.B. Lippincott.

Michlovitz, S. L. (Ed.). (1996). Thermal agents in rehabilitation (3rd ed.). Philadelphia, PA: F. A. Davis.

Minor, M. A., & Sanford, M. K. (1993). Physical interventions in the management of pain in arthritis: An overview for research and practice. *Arthritis Care and Research, 6*(4), 197-206.

Moncur, C., & Shields, M. N. (1996). Physiotherapy methods of relieving pain. *Ballieres Clinical Rheumatology, 1*(1), 183-193.

Pegg, S. M. H., Littler, T. R., & Littler, E. N. (1969). A trial of ice therapy and experience in chronic arthritis. *Physiotherapy, 55,* 51-56.

Rennie, G. A. (Sandy), & Michlovitz, S. L. (1995). Biophysical principles of heating and superficial heating agents. In S. L. Michlovitz (Ed.), *Thermal agents in rehabilitation* (3rd ed., pp. 107-138). Philadelphia, PA: J. B. Lippincott.

Sotosky, J. R., & Michlovitz, S. L. (1996). Use of heat and cold in the management of rheumatic diseases. In S.L. Michlovitz (Ed.), *Thermal agents in rehabilitation* (3rd ed., pp. 335-354). Philadelphia, PA: J. B. Lippincott.

Utsinger, P. D., Bonner, F., & Hogan, M. (1982). Efficacy of cryotherapy and thermotherapy in the management of rheumatoid arthritis pain: Evidence for endorphin effect. *Arthritis & Rheumatology, 25,* S113.

Von Nieda, K., & Michlovitz, S. L. (1996). Cryotherapy. In S. L. Michlovitz (Ed.), *Thermal agents in rehabilitation* (3rd ed., pp. 78-106). Philadelphia, PA: J. B. Lippincott.

Weinberger, A., Fadilah, R., Lev, A., & Pinkhas, J. (1989). Intra-articular temperature measurements after superficial heating. *Scandinavian Journal of Rehabilitation Medicine, 21,* 55-57.

14

THERAPEUTIC EXERCISE

Brenda M. Coppard, MS, OTR/L,
Judith R. Gale, MA, MPH, PT, OCS, and Gail M. Jensen, PhD, PT

INTRODUCTION

The primary goal in the clinical management of persons with arthritis is to improve their functional status (Semble, 1995). One essential aspect in the treatment of arthritis is establishment of an exercise program. Both occupational and physical therapists are involved in designing and implementing therapeutic exercise programs tailored for individual patients. At one time exercise was thought to increase damage to arthritic joints and often exercise was discouraged and rest was promoted. Recent research indicates that exercise has been shown to improve range of motion (ROM), strength, and functional capacity while decreasing pain in patients with arthritis and is now advocated as an essential part of the rehabilitation process (Gerber, 1990; Hicks, 1990).

This chapter provides a general discussion of the key physical elements that need to be considered when designing and implementing a therapeutic exercise program. It focuses on therapist-prescribed exercises to improve joint ROM, muscle physiology, and strength, and includes reducing stiffness and spasm, and restoring balance between muscle groups. Exercise for fitness is discussed in chapter 15 and methods for achieving adherence with home programs are described in chapter 3.

THE PHYSICAL EFFECTS OF EXERCISE

A stable skeletal base is necessary for transfer of forces through the muscular system to produce movement. The musculoskeletal system must function as an integrated unit for optimum efficiency. Skeletal muscle function is dependent on the biomechanics of the joint, the size, and number of individual muscle fibers, and the length-tension relationship of the fibers. The articular surfaces of joints are lined with hyaline cartilage that allows the bones to glide over each other. During physical activity, fluid from the underlying bone is absorbed into the cartilage and increases its thickness and its shock-absorbing ability (Shepard, 1987). In osteoarthritis, the cartilage is damaged through stress or trauma and loses this shock absorption as well as its gliding ability. The increased friction between the joint surfaces can cause further damage. Moderate loading of the joint, such as walking or lifting light weight, is essential to maintain bone and cartilage health (Gerber, 1990). In rheumatoid arthritis the synovium is involved as well as the bone and cartilage. Inflammation of the synovium, in addition to changes described above, causes pain and loss of range of motion. Joint effusion can inhibit muscle contraction and lead to decreased strength, altered joint mechanics, pain, and further inflammation. As the joint capsule and surrounding soft tissues become distended, the bones move out of normal alignment. The result is a biomechanically unstable and inefficient joint (Hicks, 1990).

Depending upon its type, frequency, and intensity, exercise training can increase the size of muscle fibers and the strength of the muscle (Jenkins, 1991; Shepard, 1987). Isokinetic and isometric exercise cause blood pressure to rise and should be used with caution for anyone with a cardiovascular condition. Isotonic exercise increases blood flow to the muscles being exercised, and peripheral resistance falls (Gerber, 1990). Generally, as the exercise intensity increases, the demand for oxygen and production of carbon dioxide increase. Chapter 12, Exercise for Health and Fitness, provides a more detailed discussion of the effects of exercise.

When a muscle is physiologically fatigued, it is unable to tolerate the activity level for a given task. Signs of fatigue may include tremors, heavy perspiration, inability to continue moving through the full available range, facial grimacing, labored breathing, and reports of exhaustion. It is important for patients to learn to recognize these signs and rest before fatigue becomes a factor. Research demonstrates that patients with rheumatoid arthritis and fibromyalgia have low exercise tolerance, decreased flexibility, and poor biomechanical efficiency (Clark, 1994; Belza, 1994); persons with these conditions should closely monitor fatigue.

RANGE OF MOTION EXERCISE

Exercise for increasing range of motion is done to lengthen soft-tissue structures such as joint capsule, tendon, ligament, and muscle. This can be accomplished through passive, active, or active-assistive exercise. The terms *passive*, *active*, and *active-assistive* refer only to how the motion should be performed, not how much force is used to complete the motion.

During passive ROM (PROM) exercise, the body part is moved through the complete available ROM by an external force. External force is provided to a joint from sources such as another person, an unrestricted limb, a splint, Coban wrapping, or continuous passive motion machines (CPMs). Passive range of motion is particularly helpful in maintaining a stretch when joints are limited in motion because of impaired tendon gliding (tenosynovitis), weakness, or soft-tissue shortening. A stretch at the end of the range is recommended to increase ROM in chronic, active, or inactive stages of arthritis. During the acute stage or when the joint is swollen, stretch is NOT recommended because it can put additional stress on the joint structures and cause additional scarring (Kendall,1965). Caution must be used when applying stretch at the end range.

Active ROM (AROM) is when the patient moves the body part through the range of motion without assistance, while active-assistive ROM (AAROM) requires some assistance from an external force to complete the entire motion. There are several ways to provide assistance for ROM such as gravity assist through positioning, equipment (e.g., pulleys, deltoid aid), water exercise, another person, or use of other extremities, as in self-ROM.

Active exercise is completed by the patient and is best for strengthening muscles. Passive exercise, on the other hand, requires no muscle contraction on the part of the patient. Although there is some evidence suggesting passive exercise may be detrimental to inflamed joints, when performed gently it can be quite helpful in decreasing edema and maintaining range of motion (Melvin, 1989; Merritt & Hunder, 1983). Active-assistive exercise allows the joint to be taken through its available range when the patient may not be strong enough to complete the motion independently.

EFFECT OF DISEASE ON JOINT ROM

Considerations for prescribing ROM exercises include (a) how the joint disease affects the ROM, (b) the type of exercise to use, (c) the minimum number of repetitions to maintain or increase mobility, (d) the time of day for doing the exercises, and (e) patient cooperation and follow-through with the program (Melvin, 1989).

Joint ROM can be limited by a number of factors including, for example, swelling, bone changes, and weakness. Intervention must be directed specifically to the limiting factor (see Table 1). The following factors are prevalent in the acute and subacute phases of arthritis. In the chronic-active stage, joints may be weak and unstable (Melvin, 1989).

• Synovitis results in lax, weak joint structures. In the presence of synovitis, exercise should be gentle to avoid further stretching from pressure during exercise.

• Periarticular or extra-articular swelling may cause joint range limitations. Edema should be reduced before the person engages in exercise. Edema reduction techniques include elevation, circular distal to proximal wrapping, and active movement.

• Pain may result in reflex spasm of the flexor-adductor muscles and limit joint extension.

• Inactivity or disuse increases the risk of soft-tissue shortening, adhesions, and muscle weakness. Protective splinting and positioning should be considered to prevent dysfunctional contractures when bed rest is required

Joint destruction resulting in limitation of joint mobility has been found to covary with poor muscle strength and may be attributable to reflex inhibition (DeAndrade, Grant, Dixon, 1965; Jayson & Dixon, 1970), muscle metabolism changes (Nordemar, Lovgran, Furst, Harris, & Hultman, 1974), atrophy of type II muscle fibers (Nordemar, Edstrom, & Ekblom, 1976), and a reduction in functioning muscle fibers and peripheral nerve impairment (Moritz, 1963).

LOSS OF ROM AND THERAPEUTIC INTERVENTIONS

PROBLEM OR CONDITION	FACTORS LIMITING ROM/ CLINICAL FINDINGS	POSSIBLE THERAPEUTIC INTERVENTIONS
Joint Effusion	Pain from distention of capsule and increased intra-articular pressure	Cold modalities; splinting; gentle AROM on small joints; PROM on large joints, joint protection
Joint Capsule Contracture	Loss of capsule length	Prolonged gentle stretching, positioning, or proning program, serial casting or splinting
Joint Capsule Pain With Stretching	Faulty posture, poor alignment	Posture retraining Mobilization, soft-tissue stretching
Loss of Joint Cartilage	Capsule at risk of shortening	AROM to maintain strength, non–weight–bearing exercises, e.g., water exercise
Loose Bodies in Joint	Sudden loss of ROM	Manual traction with rotation to free loose body; surgery
Osteophytes	Can block ROM	ROM exercise will not change limitations from bony block
Muscle Spasm Secondary to Joint or Soft-Tissue Pain	Shortening of musculotendon unit	Modalities, relaxation techniques, friction massage, manual therapy, posture education, muscle stretching
Muscle Weakness	ROM lag, incomplete AROM	Strengthening exercises
Fear of Pain, Movement, or Crepitus	Patient does not use full ROM	Patient education, cognitive reframing, relaxation training
Trigger Finger	Inconsistent AROM	Splinting to prevent triggering to reduce irritation and size of nodule; cold modalities
Wrist Flexor Tenosynovitis	Diminished AROM of fingers either in extension or flexion	Cold modalities to volar aspect of wrist, splinting if wrist motion is an aggravating factor

TYPE OF EXERCISE

The type of exercise to prescribe may be a puzzling concept for therapists. Traditionally, active-assistive exercise was preferred to passive exercise to prevent application of forces that might be too vigorous for inflamed or weakened joints. However, appropriate, gentle, passive exercise can be less damaging than active exercise. Over-ambitious patients can cause harm by exerting too much force during active exercise.

During active synovitis, passive exercise may produce greater and less painful mobility. The wrist, elbow, and ankle joints are generally easy for the patient to self-range. However, for larger joints such as hips, knees, and shoulders, passive exercise with muscle relaxation may help maintain mobility during active synovitis. In cases where there is a "lag" between active and passive motion due to impaired tendon gliding (tenosynovitis) or weakness, only passive ROM is effective in maintaining joint mobility (Melvin, 1989).

NUMBER OF REPETITIONS

There is no "cook book" that prescribes the number of repetitions for exercise programs. They need to do the number of repetitions necessary to achieve ROM goals each day. Clinical judgment is needed when developing an exercise program. For example, persons with periarticular swelling and disuse may need to perform ROM exercises twice a day. Others with stable chronic conditions may need to perform them only once daily for maintenance. Keep in mind that it may take two to five warm-up repetitions to achieve full ROM (Swezey, 1974).

The duration of pain following exercise is a guide for prescription. Joint discomfort or pain should not persist for more than 1 hour after exercise. If discomfort or pain lasts longer, the exercises are too stressful and should be reduced (Melvin, 1989).

TIME TO EXERCISE

Simple stretching exercises to help limber up can be done at any time, but specific exercises to maintain ROM should be attempted when the person feels most flexible and limber. Anti-inflammatory medications should be timed for maximum effectiveness during the exercise period. Application of heat or cold, or a warm bath or shower prior to exercise may be helpful.

CONSIDERATIONS FOR COOPERATION AND FOLLOW-THROUGH

The therapist should consider a home program that can be performed simply and efficiently in the home. There are promising data on the use of isokinetic machines by persons with osteoarthritis (Schilke, Johnson, Housh, & O'Dell, 1996). However, the therapist must weigh the advantages and disadvantages of engaging patients in clinical exercises on equipment they are not likely to have at home.

Regardless of the type of home exercise program designed, it is important to provide both verbal and written instructions. If the person's cognition is uncertain, a program may be prescribed that emphasizes the joints with the greatest impact on function.

Exercises should be demonstrated and explained, and the rationale for exercising should also be explained. Patients should be monitored when performing the exercise routine to ensure that it is done correctly.

Melvin (1989) described examples of exercises that involve patients in self-monitoring through visual feedback.

• Shoulder and elbow ROM: The patient faces the wall, raises his or her arm as far as possible. A marking tape or Post-It is placed on the wall to serve as a goal for subsequent shoulder flexion exercises.

• Finger hyperextension range: To help maintain the extensibility of volar structures, have the patient place palms together with the metacarpo-phalangeal joints touching (prayer position), and then hyperextend the fingers. A ruler can be used to measure the opening span.

• Thumb web space and finger abduction: The patient places the hand on a piece of paper and traces it with the fingers abducted and the thumb extended. Subsequent tracings can be done in different colors to mark progression.

• Temporomandibular excursion: The patient looks in the mirror while opening the mouth as far as possible. A ruler or index card is used to measure the aperture between the upper and lower teeth.

EXERCISE FOR STRENGTH AND ENDURANCE

Exercise for muscle strengthening can be either static or dynamic. Static or *isometric* exercise means "equal measure." An isometric contraction does not change the muscle length, and there is no visible limb movement; therefore, it is a static exercise. Isometric is probably the safest type of exercise for a person with arthritis because the exercise eliminates joint movement and puts less stress on the joint. Functionally, isometric contractions stabilize joints (Smith, Weiss, & Lehmkuhl, 1996). Isometric exercise can both maintain and increase muscle strength (Gerber, 1990). Maximal muscle contractions held for 6 seconds and repeated 5 to 10 times are generally recommended (Gerber, 1990). Other studies have demonstrated that a brief isometric contraction (BRIME) or one contraction held 6 seconds daily increases the strength of a muscle (Lieberson, 1984).

Patients with rheumatoid arthritis tend to tolerate isometric exercise well because it causes the least joint motion and pain. It is least likely to increase inflammation and juxta-articular bone destruction (Jayson & Dixon, 1970). However, because isometric exercise, especially upper-extremity exercise, can increase blood pressure, precautions are necessary with patients who have cardiac dysfunction. Patients should be instructed to hold isometric contractions 6 to 12 seconds to obtain maximal strengthening. To prevent a valsalva maneuver, patients should be asked to count out loud or exhale during the hold. Isometric exercise does not require a large number of repetitions to be effective; therefore, it is good for patients who fatigue easily.

Dynamic exercise is the most frequently used form of exercise when increasing strength. *Isotonic* means "equal tone." Isotonic muscle contractions produce force that causes the origin and the insertion of the muscle to shorten or lengthen while maintaining an equal amount of tension throughout the range. True isotonic contractions seldom occur in everyday activities. As the leverage changes with movement of the limb, the amount of muscle tone varies. The term is often used, incorrectly, to refer to a weight of an object remaining constant throughout the range (e.g., completing a biceps curl with a 10-lb weight in the hand). This type of exercise is dynamic as there is visible movement of the limb.

Another form of dynamic exercise is *isokinetic*, which means "equal motion." An isokinetic contraction is also dynamic as it moves a limb through its range with a consistent velocity. Instruments such as the dynamometer utilize principles of isokinetic exercise as the device limits the rate of movement to a preset velocity regardless of the force exerted by the muscles (Smith et al., 1996). Isokinetic exercises are often performed in a clinical setting using this specialized equipment because it provides constant resistance throughout the range. Some research indicates dynamic exercise that requires muscles to work during joint motion appears to be better than static or isometric exercise for patients with arthritis (Stenstrom, 1994).

METHODS OF STRENGTHENING

Voluntary exercise, where individuals voluntarily contract their muscles either isometrically or isotonically, is one of the best ways of strengthening muscles. Isometric exercises are learned quickly and can result in rapid gain in strength. The point of maximal muscle tension is when the muscle is just short of resting length (Smith et al., 1996). Isotonic exercise is commonly used for maximal strength increase or muscle hypertrophy.

A traditional method of strengthening using isotonic exercise is progressive resistive exercises (PRE). The maximum amount of weight a person can lift 10 times is the reference point. The program starts with 10 repetitions at 50% of the reference weight, progresses to 10 repetitions at 75% of reference weight, and finally to 10 repetitions at 100% of the reference weight. There is evidence of equal benefit when both the weight and the number of repetitions are decreased (Gerber, 1990).

Therapeutic exercise for patients with extreme muscle weakness or returning muscle function may include initiating active movement through facilitating voluntary muscle control. Therapeutic techniques can facilitate motor learning through use of visual cues, verbal cues, practice, and feedback to restore motor control (Winstein & Knecht, 1990).

One side effect of strengthening programs is muscle aches or postexercise soreness. These aches peak 24-48 hours after exercise (Gerber, 1990). Exercises involving eccentric, or lengthening, muscle contractions are most commonly associated with postexercise muscle aches.

EVALUATION OF MUSCLE STRENGTH

Evaluation of muscle performance has traditionally been done through muscle testing. The manual testing procedures were developed to assess the presence of muscle weakness from disease, disuse, or injury rather than to assess strength. They are most helpful for assessing 3.5 or less strength on the following scale (Daniels & Worthingham, 1986):

5 = Normal (full resistance against gravity)

4 = Good (moderate resistance against gravity)

3 = Fair (no resistance against gravity)

2 = Poor (moves part-way through range with gravity eliminated)

1 = Trace (muscle contraction palpated)

0 = Zero (no palpable contraction).

It is recommended that scores simply be reported numerically, that is, 3/5, and the descriptive terms such as "normal" be avoided. Very strong muscles can be damaged and still score 5/5. Intertester reliability data for application of this scale demonstrated that therapists score the same grade only 50% to 60% of the time (Frese, Brown, Norton, 1987).

Other methods of assessing muscle performance include dynamometers. Hand strength measured through grip and pinch dynamometers is a common assessment tool. Many claim it is vital to know the patient's strength (Vignos, 1980), while others caution that the resistance causes harm to the inflamed tissues and also causes pain. Pain during testing renders the strength test unreliable because pain inhibits a maximal contraction and strength measurements are not accurate. If muscle testing is done, it should be carried out isometrically, not isotonically (Feinberg & Trombly, 1995) and should be limited to the amount of force needed for function. Measurement of muscle performance alone will not necessarily relate to the patient's ability to function. Therefore, linking muscle performance to function is critical in terms of patient outcomes.

ENDURANCE

Endurance is the ability to repeat an activity or task over time. Endurance can be measured by the amount of oxygen consumed, the concentration of lactic acid in the blood, and pulse rate (Gerber, 1990). Improvement in endurance will increase the tolerable lactic acid concentration in the blood and increase anaerobic tolerance.

In a study by Minor, Hewett, Webel, Anderson, and Kay (1989), a group of 120 participants with rheumatoid arthritis or osteoarthritis were involved in aerobic (walking, aerobic aquatics) or anaerobic (range of motion) exercise. There were no significant differences between groups in terms of flexibility, number of joints involved, morning stiffness, or grip strength. However, the aquatics and walking exercise group showed significant improvement in aerobic capacity.

Generally, exercise programs with low resistance and high repetition demonstrate gains in strength, while those with high resistance and low repetition demonstrate gains in endurance. The number of repetitions to prescribe for an endurance program is the number of repetitions that bring on fatigue but not pain (Melvin, 1989).

EXERCISE IMPLEMENTATION

Several factors must be considered when developing an exercise program for people with arthritis. Most important, pain should be used as a guideline for the type and intensity of exercise. Severe pain during exercise or pain that persists longer than 1 to 2 hours after exercise is an indication that the program was too vigorous. Severe pain should be distinguished from normal postexercise discomfort such as muscular soreness.

The stage of the disease process is a second consideration. In acute phases, when the inflammatory process is active, exercise should be limited to a few repetitions of ROM exercises after cold modalities. As the inflammation subsides, the exercise level can be increased slowly. In chronic stages, the program can be expanded to include more vigorous exercise including aerobic, stretching, and strengthening against resistance. Resistance should be limited in the case of joint deformities, as the abnormal biomechanics can cause further damage or inflammation (Banwell, 1984; Hicks, 1990).

The age of the patient is an important factor in designing an appropriate exercise regimen. With the normal aging process, there will be decreases in strength, soft-tissue resilience, and aerobic capacity. Such changes can be accentuated in older persons with arthritis and should be considered when designing exercise programs for them (Hicks, 1990).

Excessive or improper performance of the exercises should be avoided. Signs that this has occurred include pain lasting more than 1 to 2 hours after exercise, extreme fatigue, weakness, decreased range, and increased joint inflammation.

The sequence of the exercise program is crucial. Limited range of motion should be addressed first and then strengthening exercises can be added. The last component is an aerobic program, which should be initiated once flexibility and strength have been increased (Hicks, 1990).

Because exercise can be used to affect specific musculoskeletal functions, it is essential that the program include exercises of the appropriate type, frequency, and intensity (Gerber, 1990). In the active stages of rheumatoid arthritis, movement should be limited to active range of motion. Strengthening should include only isometric exercises with few repetitions. During the subacute phase, the number of repetitions of active range of motion and isometric exercises can be increased to tolerance, and endurance exercises can be added. When the disease process is inactive, and in JRA, isotonic exercise can be initiated. Ankylosing spondylitis responds well to both active and passive movements. Isometric and endurance exercises to tolerance are appropriate. Joint mobilization can help decrease pain and stiffness. In the case of osteoarthritis, active range of motion is effectively combined with a few repetitions of isometric and isotonic exercise with low resistance. Endurance activities and joint mobilization can also be incorporated. Table 2 summarizes the exercise programs for selected rheumatological diseases.

Regardless of the treatment setting, reassessments and reviews of home exercise programs are necessary in order for patients to manage their exercise programs. Reassessments reduce the risk of harm to the patient when a program no longer reflects the capabilities of the patient. Patients should be aware of exercise precautions including the following:

- Respect pain. Stop exercising if discomfort is present. If joint pain lasts more than 1–2 hours postexercise, the exercise was too taxing.

- Exercise in such a manner that does not strain joints.

- While exercising, avoid fast, jerky movements. Exercise should be performed slowly and smoothly.

- Joints that are red, inflamed, hot, and painful should be exercised as little as possible.

- Avoid exercise that involves heavy weights.

- Change positions often; alternate between sitting, standing, and supine positions.

- Respect your limitations; do not compete against others, only yourself. The goal is to make steady progress (Simpson & Dickerson, 1983).

CLINICAL DECISION MAKING

Once the therapist has gathered evaluative data, he or she must transform that data into a workable treatment program for the patient. This is achieved through the process of clinical decision making. Experienced therapists engage in clinical reasoning and decision making every day. Clinical decision making is a goal-oriented, cognitive process that allows application of general theory to specific patients (Dutton, 1995). Clinicians should never rely on applying "cookbook" therapy regimens to all patients with similar diagnoses. Each patient, regardless of diagnosis, has varying degrees of impairment, pain, activity tolerance, and motivation.

When determining an appropriate exercise program for a patient with arthritis, the therapist calls upon general knowledge and theory about arthritis and exercise. This background information allows for a series of steps in the process of clinical decision making (Dutton, 1995). The steps include developing narrative hypotheses, devising an evaluation plan, interpreting evaluation results, defining and prioritizing a problem and asset list, and selecting a frame of reference to generate treatment goals and a treatment program (Dutton, 1995). If all steps of clinical decision making are followed, the patient benefits from a uniquely tailored program. Table 3 illustrates the critical thinking process the therapist developed for the case described.

GENERAL EXERCISE RECOMMENDATIONS FOR SPECIFIC RHEUMATIC DISEASES

DISORDER	REPETITIONS	AMOUNT OF RESISTANCE	TYPE OF ROM	TYPE OF CONTRACTION	ENDURANCE
RA **ACUTE** **SUBACUTE** **INACTIVE**	Few Few to tolerance Within tolerance	None Slight with supervision Low with supervision	Active Active Active	Isometric Isometric Isometric, isotonic	None As tolerated As tolerated
JRA	Within tolerance	Low with supervision	Active	Isometric, isotonic	As tolerated
ANKYLOSING SPONDYLITIS	Within tolerance	None	Active Passive Joint Mobilization	Isometric	As tolerated
OSTEOARTHRITIS	Few	Low	Active	Isotonic, isometric	As tolerated
FIBROMYALGIA	Within tolerance	Low	Active	Minimize use of eccentric contractions during strengthening	As tolerated, begin slow and build gradually

Table 2: General Exercise Recommendations for Specific Rheumatic Diseases

CONCLUSION

Therapeutic exercise is a valuable rehabilitation tool that physical and occupational therapists utilize for patients with rheumatic conditions. The prescription of therapeutic exercise is a collaborative effort between therapists and patients. By engaging in a critical thinking process, therapists can tailor exercise programs for their patients.

RA CASE STUDY: CRITICAL THINKING PROCESS TO DEVELOP THERAPEUTIC EXERCISE PLAN

CASE SUMMARY:
Dinah is a 47-year-old woman diagnosed with rheumatoid arthritis 1 year ago. Two weeks ago, she developed increased inflammation and swelling in the knees, ankles, elbows, wrists, and hand MCP joints. Her rheumatologist increased her medications, and she no longer experiences the exacerbation. Dinah is now being referred to occupational and physical therapy for evaluation and treatment.

Dinah has mild MCP subluxation and slight bilateral ulnar deviation and small rheumatoid nodules on her elbows. When asked about her activities and exercise, she reports that she gets enough exercise maintaining her apartment and working as an insurance salesperson. She also reports that she usually wakens with stiffness, she tires easily, and she finds walking difficult at times because of pain and stiffness. She lives alone in an apartment.

NARRATIVE HYPOTHESES:
1. Fever and fatigue may be present.
2. Joint inflammation, pain, and possible joint instability in the presence of her deformities may limit ROM, strength, coordination, function (especially in the hands) and ability to ambulate.
3. Dinah may be experiencing difficulties with ADL.
4. Dinah may lack information regarding the RA and appropriate therapeutic exercise. Resources may be limited due to lack of knowledge.
5. Dinah may have difficulty following recommendations for appropriate exercise and precautions.
6. Architectural barriers may be a hindrance.

EVALUATION PLAN:

AREA TO ASSESS	ASSESSMENT TOOL	RATIONALE FOR DATA
Fatigue or fever	Activity tolerance Self report of fever	Avoid exhaustion during evaluation and treatment
Joint Involvement	Visual observation	For baseline; to determine abilities and limitations
ROM	Observe AROM of BUEs and BLEs; Goniometric measurements	For baseline; start exercises at that resistance level to prevent fatigue and joint damage
Strength	Observe strength of BUEs and BLEs during ADL; observe grasp; Dynamometer measurements, Manual Muscle Testing	For baseline; to determine the extent of poor coordination effects on ADL

Endurance	Self report; observation of activity	For baseline performance
Dexterity	Observation of activity, standard fine motor coordination assessments	For baseline performance, to determine effects on dexterity
Gait, Mobility	Observe gait pattern, use of assistive devices	For baseline performance of mobility and ambulation
ADL	Observe performance in morning ADL (bathing, toileting, dressing)	For baseline performance; to determine ROM, strength, coordination limit patient's performance; to determine if joint protection techniques are employed
Patient's Knowledge of RA and Self-Management Skills	Interview	To determine baseline for self-management education or if nonadherence is an issue (could be because of culture, fatigue, depression, etc.)
Adherence Assessment	Interview and reassessment	Identify patient beliefs about exercise; link exercise to valued activities for the patient; identify barriers to exercising and solve problems with patient
Architectural Barriers	Interview; home visit evaluation	To determine if patient is able to complete ADL/exercise program at home and while traveling

PRIORITIZED PROBLEM AND ASSET LIST
- List all significant problems identified during evaluation process
- Prioritize problem list
- List all significant assets.

SELECTED GUIDING FRAME OF REFERENCE TO GENERATE LTGS AND STGS
- Determine which problems can be addressed through PT/OT intervention
- Determine which assets will assist in overcoming the problems
- Generate short-term and long-term goals directly related to the problems identified, patient's needs, valued activities, and resources available
- Identify treatment methods to reach goals.

Table 3: RA Case Study: Critical Thinking Process to Develop Therapeutic Exercise Plan (continued)

REFERENCES

Belza, B. (1994). The impact of fatigue on exercise performance. *Arthritis Care and Research, 7, 4,* 176-180.

Banwell, B. F. (1984). Exercise and mobility in arthritis. *Nursing Clinics of North America, 19, 4,* 605-616.

Clark, S. R. (1994). Prescribing exercise for fibromyalgia patients. *Arthritis Care and Research, 7, 4,* 221-225.

Daniels, L., & Worthingham, C. (1986). *Muscle testing techniques of manual examination.* Philadelphia, PA: W. B. Saunders.

DeAndrade, R. R., Grant, C., & Dixon, A. S. (1965). Joint distension and reflex muscle inhibition in the knee. *Journal of Bone Surgery, 47,* 312-323.

Dutton, R. (1995). Rehabilitation case simulation: Arthritis. *Clinical reasoning in physical disabilities.* Philadelphia, PA: Williams & Wilkins.

Feinberg, J. R., & Trombly, C. A. (1995). Arthritis. In C. A. Trombly (Ed.), *Occupational therapy for physical dysfunction* (4th ed.)

Frese, E., Brown, M., & Norton, B. (1987). Clinical reliability of manual muscle testing: Middle trapezius and gluteus medius muscles. *Physical Therapy, 76,* 1072-1076.

Gerber, L. H. (1990). Exercise and arthritis. *Bulletin on the Rheumatic Diseases, 39, 6,* 1-9.

Hicks, J. E. (1990). Exercise in patient with inflammatory arthritis and connective tissue disease. *Rheumatic Disease Clinics of North America, 16, 4,* 845-868.

Jayson, M., & Dixon, A. (1970). Intra-articular pressure in rheumatoid arthritis of the knee. III. Pressure changes during joint use. *Annuals of Rheumatic Diseases, 29,* 401.

Jenkins, D.B. (1991). *Hollinshead's functional anatomy of the limbs and back* (6th ed.). Philadelphia, PA: W. B. Saunders.

Kendall, P. H. (1965). Exercise for arthritis. In S. Licht (Ed.), *Therapeutic exercise.* New Haven, CT: Elizabeth Licht Publications.

Lieberson, W. T. (1984). Brief isometric exercises in therapeutic exercise. In J. Basmajian (Ed.), *Therapeutic exercise* (4th ed.). Baltimore, MD: Williams & Wilkins.

Melvin, J. (1989). *Rheumatic diseases in the adult and child: Occupational therapy and rehabilitation* (3rd Ed.). Philadelphia, PA: F.A. Davis.

Merrit, J. L., & Hunder, G. G. (1983). Passive range of motion, not isometric exercise, amplifies acute urate synovitis. *Archives of Physical Medicine Rehabilitation, 64,* 130-131.

Minor, M. A., Hewett, J. E., Webel, R. R., Anderson, S. K., & Kay, D. R. (1989). Efficacy of physical conditioning exercise in patients with rheumatoid arthritis and osteoarthritis. *Arthritis and Rheumatism, 32,* 11, 1396-1405.

Moritz, U. (1963). Electromyographic studies in adult rheumatoid arthritis. *Acta Rheumatology Scandanavia, 9,* Suppl. 6.

Nordemar, R., Edstrom, L., & Ekblom, B. (1976). Changes in muscle fibre size and physical performance in patients with rheumatoid arthritis after short term physical training. *Scandanavian Journal of Rheumatism, 5,* 233-238.

Nordemar, R., Lovgren, O., Furst, P., Harris, R. C., & Hultman, E. (1974). Muscle ATP content in rheumatoid arthritis: A biopsy study. *Scandanavian Journal of Clinical Laboratory Investigations, 34,* 185-191.

Schilke, J. M., Johnson, G. O., Housh, T. J., & O'Dell, J. R. (1996). Effects of muscle-strength training on the functional status of patients with osteoarthritis of the knee joint. *Nursing Research, 45, 2,* 69-72.

Semble, E. L. (1995). Rheumatoid arthritis: New approaches for its evaluation and management. *Archives of Physical Medicine Rehabilitation, 76, 2,* 190-201.

Shephard, R. (1987). *Exercise physiology.* St. Louis, MO: Mosby.

Simpson, C. F., & Dickinson, G. R. (1983). Exercise. *American Journal of Nursing, 83,* 272-274.

Smith, L. K., Weiss, E. L., & Lehmkuhl, L. D. (1996). *Brunnstrom's clinical dinesiology.* Philadelphia, PA: St. Louis.

Stenstrom, C. H. (1994). Therapeutic exercise in rheumatoid arthritis. *Arthritis Care Research, 7, 4,* 190-197.

Swezey, R. L. (1974). Essentials of physical medicine and rehabilitation in arthritis. *Seminars in Arthritis and Rheumatism, 3,* 352.

Vignos, P. J. (1980). Physiotherapy in rheumatoid arthritis. *Journal of Rheumatology, 7,* 269-171.

Winstein, C. E., & Knecht, H. G. (1990). Movement science and its relevance to physical therapy. *Physical Therapy, 70, 12,* 759-762.

BIBLIOGRAPHY

Furst, G. (1985). *Rehabilitation through learning: Energy conservation and joint protection.* Washington, DC: U.S. Department of Health and Human Services, Public Health Service, National Institutes of Health.

Hicks, J. E., Fromherz, W., Miller, F. et al. (1988). Cybex II strength and endurance testing in normals and polymyositis patients. *Arthritis and Rheumatism, 31,* S59.

Panush, R. S. (1990). Does exercise cause arthritis? Long-term consequences of exercise on the musculoskeletal system. *Rheumatic Disease Clinics of North America, 6, 4,* 827-836.

Williams, J. H. (1994). Normal musculoskeletal and neuromuscular anatomy, physiology, and responses to training. In S. Hanson (Ed.), *Exercise physiology.*

15

EXERCISE FOR HEALTH AND FITNESS

Marian A. Minor, PhD, PT

INTRODUCTION

Physical activity and health are clearly related. Regular levels of moderate physical activity significantly improve health for everyone. Prolonged inactivity and poor fitness are associated with increased mortality and morbidity. Whether inactivity arises from a self-selected sedentary lifestyle or arthritis, the threat to health is similar. Inactivity is as likely as smoking, obesity, and elevated cholesterol to increase the chances of coronary artery disease, atherosclerosis, hypertension, diabetes, and some types of cancer (Blair, Kohl, Paffenberger, et al., 1989). Studies have shown that increased physical activity decreases the risk of coronary artery disease, improves blood pressure, assists in weight reduction, improves mood, and enhances well-being (Pate, Pratt, Blair et al., 1995). Yet health care providers and exercise professionals often overlook the needs of people with arthritis for regular, moderate physical activity. The following chapter will present evidence of the benefit of dynamic exercise for persons with arthritis and discuss implementation and support of appropriate conditioning exercise and activity programs.

PHYSICAL ACTIVITY, EXERCISE, AND ARTHRITIS

Exercise has had a controversial role in the management of arthritis. It has been avoided and rest recommended for fear that motion or weight bearing could damage tissues and too much exertion could increase fatigue. Protecting joints from pathologic stress and increasing rest during periods of disease activity are indeed important components of good care. However, for the person with arthritis the consequences of unnecessary and prolonged inactivity add measurably to the problems of pain, stiffness, loss of motion, weakness, functional limitation, poor health, and disability. Recent studies have demonstrated the safety and efficacy of aerobic conditioning exercise for many people with arthritis (Kovar, Allegrante, MaKenzie, Peterson, & Gutin, 1992; Loeser, Messier, Gianfranco, Morgan, & Ettinger, 1995; Stenström 1994a).

The presence of arthritis can create serious health problems in ways other than direct consequences of disease and side effects of therapy. Arthritis is the primary cause for limitation in physical activity in adults. In persons over 65, 12% report limitation in physical activity due to osteoarthritis (OA; Moskowitz, 1986). Persons with a diagnosis of rheumatoid arthritis (RA) have reported that one of the first adaptations they make is to give up leisure and recreational activities (Yelin, Meenan, Nevitt, & Epstein, 1980), a primary source of physical activity for adults. Persons with longstanding or severe OA tend to be deconditioned and at increased risk for cardiovascular disease (Philbin, Goff, Ries, et al., 1995). In addition to the threat of prolonged inactivity to general health, inactivity produces many of the same signs and symptoms traditionally attributed to the arthritis disease process and subsequent disability, namely muscle weakness and atrophy, decreased flexibility, cardiovascular deficit, fatigue, incoordination, osteoporosis, depression, and lowered pain threshold.

Early reports that persons with arthritis were less fit than their nonaffected peers (Beals, Lampman, Banwell, et al., 1985; Ekblom, Lovgren, Alderin, Friedstrom, & Satterstrom, 1974; Minor, Hewett, Weber, et al., 1988) have been followed by prospective trials demonstrating that persons with both systemic inflammatory disease and OA could safely participate in appropriate aerobic exercise programs and achieve improved function, cardiovascular fitness and health (Galloway & Jokl, 1993; Kovar et al., 1992; Minor, Hewett, Webel, Anderson, & Day, 1989; Nordemar, Ekblom, Zachrisson, & Lundquist, 1981; Perlman et al., 1990; Semble, Loeser, & Wise, 1990; Stenström, 1994b).

As a result of this research, we have learned that persons with various forms of arthritis can (a) undergo meaningful diagnostic and prescriptive exercise stress testing; (b) participate in regular conditioning exercise programs of moderate intensity using exercise modes such as walking, aquatic exercise, stationary bicycle, low-impact aerobic dance, and resistance training; and (c) achieve clinically meaningful improvements in cardiovascular health and fitness, muscle strength and endurance, flexibility, function, and psychosocial status without injury or aggravation of disease.

There also may be additional arthritis-related benefits of exercise. For persons with RA, range of motion exercise performed in the evening (Byers, 1985) or aquatic aerobic exercise three times weekly (Minor et al., 1989) produced significant reductions in morning stiffness. Resistance training performed by people with well-controlled RA led to a decline in circulating inflammatory products and an increase in protein synthesis in this population with low body-cell mass (Rall, Lundgren, Reichlin, & Roubenoff, 1995). In a study of aerobic walking by persons with OA of the knees, subjects improved fitness, lost weight, and showed no biochemical signs of cartilage damage (Loeser et al., 1995). There also have been reports that individuals who maintained a regular weight-bearing exercise program exhibited less osteophyte formation at the hip (Michel, Fries, Bloch, Lane, & Jones, 1992).

A number of papers have reported reduction in joint swelling and pain in persons with RA who participated in regular dynamic or aerobic exercise (walking, low-impact aerobic dance, water aerobics) of moderate intensity (Minor et al., 1989; Perlman et al., 1990). Dynamic exercise was more effective than static exercise in improving strength, endurance, and function in persons with RA (Ekdahl, Anderson, Moritz, & Svennson, 1990) and OA of the knee (Fisher, Pendergast, Gresham, & Calkins, 1991). A recent report of the effects of various modes of exercise suggests a physiologic mechanism of action underlying this finding (James, Cleland, Gaffney, Proudman, & Chatterton, 1994). James and colleagues found that dynamic exercise, both weight-bearing (walking) and nonweight-bearing (bicycling) improved synovial blood flow in knee joints of persons with effusions secondary to arthritis, whereas static exercise such as isometric knee extension and flexion did not.

Pain, fatigue, depression, nonrestful sleep, and feelings of helplessness are often serious problems for persons with arthritis. Regular exercise of moderate intensity can raise the pain threshold, improve energy level, lessen depression, and improve physical self-concept and belief in self-efficacy (Harkcom, Lampman, Banwell, & Castor, 1985; Kovar et al., 1992; Stenström, 1994b).

In addition to arthritis-specific benefits, regular, dynamic exercise has a positive effect on bone mineralization and may improve balance and coordination. Reports from studies of growth hormone (Rall et al., 1995), cortisol (Schlaghecke, Kornely, Wollenhaupt, & Specker, 1992), endorphins (Ekdahl, Ekman, et al., 1990), and metabolism (Yocum et al., 1995) indicate that individuals with RA differ from their noninvolved peers in these physiologic parameters and suggest that these factors also may be influenced favorably by exercise.

Our current knowledge and experience support the safety, effectiveness, and importance of including appropriate conditioning exercise in the comprehensive management of persons with arthritis. Avoidance of vigorous exercise is appropriate and necessary *during periods of acute or systemic inflammation.* However, when the disease is under control or in remission, attention must be paid to helping the person with arthritis re-establish appropriate levels of physical activity. The traditional intervention—rest—which is appropriate in the acute condition, can be harmful when applied indiscriminately in the chronic state. People with arthritis should be encouraged to participate in regular physical activity or exercise.

HEALTH OR FITNESS AS AN EXERCISE GOAL

Recent studies indicate that exercise for improved health does not need to be as intense as was previously thought. This is good news for many persons with arthritis who are not able to engage safely in vigorous activities of long duration or at high intensity. It is important to recognize the distinction between exercise training to improve physical fitness and exercise habits to improve or maintain health. Early investigations in the field of exercise science often focused on persons who were already fit. Therefore, much of the information about prescribing exercise to improve fitness indicated that fairly intense exercise regimens were needed to achieve further adaptations and improvements in fitness parameters.

Persons who are extremely deconditioned can achieve significant improvements in cardiovascular capacity, muscle strength, and endurance when they participate in regular exercise at low levels of intensity. Walking, swimming, or bicycling at 60% of maximal heart rate can result in significant improvement in cardiovascular health. Persons with extreme lower-extremity muscle weakness have shown improved muscle performance and muscular hypertrophy following a moderate walking program.

Low- to moderate-intensity aerobic activities performed at least three to four times a week for at least 30 minutes a session improve weight loss and maintenance of a lower weight. A daily program that increases energy expenditure by 100 calories (equivalent to walking or jogging 1 mile) and decreases caloric intake by 100 calories (one slice of bread with pat of butter) can result in the loss of 10 pounds in 6 months.

It is not necessary for a person to participate in an intense, highly regimented exercise program or attain a high level of athletic fitness to improve health. Even persons with low fitness levels who engage in low-intensity but regular physical activity are at significantly less risk for a number of degenerative and potentially fatal conditions. Increased activity improves health status, even in the presence of other risk factors (Blair et al., 1992).

An exercise habit that accumulates 30 minutes of low- to moderate-intensity exertion in an aerobic activity, in daily 8-10 minute bouts, three or five times per week supports health and is sufficient to reduce the probability of cardiovascular illness (Pate et al.,

EXERCISE RECOMMENDATIONS

GOAL	MODE	FREQUENCY	INTENSITY	DURATION
Physical activity for general health	whole body, dynamic activity	4-7 days/wk	40-60% max VO_2 = 60-75% max HR	30 minutes accumulation
Exercise for cardiovascular fitness	dynamic, repetitive exercise of major muscle groups	3-5 days/wk	50-70% max VO_2 = 65-80% max HR	20-60 minutes continuous
Exercise for physical fitness (cardiovascular and musculoskeletal) includes a cardiovascular fitness program with flexibility exercise and resistive, strengthening program	dynamic, resistance (upper and lower body)	2-3 days/wk	8-10 exercises at 60-80% 1RM (= to moderate fatigue)	8-12 repetitions of each

Table 1: Exercise Recommendations

1995). Such a routine would be comparable to a comfortable but somewhat brisk walk, bicycle ride, or swim, or performing household tasks such as mowing the yard or raking leaves. Table 1 outlines current recommendations for physical activity to promote general health and exercise for physical fitness.

PHYSICAL FITNESS AND ARTHRITIS

Health-related physical fitness has five components: cardiovascular status, muscle strength, muscle endurance, flexibility, and body composition. This multidimensional concept of health-related physical fitness provides a comprehensive look at musculoskeletal and cardiovascular function and is particularly appropriate for assessment and exercise recommendation for persons with arthritis. This comprehensive yet categorical perspective allows specificity and grading of the exercise program to meet current needs and respond to changes in disease status. Assessment of physical fitness and exercise status, in addition to disease-related considerations, is the foundation for the prescription of safe and effective exercise. Assessment also provides a baseline from which to monitor for harm and measure progress.

Physical fitness also offers a popular health- and wellness-oriented framework into which therapeutic exercise can be incorporated. This can be especially important for the acceptance and adoption of healthy exercise behaviors by the person with arthritis. A case has been made to include physical fitness as an outcome measure in rheumatology (Burckhardt, Moncur, & Minor, 1994).

THE EXERCISE PRESCRIPTION

Research reports of the efficacy and safety of conditioning exercise are based on clinical trials that have used stationary bicycle, walking, aquatic exercise, low-impact aerobic dance, dynamic resistive and flexibility exercise (Harkcom et al., 1985; Kovar et al., 1992; Minor et al., 1989; Nordemar et al., 1981; Perlman et al., 1990; Stenström, 1994a). Intensity of the aerobic stimulus has been reported as 60% to 80% of age-predicted maximal heart rate. Duration of the aerobic stimulus has been from 15 to 30 minutes. Frequency generally has been 3 to 4 times a week. The majority of subjects have been persons with either RA or OA, ACR Functional Class I-III, between the 20th and 80th decade. Physiologic measures have shown 12% to 21% improvement in cardiovascular performance and up to 55% increase in muscle strength as well as significant increases in flexibility.

An exercise prescription or activity recommendation should suggest modes of exercise, frequency, intensity, and duration appropriate to the individual's cardiovascular health and current physical fitness as well as arthritis-related needs. The major impact of joint disease on the exercise prescription is to take into account the need for (a) joint protection, (b) individualized progression of intensity and duration, (c) appropriate exercise/fitness goals, and (c) education for self-management.

EXERCISE CHOICES

The type of exercise depends upon individual preference, exercise goals, musculoskeletal impairment, and available resources. It is wise to help the person identify and learn to be comfortable in performing at least two activities that require rhythmic, repetitive muscular work of large muscle groups. These activities should vary in requirements for weight bearing and joints used to perform the activity. Other considerations might be activities for both indoors and outdoors, for changes in weather, and for solitary or group exercise.

INTENSITY

Exercise intensity is defined by the exertion or effort expended. The recommendation for intensity is based on the pre-exercise fitness assessment. Persons who are deconditioned or who have not exercised for 3 months or more should begin at a low intensity. In persons with low initial capacity, intensity of 50-60% of maximal heart rate (MHR) is both safe and adequate to produce a training effect. For persons with average levels of cardiovascular and neuromusculoskeletal fitness, intensity of 60-80% of MHR will be appropriate and probably well tolerated.

Intensity is most often monitored by heart rate or self report of perceived exertion. It is useful to prescribe an exercise range with a lower intensity as the threshold for training and the higher intensity as the "not-to-exceed" level. Individuals can learn to regulate activity within the range by modifying exertion as desired. Heart-rate response may not be an appropriate measure of intensity if the person is taking medications to regulate

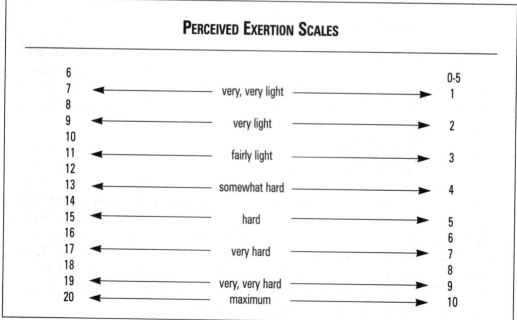

PERCEIVED EXERTION SCALES

		0-5
6		
7	very, very light	1
8		
9	very light	2
10		
11	fairly light	3
12		
13	somewhat hard	4
14		
15	hard	5
16		6
17	very hard	7
18		8
19	very, very hard	9
20	maximum	10

heart rate. It is often desirable to prescribe and teach exercise-intensity regulation with the rating of perceived exertion scale. Figure 1 displays commonly used ratings of perceived exertion that can easily be used by the exerciser to assess exertion.

For some people the simple "talk test" may be the most useful way to make sure that exercise intensity does not exceed a moderate level. The talk test requires only that the person be able to speak normally and converse while exercising. If the exerciser is short of breath or cannot speak in comfortable sentences, the exercise is too intense and effort should be decreased.

DURATION

Duration of the exercise session can be manipulated with intensity to provide the desired exercise stimulus. The aerobic portion of the exercise period probably needs to comprise at least 30 minutes of dynamic activity at a moderate level of intensity. There is evidence that exercise may be accumulated in two or three bouts throughout the day to achieve this 30-minute goal.

FREQUENCY

Frequency of exercise depends on the exercise goal and mode of exercise. A frequency of 3 to 4 times a week for an aerobic stimulus appears to produce optimal results in terms of cardiovascular benefit with a minimal risk of injury or fatigue. A frequency of 5 days per week is safe and effective when the exercise intensity is low. Resistance training to improve strength should be performed no more often than 2-3 days a week to allow the muscles adequate time to repair and adapt.

RESISTANCE TRAINING

Recommendations for physical fitness for the general population now include guidelines for muscle strengthening. Maintaining muscle mass and strength is important for good health and fitness. Appropriate resistance training in persons with RA and OA can result in muscle strengthening, improved function and independence, and increased lean body mass without increased joint pain or disease activity.

Knowledge of disease process, biomechanics, and joint protection principles must form the foundation for any weight-training program for persons with arthritis. Eight to 10 exercises of 8-12 repetitions each performed twice a week is the recommendation for health-related strength training. The principles of circuit resistance training appear to be appropriate for persons with arthritis. This mode of exercise, designed to improve upper- and lower-body strength and provide a cardiovascular training effect, employs moderate resistance and is easily graded and progressed. Research in resistance training in OA and RA has reported positive results using weight loads of 60-80% of one-repetition maximum (1 RM), light- to moderate-weight elastic bands, and approximately 60% of maximal voluntary contraction (MVC) for isometric exercise.

EXERCISE PROGRAM COMPONENTS

A comprehensive exercise program has three parts: warm-up, aerobic exercise, and cool-down. Within this framework it is possible to include exercises to improve or maintain flexibility, range of motion, and muscle strength and endurance as well as cardiovascular fitness and health. Specific therapeutic goals and considerations of disease activity, joint protection, progressive grading, and self-management strategies also are easily accommodated. This compartmentalized approach to the exercise prescription gives the health professional and the person with arthritis an exercise program that is easy to individualize and modify.

WARM-UP OR PREAEROBIC COMPONENT

This component provides an essential neuromuscular and cardiovascular warm up. The warm-up routine can be designed to incorporate individualized range of motion and strengthening exercises and may serve as a traditional home exercise program. The warm-up can be progressed to include 12-15 exercises performed 5 to 10 repetitions each. The goal may be 15 minutes of continuous low-intensity exercise, which is an indication of readiness to proceed to an aerobic stimulus activity.

AEROBIC EXERCISE

The aerobic-exercise component provides the stimulus for cardiovascular fitness, muscular endurance, and activity tolerance. It is this dynamic, repetitive exercise requiring the use of large muscle groups that appears to be of most benefit to general health, emotional status, weight management, self-concept, and fatigue.

The aerobic component can be designed to meet individual needs and variations in disease activity. Experience with and availability of a variety of aerobic activities gives the exerciser freedom to alternate modes. A flexible prescription of intensity, duration, and frequency, which the client understands and can adjust to meet daily needs, promotes self-management skills and appropriate activity levels. The utilization of *interval training techniques* (i.e., alternate bouts of brisk and low-intensity activity) and *additive bouts of exercise* (i.e., add three 10-minute exercise bouts during the day for 30 minutes of exercise) enables even the most deconditioned person to engage safely in health-promoting physical activity. Alternating exercise intensity within an exercise session or performing several short sessions during the day also provides the person with vulnerable joints and fluctuating disease activity a way to establish an appropriate exercise habit.

Exercise success and maintenance appear to be enhanced by using time rather than distance as the aerobic exercise goal. For example, 20 minutes of walking, biking, or swimming is easier to maintain successfully than a set mileage or number of laps. Using alternate forms of exercise that vary weight-bearing and joints involved also fosters maintenance of the exercise habit. A stationary bicycle is a good alternative to walking on days when knees are sore and a walk may be a better exercise choice than swimming on a day when hands, wrists, and shoulders are painful.

COOL-DOWN

Once a person is performing 10 minutes or more of aerobic activity at an intensity of 70% or more of age-predicted heart rate (moderate intensity), a 3- to 5-minute cool-down period is recommended. During this time, exertion is reduced to a low intensity and gentle, static stretching of exercised muscles is performed. The goal of the cool-down period is to allow the cardiovascular response to adjust to less demand, to allow the body to return to resting levels, and to gently stretch muscle to minimize the possibility of delayed-onset muscle soreness.

As with the warm-up routine, low-intensity cool-down activities can be designed and used in a daily program that provides general as well as therapeutic benefit. The warm-up and cool-down may be combined to form a 25-30 minute exercise routine for flexibility, strength, and pain management without the more intense aerobic period. These routines can be used on days when aerobic exercise is not done.

PRECAUTIONS

Inflammatory rheumatic diseases may affect cardiac and pulmonary function and may cause widespread vasculitis. These possibilities must be considered in the decision whether anyone with a systemic rheumatic disease ought to perform vigorous exercise. Vigorous exercise is contraindicated in the presence of acute joint inflammation (red, hot, swollen, painful) or uncontrolled systemic disease. However, the more common presentation and challenges are subacute or chronic joint symptoms and possible sequelae of previous systemic inflammation.

Safe and clinically meaningful exercise testing can be performed in most cases. Submaximal and subjective symptom-limited treadmill tests requiring less than 3 mph walking speed are well tolerated and informative of aerobic capacity. Early-onset muscle fatigue may limit information regarding cardiopulmonary disease. Guidelines for exercise stress testing and cardiovascular disease are described in Table 2.

Cardiovascular and pulmonary complications may limit exercise capacity, particularly in diseases with a major systemic component such as systemic sclerosis, systemic lupus erythematosus, and RA. The seronegative spondyloarthropathies (ankylosing spondylitis, and psoriatic arthritis) may be associated with heart involvement and conduction defects. In general, these limitations do not interfere except during high-intensity exercise, which is not appropriate for this type of patient. It is necessary, therefore, to make sure that people are not working too vigorously. It is important to keep in mind that elderly, deconditioned, and biomechanically inefficient people are working much harder than younger, fit, and agile people to accomplish the same task. Even walking at a slow speed (2 mph) requires significantly greater exertion than might be expected.

Painful, swollen joints need to be protected from deforming forces and unnecessary joint stress. Acute joint effusions should be controlled prior to performing conditioning levels of exercise. This may require a course of drug therapy and/or joint aspiration. Joint effusion increases intra-articular pressure during joint motion and may lead to pain and

GUIDELINES FOR EXERCISE TESTING AND CORONARY ARTERY DISEASE (CAD)

PERFORM SUPERVISED EXERCISE STRESS TEST FOR:

1. Apparently healthy:
    – men ≥ 40; women ≥ 50 for vigorous exercise only

2. Persons at risk with no symptoms:
    – all ages for vigorous exercise only

3. Persons at risk for CAD with symptoms and with disease:
    – all ages for moderate and vigorous exercise

    > CAD risk factors (2 or more = at risk):
    > – HTN, BP ≥ 160/90 mmHg
    > – Serum cholesterol ≥ 240 mg/dl (6.2 mmol/L)
    > – Cigarette smoking
    > – Diabetes mellitus
    > – Family history

EXERCISE INTENSITY

1. Moderate exercise
    – 40-60% max VO_2 = 60-75% max heart rate
    – well within current capacity
    – sustainable comfortably for 60 minutes
    – slow progression
    – noncompetitive

2. Vigorous exercise
    – >60% max VO_2 = >75% max heart rate
    – substantial challenge
    – fatigue within 20 minutes

Table 2: Guidelines for Exercise Testing and Coronary Artery Disease (CAD). Source: Gordon, N. F., Kohl, H. W., Scott, C. B., Gibbons, L. W., Blair, S. N. (1992).

DISEASE-SPECIFIC CONSIDERATION IN AEROBIC EXERCISE

OSTEOARTHRITIS (OA)

- alter duration and intensity of joint loading. Continual weight-bearing should last no longer than 2-4 hours, followed by at least 1 hour of non–weight-bearing.
- strengthen muscles that cross and support joints.
- do not overstretch around lax joints.

RHEUMATOID ARTHRITIS (RA)

- protect vulnerable joints from unnecessary stress and impact.
- support for ankle/foot stability and position with orthoses as needed.
- be aware of signs for cervical instability, cord, or nerve-root involvement.

ANKYLOSING SPONDYLITIS (AS) AND PSORIATIC ARTHRITIS

- emphasize hip and spinal extension, flexibility, posture, and chest expansion.
- use gentle, static stretching daily.
- use low-impact activities to preserve musculoskeletal and cardiovascular fitness.
- swim with mask and snorkel to reduce the need for cervical rotation.

SYSTEMIC LUPUS ERYTHEMATOSUS (SLE)

- use regular moderate activity to decrease fatigue and improve mood.
- be aware of increased risk of osteoporosis, stress fractures, avascular necrosis of the femoral head, and myopathy with prolonged use of corticosteroids.

FIBROMYALGIA

- encourage a progressive program of dynamic, low-intensity exercise.
- use heat, cold, massage, and relaxation techniques as exercise adjuncts.

Table 3: Disease-Specific Consideration in Aerobic Exercise

joint damage. Rest in the form of protective splints and activity modification also may be recommended.

For a disease flare in one or a few joints, it is often possible to alternate modes of exercise to maintain the exercise habit and protect joints. For example, a painful and swollen knee may be protected by a change from a 30-minute walking routine every other day to 10 minutes twice daily on the stationary bicycle with no resistance.

Joints with loss of joint space, damaged cartilage, laxity, or tightness in periarticular tissue, chronic effusion, or malalignment are highly susceptible to activity-related injury. Joint pain and swelling following activity should be treated as an "overuse" or athletic injury. In addition to immediate care with ice and rest, preventive steps should be taken to strengthen the joint in preparation for a safe return to the activity.

If joint integrity or stability is not amenable to change, activity modifications can decrease the amount of joint stress incurred. A clinical knowledge of biomechanics is essential. For example, intra-articular pressure in the hip can be reduced up to 50% by use of a cane in the contralateral hand during ambulation. Suggestions for exercise considerations in specific diseases are given in Table 3.

SUMMARY: WHY PEOPLE WITH ARTHRITIS SHOULD EXERCISE

People who are physically active are healthier and live longer than people who are sedentary. This is true for everyone, especially people with arthritis. In addition to the general benefits of regular exercise, certain kinds of exercise have shown important benefits for people with arthritis.

Arthritis is one of the most common reasons people give for limiting physical activity. Being inactive may increase arthritis problems, and many people are deconditioned, weaker, less flexible, and have more pain than necessary due to the complications of inactivity. Pain, stiffness, fatigue, and the fear of doing harm can make it difficult to be physically active with arthritis. However, for persons with arthritis to be as healthy, capable, and comfortable as possible, an appropriate exercise program is extremely important.

WHAT KINDS OF EXERCISE ARE HELPFUL AND SAFE?

Research shows that many people with arthritis can safely participate in appropriate, regular exercise programs and can achieve better aerobic fitness, improve strength, endurance, and flexibility, and improve their ability to walk and perform daily tasks. They also experience less pain and depression. There are three major types of exercise, and each plays a role in maintaining or improving health and fitness and reducing arthritis-related disability and pain.

Flexibility or stretching exercises are gentle, low-intensity exercises performed daily to maintain or improve range of motion. These exercises are the foundation of most therapeutic exercise programs and are also important in recreational or fitness exercise. Adequate flexibility improves function and reduces the chance for injuries.

EXAMPLE OF AN EXERCISE PROGRAM

EXERCISE GOALS:

1. Improve general flexibility, strength, and endurance

2. Improve posture

3. Develop life-long exercise habits

EXERCISE PLAN:

PHASE	MODE	FREQUENCY	INTENSITY	DURATION
PHASE I Pre-aerobic conditioning program	Active range of motion; gravity-resisted and isometric strengthening	Daily	Start with 3-5 repetitions of 12 exercises; increase to 10 repetitions	Progress to 15 minutes of continuous, comfortable activity
PHASE II Add aerobic component, alternate aerobic activities	Walking and/or stationary bicycle	Start with 3 times a week; may increase to 5 days as tolerated	Low to moderate (60-75% max HR; 3-4 RPE)	Start with 5-10 minutes walking or pedaling at a comfortable speed
PHASE III Total physical fitness program: 1. Daily flexibility routine of 15-20 minutes 2. Aerobic exercise of choice 3-4 times per week. May add swimming and water aerobics as alternate forms of aerobic activity 3. Add resistive strengthening component	Resistance exercise (free weights, elastic bands, or equipment.) Use wrist weights or equipment that does not require gripping to avoid hand and wrist stress if necessary	2 times a week	60-70% 1 RM	8-10 exercises, progressing to 10 repetitions each

Note: maxHR = age-predicted maximal heart rate; RPE = rating of perceived exertion; 1 RM = one-repetition maximum)

Table 4: Example of an Exercise Program

EXERCISE TIPS FOR THE NEW EXERCISER

WALKING

- Start on flat, level surface.
- Stretch out heel and calf muscles.
- Warm up and cool down with 3-5 minutes of slow walking.
- Walk at a comfortable pace, sing, or talk as you go along.
- If knees get sore, walk more slowly.
- Wear supportive shoes with good soles and shock-absorbing insoles.

SWIMMING OR WATER AEROBICS

- Swim only with lifeguard present.
- Vary strokes for comfort and overall conditioning.
- Regulate exercise intensity by changing the speed, arc of movement, and length of lever arm.
- Slower and smaller motions use less energy and cause less stress.
- Use mask and snorkel if head turning is a problem.
- Begin and end at a slower pace.
- If water is cool, finish with a warm shower or soak.
- Wear tights, t-shirt, and disposable latex gloves to retain body heat in the water.
- Protect your feet with water shoes or slippers for aerobics or walking.

BICYCLE (OUTDOOR OR STATIONARY)

- Start and end with no resistance or on flat ground.
- Pedal with ball of foot.
- Make sure seat height allows knee to get comfortably straight.
- Feet should be able to swivel freely within pedal straps.
- Keep speed of pedaling at or below 60 rpm. Use gears as applicable to protect knees.

LOW-IMPACT AEROBIC DANCE

- Wear shoes and exercise on a hard floor or firm carpet.
- Don't bounce, lunge, or do low squats.
- Control your movements. Don't move too fast at the outer range of your movements.
- Change movements frequently if you start to feel muscle fatigue or joint soreness.
- Avoid prolonged exercise with arms above shoulder level.

Table 5: Exercise Tips for the New Exerciser

Muscle conditioning (strength and endurance) exercises are more vigorous than flexibility exercises. These exercises are usually done every other day and are designed to ask the muscle to work harder than usual. This extra workload may come from lifting the weight of the arm, leg, or trunk against gravity, or using weights, elastic bands, or weight machines for more resistance. Muscles adapt to the new demands by getting stronger and becoming capable of working longer.

Cardiorespiratory or *aerobic exercise* includes activities that use the large muscles of the body in rhythmic, repetitive movement. Aerobic exercise improves heart, lung, and muscle function, and it has benefits for weight control, mood, and general health. Examples of aerobic exercise are walking, swimming, aerobic dance or aquatics, bicycling, or exercising on equipment such as treadmills or rowing machines. Daily activities such as mowing the lawn, raking leaves, sweeping the driveway, playing golf, and walking the dog are also aerobic exercise. Table 4 displays an example of an exercise program progression. Tips for beginning exercisers are shown in Table 5.

CONCLUSION

Persons with arthritis are a heterogenous population ranging widely in age, disease, impairments, functional goals, and interests. Some are interested in and capable of performing exercise programs to improve physical fitness. Others may need instruction and support to participate in cardiovascular- or pulmonary-rehabilitation programs. Others may not be candidates for fitness-training programs but can be educated and encouraged to adopt appropriate activity habits to improve or maintain health and reduce the risk of inactivity-related illness.

REFERENCES

Beals, C. A., Lampman, R. M., Banwell, B. F., et al. (1985). Measurement of exercise tolerance in patients with rheumatoid arthritis and osteoarthritis. *Journal of Rheumatology, 12,* 458-461.

Blair, S. N., Kohl, H. W., Paffenbarger, R. S., et al. (1989). Physical fitness and all-cause mortality: A prospective study of healthy men and women. *Journal of the American Medical Association, 262,* 2395-2401.

Blair, S. N., Kohl, H. W., & Gordon, N. F. (1992). How much physical activity is good for health? *Annual Review of Public Health, 13,* 99-126.

Burckhardt, C. S., Moncur, C., & Minor, M. A. (1994). Exercise tests as outcome measures. *Arthritis Care and Research, 7,* 169-175.

Byers, P. H. (1985). Effect of exercise on morning stiffness and mobility in patients with rheumatoid arthritis. *Research in Nursing and Health, 8,* 275-281.

Ekdahl, C., Andersson, S. I., Moritz, U., & Svensson, B. (1990). Dynamic versus static training in patients with rheumatoid arthritis. *Scandanavian Journal of Rheumatology, 19,* 17-26.

Ekdahl, C., Ekman, R., Andersson, S. I., Melander, A., & Svensson, B. (1990). Dynamic training and circulating levels of corticotrophin-releasing factor, beta-lipoprotein and beta-endorphin in rheumatoid arthritis. *Pain, 40,* 35-42.

Fisher, N. M., Pendergast, D. R., Gresham, G. E., & Calkins, E. (1991). Muscle rehabilitation: its effect on muscular and functional performance of patients with knee osteoarthritis. *Archives of Physical Medicine and Rehabilitation, 72,* 367-74.

Galloway, M. T., & Jokl, P. (1993). The role of exercise in the treatment of inflammatory arthritis. *Bulletin of Rheumatic Disease, 42,* 1-4.

Gordon, N. F., Kohl, H. W., Scott, C. B., Gibbons, L. W., Blair, S. N. (1992). Reassessment of the guidelines for exercise testing. *Sports Medicine, 13,* 293-302.

Harkcom, T. M., Lampman, R. M., Banwell, B. F., & Castor, C. W. (1985). Therapeutic value of graded aerobic exercise training in rheumatoid arthritis. *Arthritis and Rheumatism, 28,* 32-39.

James, M. J., Cleland, L. G., Gaffney, R. D., Proudman, S. M., & Chatterton, B. E. (1994). Effect of exercise on 99mTc-DPTA clearance from knee with effusions. *Journal of Rheumatology, 21,* 501-504.

Kovar, P. A., Allegrante, J. P., MacKenzie, C. R., Peterson, M. G., & Gutin, B. (1992). Supervised fitness walking in patients with osteoarthritis of the knee. A randomized, controlled trial. *Annals of Internal Medicine, 116,* 529-534.

Loeser, R., Messier, S., Gianfranco, V., Morgan, T., & Etttinger, W. (1995). The effects of an exercise and weight loss intervention on osteoarthritis of the knee. *Arthritis and Rheumatism, 38,* S268.

Michel, B. A., Fries, J. F., Bloch, D. A., Lane, N. E., & Jones, H. H. (1992). Osteophytosis of the knee: Association with changes in weight-bearing exercise. *Clinical Rheumatology, 11,* 235-238.

Minor, M. A., Hewett, J. E., Webel, R. R. et al. (1988). Exercise tolerance and disease related measures in patients with rheumatoid arthritis and osteoarthritis. *Journal of Rheumatology, 15,* 905-911.

Minor, M. A., Hewett, J. E., Webel, R. R., Anderson, S. K., & Day, D. R. (1989). Efficacy of physical conditioning exercise in patients with rheumatoid arthritis or osteoarthritis. *Arthritis and Rheumatism, 32,* 1396-1405.

Moskowitz, R. W., & Haug, M. R. (Eds.) (1986). *Arthritis and the elderly.* New York: Springer Publishing.

Nordemar, R., Ekblom, B., Zachrisson, L., & Lundquist, K. (1981). Physical training in rheumatoid arthritis: A controlled long-term study. I. *Scandanavian Journal of Rheumatology, 10,* 17-23.

Pate, R. R., Pratt, M., Blair, S. N., et al. (1995). Physical activity and public health: a recommendation from the Centers for Disease Control and Prevention and the American College of Sports Medicine. *Journal of the American Medical Association, 273,* 402-407.

Perlman, S. G., Connell, K. J., Clark, A., Robinson, M. S., Conlon, P., Gecht, M., Caldron, P., & Sinacore, J. M. (1990). Dance-based aerobic exercise for rheumatoid arthritis. *Arthritis Care Resources, 3,* 29-35.

Philbin, E. F., Groff, G. D., Ries, M. D. et al. (1995). Cardiovascular fitness and health in patients with end-stage osteoarthritis. *Arthritis and Rheumatism, 38,* 799-805.

Rall, L. C., Lundgren, N., Joseph, L., Dolinikowski, G., Kehayais, J. J., & Roubenoff, R. (1994). The metabolic cost of rheumatoid arthritis: reversal with progressive resistance exercise. *Arthritis and Rheumatism, 37,* S222.

Rall, L. C., Lundgren, N., Reichlin, S., & Roubenoff, R. (1995). Evidence for growth hormone deficiency in rheumatoid arthritis: Assessment by deconvolution analysis. *Arthritis and Rheumatism, 38,* S289.

Schlaghecke, R., Kornely, E., Wollenhaupt, J., & Specker, C. (1992). Glucocorticoid receptors in rheumatoid arthritis. *Arthritis and Rheumatism, 35,* 740-744.

Semble, E. L., Loeser, R. F., & Wise, C. M. (1990). Therapeutic exercise for rheumatoid arthritis and osteoarthritis. *Seminars in Arthritis and Rheumatism, 20,* 32-40.

Stenström, C. H. (1994a). Therapeutic exercise in rheumatoid arthritis. *Arthritis Care Resources, 7,* 190-197.

Stenström, C. H. (1994b). Home exercise in rheumatoid arthritis functional class II: Goal setting versus pain attention. *Journal of Rheumatology, 21,* 627-634.

Yelin, E., Meenan, R., Nevitt, M., & Epstein, W. (1980). Work disability in rheumatoid arthritis: Effects of disease, social, and work factors. *Annals of Internal Medicine, 93,* 551-556.

Yocum, D. E., Zautra, A., Matt, K. S., Castro, L., Potter, P., Nordensson, K., Hoffman, J., & Cornett, M. (1995). Exercise and stress reduction result in positive changes in prolactin, cortisol and immune function in rheumatoid arthritis. *Arthritis and Rheumatism, 38,* S384.

BIBLIOGRAPHY

American College of Sports Medicine Position Stand (1990). The recommended quantity and quality of exercise for developing and maintaining cardiorespiratory and muscular fitness in healthy adults. *Medicine and Science in Sports and Exercise, 22,* 265-274.

Ekblom, B., Lovgren, O., Alderin, M., Friedstrom, M., & Satterstrom, G. (1974). Physical performance in patients with rheumatoid arthritis. *Scandanavian Journal of Rheumatology, 3,* 121-25.

Houlbrooke, K., Vause, K., & Merrilees, M. J. (1990). Effects of movement and weight bearing on the glycosamineglycan content of sheep articular cartilage. *Australian Physiotherapy, 36,* 88-91.

16

ASSISTIVE TECHNOLOGY FOR PERSONS WITH ARTHRITIS

William Mann, PhD, OTR

ASSISTIVE TECHNOLOGY

The terms *assistive device* and *assistive technology* are used interchangeably. Assistive technology is "any item, piece of equipment, or product system whether acquired commercially off the shelf, modified, or customized, that is used to increase, maintain, or improve functional capabilities of individuals with disabilities" (Technology Related Assistance for Individuals with Disabilities Act of 1988, PL 100-407). This is a broad definition that encompasses many basic consumer products such as garage-door openers and microwave ovens, special-needs products such as walkers and button hooks, and specially modified devices such as a TV remote control with large buttons. Some assistive devices are found in specialty stores such as suppliers of durable medical equipment, and others can be purchased in department stores, electronics stores, or pharmacies.

Physical therapists have traditionally provided assessment and recommendations for assistive devices related to mobility, and occupational therapists addressed devices for other activities of daily living (ADL), instrumental activities of daily living (IADL), and leisure. The past decade has seen the development of many new assistive devices that are based on microprocessor technology, and a number of these are not familiar to occupational and physical therapists. This chapter will present and discuss the range of assistive devices available and their applications for persons with arthritis. Computers and ways to make them more accessible, and environmental-control devices are discussed in separate sections inasmuch as their use encompasses many ADL, IADL, and leisure activities. This chapter first reviews important considerations in the use of assistive devices for persons with arthritis and then suggests resources for assistive devices. Next, the chapter discusses assistive devices for persons with arthritis and considers them relative to ADL, IADL, and leisure. This chapter concludes with a discussion of special considerations in the use of assistive technology by the frail elderly with arthritis.

SPECIAL CONSIDERATIONS FOR PERSONS WITH ARTHRITIS

For persons with arthritis, careful assessment must precede recommendations for assistive devices. That assessment must consider the physical condition of the person, especially the status of each affected joint. It is equally important to consider the tasks that the person performs—or would like to perform—and the environment in which those tasks will be carried out. Are there others who can provide assistance with certain tasks? All such considerations have an impact on the selection of appropriate assistive devices.

The symptoms associated with arthritis are not constant and vary with the type of arthritis and the specific joints affected. A person may experience more pain and joint stiffness in the morning than later in the day. Inflammation and pain may also vary over days, weeks, and months. For some, symptoms will become more severe over a period of years.

It is very important to consider joint protection in recommending assistive devices. While many devices will make tasks easier and protect joints from excessive strain, other devices may actually stress joints. For example, a reacher may make it possible for a person with shoulder pain and limitation in ROM to reach items high in a cabinet. However, if this person also has arthritis in the hands and must apply a strong grip to operate the reacher, joints of the hands could be stressed.

In assessing the needs of a person with arthritis, it is very helpful to have several different assistive devices available for each task for which the person might benefit from using a device. For example, a person may find one type of reacher difficult to grasp but could easily use another.

In addition to careful assessment and providing recommendations, therapists play another critical role with assistive devices: training. While some devices are easily used by most people immediately and without modification, others require explanation, modification, and training. For example, many people have difficulty programming the memory feature on phones. While not a traditional role for a therapist, teaching the person with arthritis how to program the phone for one-button operation will ensure its successful use. Training often involves not only the person with arthritis but also family members and other care providers. Since a parent or spouse may program the memory phone in the example above, he or she could benefit from the therapist's instruction.

RESOURCES ON ASSISTIVE TECHNOLOGY

No single chapter or book could describe all available assistive devices. Even if such a book were written, it would quickly require updating. This chapter will provide many examples of devices for use with different tasks, but therapists must utilize other resources in searching for appropriate devices in individual situations. Several resources are listed below.

Abledata is a database of over 20,000 assistive devices available from approximately 2,500 manufacturers. Detailed information and, for many devices, pictures are provided for each. Abledata is available on CD-ROM or 3.5" disks from Trace Center, University of Wisconsin, 1500 Highland Avenue, Room 5-151, Madison, WI 53705. It is also available on the World Wide Web at <http://trace.wisc.edu>. Abledata is very user friendly. It will even prepare letters to manufacturers to request more product information.

Programs funded under the Technology Related Assistance for Individuals with Disabilities Act (Tech Act, 1988) are now providing information and referral services in every state. Most programs offer Abledata searches as a free service. For information on the Tech Act program in your state, contact the RESNA Technical Assistance Project at (703) 524-6686.

The American Occupational Therapy Association publishes the textbook, *Assistive Technology for Persons With Disabilities*, now in its second edition (1995). This book provides information on assistive devices and many case studies, and it devotes a whole chapter to assistive-technology resources.

At the end of this chapter is a list of companies that publish catalogs of assistive products (see appendix 1). It is often helpful to show the person a picture of a device from a catalog if you do not have the device on hand. Catalogs are grouped into those targeted directly for consumer purchase and those aimed at therapists who assess and recommend devices.

Maintaining and using resources is essential with assistive technology. With the number of devices currently on the market and the number of new devices entering the marketplace each year, therapists must have up-to-date information to ensure that they are recommending optimal interventions.

USING ASSISTIVE TECHNOLOGY

This section will discuss the use by persons with arthritis of assistive devices for a number of tasks. Therapists need to view assistive technology in its broadest sense and ask, "What devices might make it easier or possible for this person to complete important tasks?" Thus, listening to the consumer's perspective on relevant tasks will help delineate the specific areas to consider in recommending assistive technology. Some assistive devices such as reachers, grab bars, canes, and computers can be used for a number of tasks. Computers and their configuration for persons with arthritis are discussed as a separate section.

ACTIVITIES OF DAILY LIVING

Activities of daily living include bathing, dressing, grooming, eating, using the toilet, and walking. Each will be discussed separately and examples of assistive devices presented. Bear in mind that everyone uses a variety of tools to accomplish activities of daily living, and some of these tools can be adapted without replacing the device. For example, most people use knives, spoons, and forks for eating. The handles of these utensils can be built up with low-cost materials. Abledata lists 21 different padding products including cushioned tape, cylindrical foam padding, preconstructed adaptors, plastic coating, spray-on nonslip grip, and vinyl coating. Some of the assistive devices discussed below may be difficult to use for some persons with arthritis, and even these devices may require adaptation or modification.

BATHING

In the United States, most homes have bathtubs. While sponge bathing is an alternative method for cleaning oneself, Americans typically prefer to shower or to bathe. Bathtubs were not designed for persons with physical limitations such as those that result from arthritis. There are a number of assistive bathing devices to address the challenges bathtubs pose. For those who have difficulty getting into or out of a tub, or who have trouble standing during a shower, there are bath stools, seats, and chairs. Abledata lists 291 such items. A bath bench that extends over the outside of the tub can be used for seated transfers (Figure 1). There is a wide variety of shapes and styles, and a number of issues arise in selecting the most appropriate device. If the person with arthritis is the only member of the household using the bathtub, then once it is installed, its weight and size are not an issue. However, if other members of the household also use the tub and do not want to use the bath bench, seat, or stool, then weight becomes an important consideration because of the necessity to move the device each time it is used. Size also becomes important if there is no appropriate place for storage.

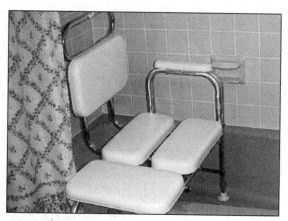

Figure 1. This bath bench enables seated transfers into the tub.

If the person with arthritis requires back support, then a bath chair, which has a back, is probably a better choice than a stool. On the other hand, if this person receives assistance with bathing, then it might be easier to wash the person's back with the person seated on a stool. Some tubs are too narrow for some bath seats and benches, so it is important to measure the tub and determine the fit of the device recommended. Bath benches, stools, and chairs provide a good example of the complexity of decision making in selecting the best device to fit the person, the environment, and the other members of the household. A recent study of dissatisfied owners of bath devices suggested that the dissatisfaction might be due to a mismatch between the owners' functional status and the type of device (Mann, Hurren, Tomita & Charvat, in press).

Grab bars are another useful device for persons who have difficulty getting into and out of the shower head. A portable grab bar that can be attached to the side of the tub is pictured in Figure 2. Individuals who bathe in a seated position often use a hand-held

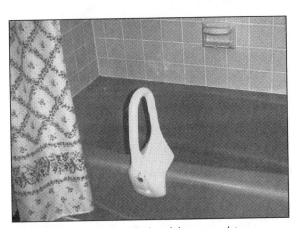

Figure 2. This easy-to-attach bath grab bar can assist a person making a standing transfer into the tub.

shower head, but this can be a problem for persons with limited or painful grasp. The weight of hand-held shower heads varies, and plastic is generally lighter than metal. Handles can also be built-up to make grasping easier. Using the water controls can be difficult for a person with limited hand strength, and lever-type faucet handles are much easier to operate. For people with hand involvement it is a worthwhile investment to install lever faucet handles throughout their homes.

There is a variety of other devices for bathing, most low-cost but very useful. Bath caddies placed in a convenient location eliminate the need to reach for soap, shampoo, and related items. There are devices that can dispense soap (Figure 3) and shampoo at the push of a large button; they can be placed conveniently on the shower wall. Soap-on-a-rope works very well for many persons with arthritis. Back brushes and hand brushes come in a variety of styles and shapes. For persons with arthritis, cloth or loofa slings that can be pulled with both hands are often the best choice for washing the back. Brushes and sponges on long handles can cause excessive force on the wrist. Wash mitts can also pose a problem: when wet they can become heavy and increase stress to the wrist. Figure 4 illustrates just one of the 23 bath brushes listed in Abledata.

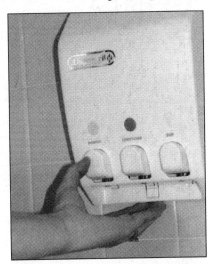

Figure 3. Soap dispensers can be placed on the wall in the tub or shower.

The time of day the person bathes can have an impact on the level of difficulty. If the person is more limber later in the day, it might be best to bathe at that time, and perhaps there will be less need for some of these assistive devices. On the other hand, some individuals prefer to bathe first thing in the morning, perhaps simply because it is a familiar routine or because the warm water has a therapeutic effect and helps to get the day off to a good start. When a person bathes or showers, and where, and with what level of assistance, have an impact on selecting appropriate devices to recommend.

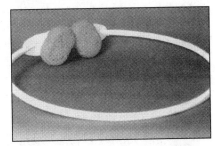

Figure 4. This device assists with washing body parts that are difficult to reach, especially the back.

BATHING DEVICES

DEVICE TYPE	NUMBER[*]
Bath lifts	24
Back brushes	23
Hand brushes	1
Foot brush	1
Safety treads	12
Wash mitts and Washcloths	6
Water temperature control	5
Bathroom caddy	1
Bath seats, chairs, stools	291

* Number of devices listed in HyperAbledata, 1995

Table 1: Bathing Devices

The complexity of issues involved with selecting assistive devices—those surrounding the status of the person, the environment, and the other people involved—are well illustrated with bathing devices. There is no simple formula, no simple list of assistive devices for all people with arthritis, and "high-tech" devices are not necessarily more or less effective than "low-tech" devices. For the therapist, the judgment involved in sorting out the complexity of variables and making recommendations is of utmost importance. All too often individuals end up with devices that are partially or totally inappropriate for them, and it is usually the result of failure to take into account all relevant factors and consider all possible products or environmental modifications. Table 1 lists the types of assistive devices for bathing and the number available as listed in Abledata.

DRESSING

Dressing requires movement of virtually every joint in the body. For example, trunk flexion (gross movement) is required in putting on socks and shoes. Gross movement is also required in getting items from closets. Putting on pullover tops such as sweaters requires significant shoulder extension and rotation. Fine motor activities include buttoning, zipping zippers, and tieing shoes. Fortunately there are a number of devices that can help with or substitute for both fine and gross motor tasks.

Changing the time of day to begin dressing may be helpful for some persons with arthritis. One's day typically begins with getting dressed. If this can be delayed until after breakfast, perhaps after a warm bath or shower, joints may be more limber and the task of donning clothes may be easier.

Persons with arthritis who have difficulty dressing may benefit from clothing designed especially for persons with physical limitations. Velcro® fasteners are often a good substitute for buttons or zippers. Clothes that fasten in front are much easier to put on and take off than those with fasteners in the back. Clothes that are loose-fitting will be more comfortable, especially when one sits. Clothes must be able to fit over whatever splints the wearer may use. A good question to ask about any item of clothing is, "How much fatigue and/or pain is caused by putting this clothing on or taking it off?" If there is significant fatigue or pain, consider a substitute for or modification of that piece of clothing. A wide variety of special clothing is now available, and a person with arthritis need not sacrifice attractiveness for ease of dressing. Therapists must consider the psychological and social aspects of clothing and direct the person with arthritis not only to solutions that make dressing easier (or, indeed, possible) but also to solutions that fit the way the person wishes to present him or herself.

It is not necessary to replace every item of clothing. Clothes the person owns can often be adapted: adding zippers to the front of garments can eliminate the shoulder movement required to don pullover items, and replacing buttons with Velcro® can make a favorite shirt easy to manage. Using elastic thread on cuff buttons can eliminate the need for buttoning and unbuttoning them.

Assembling an appropriate wardrobe should precede considerations for assistive devices. The items of clothing that are still difficult to manage can then be considered. If putting on pants or shoes is difficult, a dressing stick or trousers' aid could make these tasks easier. Figure 5 illustrates the use of a dressing stick in putting on a shoe. Zipper pulls and button hooks can ease the use of zippers and buttons. Figure 6 illustrates the use of a button hook to button a sweater. There are many different dressing aids; therapists can keep a supply on hand to provide persons with arthritis the opportunity to try several different items. The use of some of these devices may be difficult to understand at first; sock aids are a good example. Instructions that come with the devices are often difficult to follow. The therapist needs to teach persons with arthritis to use these devices. Figure 7 shows the sock aid being used and the sock close to being fully on the person's foot.

Storage of clothing also requires careful consideration. Lowering the clothes bar in closets makes access easier. Changing the handles on drawers may make it possible to get to clothing that would otherwise be inaccessible. If drawers are too difficult to pull open

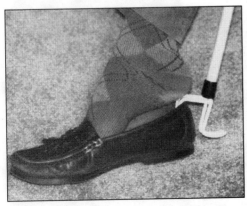

Figure 5. Dressing sticks can be used to assist with putting on shoes.

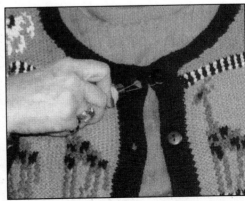

Figure 6. Button hooks are low cost and quite effective for many persons with arthritis.

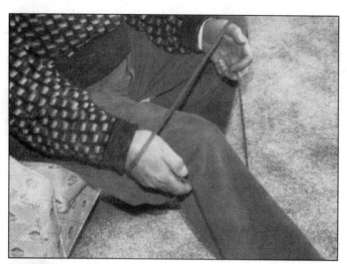

Figure 7. The sock aid in use.

or push shut, add new glides; this may greatly reduce friction and lower the energy required to open and shut the drawer. Knobs on closet doors can be replaced with levers. Table 2 lists types of assistive devices for dressing and the number of products listed in HyperAbledata.

GROOMING

Dental care can be made easier simply by building-up the handle of the toothbrush. Toothbrushes with built-up handles can be purchased from a number of sources, or foam tubing can be added. Electric toothbrushes and water-cleansing devices (oral irrigating aids) may also make dental care easier, but the weight of the device is an important consideration. Dental floss holders make flossing easier and can be found in most pharmacies. For persons who find toothpaste difficult to remove from the tube, tube squeezers are available to assist with this task. Pump dispensing toothpaste containers may be easier than a tube for many persons to operate.

DRESSING DEVICES	
DEVICE TYPE	**NUMBER***
Special clothing	1051
Button aids	26
Shoe aids	46
Stocking aids	36
Dressing stick	12
Leg positioning aid	4
Trouser aids	3
Zipper pull	9

* Number of devices listed in HyperAbledata, 1995

Hair care can be made easier by building up handles of brushes and combs. Combs and brushes with straps can eliminate the need to maintain a grasp. Long-handled brushes and combs can reduce the amount of gross movement required. Hair dryers on stands or mounted on a wall also reduce the need to grasp the dryer. Select dryers with large control buttons to turn the dryer on and off and adjust the heat.

Nail care can be made easier with hand brushes that have suction cups and can be attached to the sink to eliminate the need to grasp. Nail clippers with longer handles require less fine-motor movement. Even better, nail clippers on a stand eliminate the need for grasping.

Shaving may be easier for many persons if they use an electric razor. There are many electric razors available. Select one that has a large handle and is lightweight. For those who prefer a blade, use foam tubing to build up the handle. Table 3 lists assistive devices for grooming and hygiene and the numbers of devices available.

EATING AND DRINKING

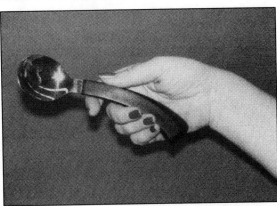

Figure 8. These eating utensils are easier to grasp than most dinnerware and more attractive than most specialty item eating utensils.

A variety of simple devices can make eating easier: utensils with built-up handles and/or straps (see Figure 8); plates with rims; materials to stabilize plates and prevent them from sliding; knives that permit one-handed cutting; and cups with handles that are easy to grasp. Therapists can offer persons with arthritis the opportunity to try out a number of devices to discover which work best for them and which are what they wish to use at the table. Mechanical feeders are available for persons with very severe arthritis who have little or no joint movement of the upper extremities. Mechanical feeders are slow and relatively expensive, and the person who uses one requires assistance with set-up. Many people prefer personal assistance to mechanical feeders. Table 4 lists assistive devices for eating and drinking that are available from Abledata.

TOILETING

For hygiene, tong-like devices are available to assist in wiping. Premoistened wipes may also make toilet hygiene easier. Use of a bidet for washing and drying the perianal area is an excellent solution for many people who cannot manage toilet paper. Bidets can be quite expensive, but add-on washing devices are available at much lower cost. Another device useful to many persons is a toilet-tissue holder that does not require the roller to be snapped into place.

GROOMING AND HYGIENE DEVICES

DEVICE TYPE	NUMBER*
Dental care	
Special toothbrushes	17
Dental floss holders	3
Denture washing devices	5
Toothpaste dispenser	1
Hair care	
Special combs	7
Hair brushes	12
Shampoo aids	20
Special mirrors	31
Devices for nail care	8
Devices for shaving	2

* Number of devices listed in HyperAbledata, 1995

Table 3: Grooming and Hygiene Devices

EATING AND DRINKING DEVICES

DEVICE TYPE	NUMBER*
Drinking devices	
Special cups	36
Special glasses	11
Special straws	11
Special dishes	57
Feeders	16
Special utensils	180

* Number of devices listed in HyperAbledata, 1995

Table 4: Eating and Drinking Devices

Toilet handles can be modified (built up or extended) to make flushing easier. Raised toilet seats make getting on and off the toilet less difficult. Those made from plastic may be somewhat easier to clean and remove. A wide variety of grab-bars can assist with getting on and off the toilet.

Use of bedpans or urinals may be necessary. Their size, shape, and weight must be considered in selecting one that can be used independently. Some urinals are designed for

TOILETING DEVICES

DEVICE TYPE	NUMBER[*]
Commodes	142
Incontinence supplies	210
Toilet safety frames	58
Toilet seats	95
Urinals	30
Suppository inserters	6
Toilet paper holders for commode	2
Toilet paper holding devices	10

* Number of devices listed in HyperAbledata, 1995

Table 5: Toileting Devices

one sex, and others are designed for both. Table 5 lists the types of assistive devices for toileting, and the number of products listed in Abledata.

WALKING AND MOBILITY

There is a variety of mobility aids for persons who require support or assistance with balance. Mobility devices are used by more people than any other type of assistive device. The simplest device is the cane. More than 4 million Americans use canes (LaPlante, Hendershot, & Moss, 1992). Canes can support up to 25 percent of an individual's weight. In addition, almost 1.5 million people use walkers. A large percentage of these individuals have arthritis. Walkers can support up to 50 percent of a person's weight.

There are hundreds of different kinds of canes and walkers. For persons with difficulty grasping, cane handles can be built up. There is one cane handle on the market specifically designed for persons who have difficulty grasping, the Orthoease® cane available from Cleo (800) 321-0595. A trough design allows the forearm to bear some of the weight and reduces the stress on painful hands and wrists. There are also walkers available with the trough handle design. Walkers with wheels may be easier to use than the standard walker, which requires lifting. Two recent articles provide an overview of cane and walker designs and point out some problems with their use (Mann, Granger, Hurren, Tomita, & Charvat, 1995; Mann, Hurren, Tomita, & Charvat, 1995). Canes, for example, vary greatly in weight. For a person who has had a stroke and also has arthritis, a quad cane may be needed for support, but the greater weight of this type of cane may preclude its use. In such a case, a wheeled walker might provide optimal support and ease of use, if the person is able to push it.

"Add-on" devices for canes and walkers can provide more convenience for persons with arthritis. Bags or baskets for carrying items when shopping make a walker more functional but can add weight and put additional stress on the wrists. Walkers with seats allow rest stops and can reduce overall fatigue.

For persons with arthritis, wheelchairs may be helpful. Many people with arthritis will use a wheelchair on longer trips outside the home but do not require one in the house. Powered wheelchairs can provide independent mobility for persons with very severe arthritis. A wide variety of wheelchair designs, cushions, and accessories is available. It is essential that persons with arthritis consult professionals before purchasing a wheelchair. A recent study found a significantly higher rate of wheelchair problems when the user did not seek help from professionals in selecting a wheelchair (Mann, Hurren, Charvat, & Tomita, in press).

Scooters provide powered, wheeled mobility at a much lower cost than powered wheelchairs, although they might not provide optimal support for some persons. Many supermarkets now provide scooters with baskets for customers who require them. Motorized carts like the Amigo® can be rented by the day or week. For traveling to another city, this makes a mobility device available without carrying one's own, which in the case of a scooter would be very heavy to transport.

Maintenance is critical with mobility devices. A poorly maintained mobility device could cause a fall. Therapists must instruct their patients not only in the use of mobility devices but also in their long-term maintenance. When initiating services for a newly referred patient, therapists should routinely check all mobility devices the person uses to be sure that the devices are properly maintained. Table 6 lists types of mobility devices and the number of products listed in Abledata.

INSTRUMENTAL ACTIVITIES OF DAILY LIVING

Instrumental activities of daily living include such activities as using the telephone, taking medications, food preparation, money management, household maintenance, and shopping.

TELEPHONE

The telephone is one of our most important tools for work, leisure, shopping, banking, and calling for help. Therapists should assess phone needs routinely. There is a wide variety of commercially available products to assist persons with arthritis in using the phone.

For persons with joint pain or limitations in the hands, a number of options may be considered. Phones with large buttons can be easier to operate. A redial feature or memory function can permit one-button dialing. Voice-activated phones provide total freedom from use of hands. For persons who have difficulty holding the receiver, phone holders are available for hands-free operation; speaker phones also eliminate the need to hold the receiver. Cordless phones kept within easy reach can eliminate the need to get up and move to answer the phone, thus reducing fatigue. The pager feature on many cordless

WALKING DEVICES

DEVICE TYPE	NUMBER *
Canes	139
Crutches	124
Standing	121
Walkers	358
Manual wheelchairs	447
Powered wheelchairs	320
Sport wheelchairs	84
Wheelchair accessories	895

* Number of devices listed in HyperAbledata, 1995

Table 6: Walking Devices

phones can reduce the amount of energy spent searching for the phone, should it be misplaced. Answering machines are useful in screening out nuisance calls and eliminating the need to hurry to pick up a call.

Furniture arrangement can also make a difference. It may help to place a small table next to a favorite chair for a phone, and a table for a phone next to the bed may prove helpful. Additional phone jacks and extension phones are additional options for persons with arthritis.

MEDICATIONS

Opening medicine bottles can be difficult; devices are available to assist with getting lids off. Persons with arthritis can request screw tops (as opposed to child-proof caps) from the pharmacy. Some persons with arthritis have to cut or crush medications, and special devices are available for this at drug stores. Using a medicine organizer or a dispenser may require some help with filling the device, but it can promote independence each time medicine needs to be taken. Asking people with arthritis about difficulties opening, taking, or cutting medications should be a routine ADL question for therapists.

FOOD PREPARATION

Before looking at devices, consider the area in which a person will be working. Is it possible for the person to sit and reduce the potential for fatigue? Would adding a stool near the food preparation area be possible? Food items and cooking utensils should be stored where they can be reached easily. Adding pull-out racks in lower cabinets can eliminate some of the need for reaching, and the use of swivel trays can also make it easier to get to stored food items.

There is a wide variety of tools for making cooking easier: cooking utensils with large handles (Figure 9), cutting boards to hold items to be cut, openers for milk containers,

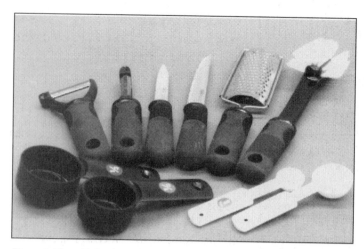

Figure 9. These kitchen utensils have lightweight, easy to grip and hold handles, making food preparation easier for many persons with arthritis.

boxes, cans, and jars (Figures 10 and 11), milk carton holders, and devices for cleaning up. Reachers can be helpful for removing items from upper cabinets as well as for items below the counter, but they are not generally recommended for persons with RA of the hands. Carts are helpful in moving items around in the kitchen. Aprons with pockets can also help in carrying items. Food processors can perform a number of food preparation tasks, but they require extra clean-up and the ability to handle the sharp blade safely. Keeping knives and vegetable peelers sharp can make food preparation easier, and people are often unaware that washing these items in a dishwasher dulls their blades. Another helpful device that assists with stove and oven controls is illustrated in Figure 12.

Using lightweight pots, pans, and dishes is often helpful. Larger handles on pots and pans can also help persons with arthritis. Handles can be built up by using pan-handler mitts that fit over the handles of pots and pans. There are also pan holders that allow one-handed stirring.

An excellent cooking device is the microwave oven. Food preparation time and chances of burns during cooking are reduced, food can be heated in lightweight containers, controls are usually easy to manipulate, and food can be purchased ready to place in the microwave or prepared in larger batches on conventional stoves and ovens and reheated in the microwave oven. Some sacrifice is made in texture of certain foods when they

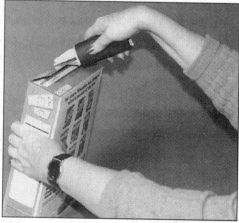

Figure 10. This device assists with opening boxes.

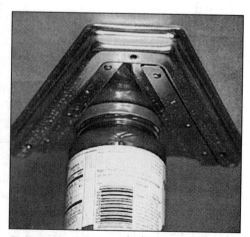

Figure 11. This device assists in opening jars.

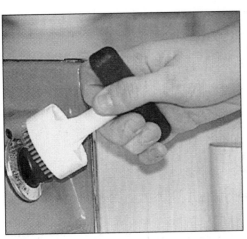

Figure 12. This device assists with the controls on a stove.

are cooked in a microwave oven. Many people combine microwave oven and other counter-top cooking devices such as toaster ovens to prepare meals.

MONEY MANAGEMENT

A variety of money-management tasks can now be done from home. Most banks, in cooperation with a number of employers, offer direct deposit for paychecks. Banks offer phone services to check account balances and retrieve other detailed information on checking and credit-card accounts. Many people are now using computers for money management. One popular software program, Quicken, will even provide electronic fund transfers where available and prepare checks for paying bills. As discussed below, computers can be configured for access by persons with all types of physical limitations, and the computer offers a good option for handling many money-management tasks; we can expect to see it used for many more money-management tasks in the near future.

SHOPPING

Some shopping can be done by phone, and like money management, shopping can also be done by computer. Cable TV also offers shopping stations. Of course, not all shopping can be done by phone or computer. For going to stores, devices already mentioned can be helpful: walkers with seats and baskets and scooters with baskets in grocery stores. Using a pull cart, backpack, or belt pack can also make it easier to carry purchases.

LEISURE

Leisure is all too often overlooked as an area for assistive devices. Yet Abledata lists over 1,000 different leisure products. A good occupational therapy assessment will determine the leisure interests of the person with arthritis, and the therapist should make suggestions about leisure-time assistive devices. However, most third-party payers will not reimburse for those devices. Some leisure assistive devices include card shufflers, TV remote controls with large buttons

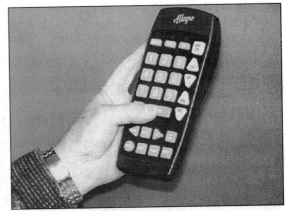

Figure 13. This TV remote control device offers larger-than-usual buttons for easier operation.

(Figure 13), pen holders, and steering wheel covers that make driving more comfortable.

Driving may at times be recreational but has important implications for IADL, work, and educational activities as well.

THE COMPUTER

We have already mentioned several applications of the computer: at work, at school, and at home. Computers have increased productivity and made it possible to do many tasks more quickly and easily: writing, banking, educational activities, searching for information, leisure activities, and controlling virtually every electronic device in the home. Computers can be configured so that individuals with even the most severe physical impairments can use them. Computer access has become an area for service provision, but at this point there are no clear guidelines for training and credentials for those who provide computer access services. While many occupational therapists provide computer access services, many other individuals outside the health professions are claiming expertise in this area.

Computer access involves (a) methods for "inputting" to the computer and (b) options for "output" from the computer. The most common input devices are the keyboard and the mouse, and output devices include the computer screen and printers. Persons with arthritis typically have more difficulty with input devices than with output devices. A detailed description of alternative input options is provided in *Assistive Technology for Persons with Disabilities* (Mann & Lane, 1995). Several examples of input devices for persons with arthritis are provided below.

Personal computers are typically sold with a keyboard and mouse. There are substitutes for both the keyboard and mouse that can make it easier for a person with arthritis to interact with a computer. For example, a reduced, or small, keyboard that uses a striking pen requires less gross and fine movement. The striking pen can be placed in the pen holder, eliminating the need to grasp. There are also keyboards whose position can be adjusted for each hand or that offer more wrist support. This is especially helpful for people with limited pronation and wrist motion. IBM, Apple, and a number of other companies sell such keyboards. For individuals with arthritis who use a computer for long periods of time, these ergonomically designed keyboards, with appropriate setup, can reduce fatigue and stress on joints.

Persons who use a modified keyboard will most likely need a mouse or some alternative, especially if they are using a graphical operating system. Trackballs offer an inexpensive option. With a trackball, the individual does not have to move the whole device to achieve cursor movement; rather, the ball is moved on the stationary device to accomplish the cursor movement. The ball can be moved with the palm of the hand, with relatively little movement.

For persons with very severe arthritis and very limited hand movement, there are a number of input options. Computers can be set up to operate with single switch control. There are a wide variety of switches that can be operated with very minimal hand, head, chin, or tongue movement, or even sipping and puffing.

DEVICES FOR LEISURE

DEVICE TYPE	NUMBER*
Arts and crafts	153
Electronics	99
Games	227
Gardening	51
Music	11
Photography	10
Play	99
Sewing	31
Sports	335

* Number of devices listed in HyperAbledata, 1995

Table 7: Devices for Leisure

Voice-recognition systems offer another alternative for input. While still relatively expensive and slower than keyboard input, prices continue to fall, and for many individuals voice input is a faster, easier method than a switch option. Dragon Dictate for Windows is one of the most popular and powerful programs (available from Voice Recognition Systems, Inc., 1-800-624-7987).

A number of additional accessories are available for computers to assist with getting floppy disks in and out of the computer, holding print material that is being viewed while using the computer, and positioning the monitor and keyboard. Therapists who specialize in computer access face the challenge of keeping up to date on the large number and variety of new products and services available for computer access: both "special" products, which tend to be more expensive, and mainstream-market products, which often achieve goals at lower cost than the special products. Both Abledata and some of the companies listed at the end of this chapter offer information on computer-related products that can assist persons with arthritis.

Good seating and positioning are extremely important for anyone using a computer for long periods of time, and even more important for persons with arthritis. There must be careful selection and adjustment of the chair, feet must firmly reach the floor, the back must be supported, and the seat should be comfortable. Adjustable arm rests can help reduce shoulder and neck strain. The keyboard placement should allow the elbows to be at 90 degrees. The monitor should be positioned approximately at eye level. Footrests may help when adjusting chair and monitor position. Monitor stands can be used to achieve optimal position of the computer monitor. Computer chairs range in price from under $100 to over $400 and can have features such as adjustable arm rests, high backs, adjustable seat height, adjustable back height and angle, and pneumatic lift. These features will increase the price, but they make many adjustments possible. This is a particularly important consideration if more than one person is using the chair.

ENVIRONMENTAL CONTROL

Devices that permit operation of lights and appliances from a distance, typically without a wire connection, are considered remote-control devices. One of the simplest environmental-control devices is the timer. Setting up lights in the home to come on and go off at preset times eliminates the need to get up and turn them on each day. This can reduce fatigue and eliminate the need to manipulate small, difficult-to-handle switches. Seasonal changes in the sunrise and sunset require changes in setup, for which the person with arthritis may require assistance.

X-10 type devices offer an alternative to timers. Lights and some small appliances can be plugged into inexpensive plug-in modules, which in turn are plugged into an electrical wall outlet. A base unit can control all lights and appliances at once or groups at different times. This can be done manually from the base unit or a timer function can be added. These remote-control devices are low-cost, offer significant control and flexibility and can reduce stress and fatigue.

Computers can be used for remote control with the appropriate software and can be used in conjunction with X-10 modules. Systems are available that will even allow adjustments in the heating and cooling system from the computer. Computers can also be used to answer and make phone calls. Thus, once the appropriate input mechanisms are set up, control of most of the home functions can be accomplished with the computer.

Another form of remote control is represented by hand-held remotes for TVs, VCRs, and stereos. These offer many more features than the X-10 devices and can save energy for the user. Remotes with larger buttons are beginning to appear in stores, although this is often at the sacrifice of features. A recent study of frail elders' use of TV remotes found that they preferred remotes with larger buttons over remotes with more features (Mann, Ottenbacher, Tomita, & Packard, 1994).

A number of other devices offer a form of remote control. Voice-activated and movement-activated switches can turn lights on and off. One device will turn lights on or off in response to a hand-clapping, although this is not recommended for persons with arthritis in the hands. Another device enables metal lamps to be turned on by simply touching any metallic part of the lamp. Voice-activated phones also permit hands-free operation. Answering machines can serve as remote control devices by providing a means for screening nuisance calls.

As mentioned in discussing TV remotes, the design of the control unit of remote-control devices may not be optimal for persons with arthritis, who may need assistance in setting up some devices such as X-10 systems. Other devices such as TV remotes can be replaced with better devices or adapted by gluing on larger buttons.

SPECIAL CONSIDERATIONS FOR OLDER PERSONS

Arthritis is disproportionately distributed in the population, with the elderly having the highest incidence; reports suggest that 55% of elderly persons have arthritis (Yelin,

1992). Yelin and Katz (1990) used data from the Longitudinal Study on Aging to estimate that for those elderly persons who had arthritis and no other chronic conditions, 66% had limitations in physical activities; for those who had arthritis and at least one other chronic condition, 82% had limitations in physical activity.

Many elder persons have multiple chronic conditions. The noninstitutionalized frail elderly, about 8-10% of the population over 65, experience, on average, more than four chronic conditions and take several different medications. Those multiple chronic conditions and side effects of medications can have an impact on hearing, vision, balance, strength, pain, respiration, and fatigueability. In considering the needs of elders with arthritis for assistive devices, the impact of these multiple chronic conditions must be taken into account. For example, consider someone who has arthritis and severe low vision. A high-powered magnifier may enable this person to see, but if, because of arthritis, he or she cannot grasp the magnifier, the person will be unable to use it. Selecting a magnifier that can be worn around the neck or that sits on a stand provides a possible alternative solution. Careful assessment of all strengths and limitations, thoughtful selection of appropriate devices, and thorough training and follow-up all require very careful consideration in the presence of multiple chronic conditions.

Assistive-device use was studied by Haworth (1990), who followed 163 patients with arthritis at 2, 6, and 10 weeks following hospital discharge (hospitalized for hip replacement) and found that patients used 2.2 devices at admission, 5.8 devices 2 weeks after discharge, and 2.3 devices 10 weeks after discharge. Mann, Hurren, & Tomita (1995) found that home-based frail elders with arthritis use a mean of about 10 assistive devices per person and that the devices generally work satisfactorily. More than half of these devices addressed physical impairment. Almost three quarters of this sample experienced arthritis (Mann, Hurren, & Tomita, 1993). While frail elders own and use a rather large number of assistive devices, another recent study demonstrated that they lack up to-date information on assistive devices (Mann, Hurren, Tomita, Packard, & Creswell, 1994). When asked, "Can you think of a device you would like to have that you haven't been able to find, a device that may not have yet been developed?" The suggestions of 110 elders were found to be available in the form of one or more products in the marketplace. Elders are willing users of assistive devices, but they require assistance in identifying sources for appropriate assistive technology solutions.

Frail elders are generally isolated. More than half live alone and make few trips outside the home. The telephone becomes an important device to maintain communication with friends and relatives and to call for help. Careful assessment of phone-related needs that addresses the physical limitations of arthritis and limitations in hearing, vision, and cognition is an essential component of occupational therapy interventions in home care. Phone-related needs should also be considered in institutional settings.

Although most elders, especially the frail elderly, are not working older persons with arthritis may still be working, and interventions relating to the workplace need to be considered. While therapists should not ignore assistive technology interventions for ADL and IADL, from the consumer's perspective leisure pursuits are also very important. There is a wide variety of devices for leisure activity that can address arthritis-related limitations. The computer can be used for game playing and communication as well as for exploring for information. Low-tech devices include card holders, card shufflers, and games with larger playing pieces, to name a few.

SUMMARY

Assistive devices can make a major difference in the ability of people with arthritis to perform daily tasks. Therapists play a very important role in assessing these individuals for appropriate devices, including offering the opportunity to try various products. Therapists also assess the environment and the role of other persons and use this information in making recommendations. Training is important with many assistive devices, and follow-up is essential.

REFERENCES

Haworth, R. J. (1990). Use of aids during the first three months after total hip replacement. *British Journal of Rheumatology, 22*(1), 29-35.

HyperAbledata. Madison, WI: Trace Research & Development Center. For information, telephone (608) 262-6966.

LaPlante, M. P., Hendershot, G. E. & Moss, A. J. (1992). Assistive technology devices and home accessibility features: Prevalence, payment, need, and trends. In *Advance Data*. United States Department of Health and Human Services, Public Health Service, Centers for Disease Control, National Center for Health Statistics.

Mann, W. C., Granger, C., Hurren, D., Tomita, M., & Charvat, B. (1995). An Analysis of Problems with Canes Encountered by Elderly Persons. *Physical & Occupational Therapy in Geriatrics, 13,* 25-49.

Mann, W. C., Hurren, D., Charvat, B. & Tomita, M. (in press). Problems with wheelchairs experienced by frail elders. *Technology and Disability, 5,* 1.

Mann, W. C., Hurren, D., & Tomita, M. (1993). Comparison of Assistive Device Use and Needs of Home-Based Seniors With Different Impairments. *The American Journal of Occupational Therapy, 47,* 980-987.

Mann, W.C., Hurren, D., & Tomita, M. (1995). Assistive devices used by home-based elderly persons with arthritis. *The American Journal of Occupational Therapy, 49,* 810-820.

Mann, W. C., Hurren, D., Tomita, M., & Charvat, B. (1995). An Analysis of Problems with Walkers Encountered by Elderly Persons. *Physical & Occupational Therapy in Geriatrics, 13,* 1-23.

Mann, W. C., Hurren, D., Tomita, M., & Charvat, B. (In press). Use of Assistive Devices for Bathing by Noninstitutionalized Elderly. *The Occupational Therapy Journal of Research.*

Mann, W. C., Hurren, D., Tomita, M., Packard, S., & Creswell, C. (1994). The Need for Information on Assistive Devices by Older Persons. *Assistive Technology, 6,* 134-139.

Mann, W. C., & Lane, J. (1995). *Assistive Technology for Persons with Disabilities.* Bethesda, MD: American Occupational Therapy Association.

Mann, W., Ottenbacher, K.J., Tomita, M.R., & Packard, S. (1994). *Design of Hand-Held Remotes for Older Persons with Impairments, 6,* 140-146.

Yelin, E. (1992). Arthritis: The cumulative impact of a common chronic condition. *Arthritis Rheumatism, 35,* 489-497.

Yelin, E., & Katz, P. P. (1990). Transitions in health status among community-dwelling elderly people with arthritis: A national, longitudinal study. *Arthritis Rheumatism, 33,* 1205-15.

COMPANIES OFFERING CATALOGS THAT INCLUDE ASSISTIVE DEVICES FOR PERSONS WITH ARTHRITIS

Ableware Maddak, Inc.
6 Industrial Drive
Pequannock, NJ 07440-1993
(201) 628-7600

Accessible Services, Inc.
142 North Fairview Avenue
Upper Darby, PA 19082
(610) 446-5206

AdaptAbility
PO Box 513
Colchester, CT 06415-0515
(800) 288-9941

AliMed Rehab Products, Inc.
297 High Street
Dedham, MA 02026-9135
(800) 225-2610

American Orthopedic Supply Co. Inc.
PO Box 148
Cleveland, AL 35049
1(800) 421-7344

Amigo Mobility International, Inc.
6693 Dixie Highway
Bridgeport, MI 48722
(517) 777-0910

Back Designs
1045 Ashby Avenue
Berkeley, CA 94710
(510) 849-1923

Bruce Medical Supply
411 Waverly Oaks Road
PO Box 9166
Waltham, MA 02254
(800) 225-8446

Care Catalog Services
1877 NE Seventh Avenue
Portland, OR 97212
(800) 443-7091

Charisma Canes
6010 Highway 9
Felton, CA 95018
(408) 335-9164

Cleo, Inc.
PO Box 1076
White Plains, NY 10602
(800) 321-0595

Clarke Health Care Products, Inc.
1003 International Drive
Oakdale, PA 15071-9226
(412) 695-2122

Columbus McKinnon Corporation
Mobility Products Division
140 John James Audubon Parkway
Amherst, New York 14228-1197
(800) 888-0985

Core Products International, Inc.
808 Prospect Ave
Osceola, WI 54020
(800) 365-3047

Dr. Leonard's Healthcare Products
Catalog Orders
42 Mayfield Avenue
PO Box 7821
Edison, NJ 08818-7821
(800) 785-0880

APT Technology, Inc.
8765 Township Road 513
Shreve, Ohio 44676-9421
(330) 567-2001

Duro-Med Industries, Inc.
1788 West Cherry Street
Jesup, GA 31545-4464
(800) 526-4753

Enrichments
PO Box 5071
Bolingbrook, IL 60440-5071
(800) 435-8573

The Kiwi Connection
EzyFold Door Control Units
82 Shelburne Center Road
Shelburne, MA 01370
(413) 625-9506

Griptex Industries, Inc.
63 Industrial Drive
Cartersville, GA 30120
(800) 997-0400

Wheelchair Carrier, Inc.
726 Farnsworth Road
Waterville, Ohio 43566-0079
(800) 541-3213

Direct Market Enterprises
Health House USA
Box 85
Westbury, NY 11590
(516) 334-9754

Independent Living Aids, Inc.
27 East Mall
Plainview, NY 11803
(800) 537-2118

Innovative Products Catalogue
c/o Innovations for Enhanced Senior Living
2847 Quarry Heights Way
Baltimore, MD 21209-1064
(410) 653-6288

Invacare Corporation
899 Cleveland Street
Elyria, OH 44036
(800) 333-6900

Futuro, Inc.
5405 Dupont Circle
Suite A
Milford, Ohio 45150-2735
(513) 576-8000

Lakeland Protective Wear, Inc.
5109 Harvester Road
Unit B 14
Burlington, Ontario L7L 5Y9
1(800)489-9131

DeRoyal/LMB, Inc.
PO Box 1181
San Luis Obispo, CA 93406
(800) 541-3992

Lumex Medical Products
100 Spence Street
Bay Shore, New York 11706-2290
(516) 273-2200

Maddak, Inc.
PO Box 384
Pequannock, NJ 07440-1993
(800) 443-4926

Maxi Aids
PO Box 3209
42 Executive Boulevard
Farmingdale, New York 11735
(800) 522-6294

Nor-Am Patient Care Products, Inc.
PO Box 543
Lewiston, New York 14092
(716) 285-7548

NorthCoast Medical, Inc.
187 Stauffer Boulevard
San Jose, CA 95125-1042
(800) 821-9319

Omron HealthCare, Inc.
300 Lakeview Parkway
Vernon Hills, Illinois 60061
(847) 680-6200

Pressalit Products for
American Standard, Inc.
PO Box 6820
Piscataway, NJ 08855
(908) 980-3000

S&S AdaptAbility
PO Box 513
Colchester, CT 06415-0515
(800) 266-8856

Sammons Preston
PO Box 5071
Bolingbrook, IL 60440-5071
(800) 323-5547

Sears Health Care
9804 Chartwell Drive
Dallas, TX 75243
(800) 326-1750

Soho, Inc.
258 Milford Commons
Milford, MA 01757
(508) 634-2657

Smith & Nephew, Inc.
Rehab Division
PO Box 1005
One Quality Drive
Germantown, WI 53022-8205
(800) 558-8633

Sportime
Abilitations
One Sportime Way
Atlanta, GA 30340
(800) 850-8602

Sportime
Senior Products
One Sportime Way
Atlanta, GA 30340
(800) 428-5127

Susquehanna Rehab Products
RD 2, Box 41
9 Overlook Drive
Wrightsville, PA 17368
(800) 248-2011

Urocare Products, Inc.
2735 Melbourne Avenue
Pomona, CA 91767-1931
(909) 621-6013

COMMUNITY RESOURCES IN COMPREHENSIVE REHABILITATION

Kathleen M. Haralson-Ferrell, MLA, PT

INTRODUCTION

Comprehensive care for patients with chronic diseases should not end with the patient's discharge from the clinical setting. Community resources offer therapists a broad diversity of programs and materials to enhance the health care that we traditionally provide, and referral to community resources is an important part of the role of the therapist in the treatment of rheumatic disease (Moncur, 1988). The chronicity of arthritis makes it especially important for patients to engage in positive self-management in their homes and communities. Research has demonstrated that patient education focused on self-management (Lorig, Lubeck, Seleznick, Drqines, & Holman, 1985; Lorig, Holman, O'Leary, & Shoor, 1986; Mullen, Laville, Biddle, & Lorig, 1987) and general fitness exercise programs (Danneskiold-Samsoe, Lynberg, Risum, & Telling, 1987; Minor, Hewett, Webel, Anderson, & Kay, 1989; Zischke, 1986) can significantly reduce pain, increase function, and enhance overall quality of life. Guidelines for comprehensive medical management of osteoarthritis call for patients to participate in arthritis self-management programs (Hochberg et al., 1995).

Appropriate use of community resources has become even more important in recent years. The ever-increasing limitations on delivery of services and duration of care make it impossible to address the long-term needs of rheumatology patients adequately in the clinic. Fortunately, numerous and varied federal, state, and local community resources are readily available and provide a valuable adjunct to clinic rehabilitation. By providing patients with information about services and materials available to them and, if necessary, helping them to gain access to these resources, therapists can provide a more complete rehabilitation experience.

Use of community resources may extend or supplement treatment provided in the clinical setting; for example, a community exercise program may complement a home physical therapy program, or an arthritis support group may offer ongoing emotional support, advice, and information. Community resources may need to substitute for traditional health care if services such as physical therapy, occupational therapy, counseling, or social services are not covered or are limited by reimbursement policies. Patients in rural areas may need to depend on community resources to replace care that is not available locally. Occupational and physical therapists must be sensitive both to the limitations of our clinical settings and to the needs of arthritis patients so that we can refer them to appropriate community resources. We have not provided complete and comprehensive care unless we have provided those referrals.

This chapter provides an overview of local and national resources including state and federal resources that are usually available to persons with arthritis. The availability and types of services vary widely and depend on many factors including rural versus metropolitan locations, the individual state and county, the economic resources of the community, delivery mechanisms, and so on. In addition, there are numerous types or categories of resources such as educational programs, exercise classes, and print and audiovisual materials. The emergence of the "information superhighway" has resulted in a virtual explosion of home pages on arthritis on the World Wide Web. "Chat rooms," on-line meetings, support groups, and educational programs increasingly are available on the internet, and many materials are available on CD-ROM. It is important to note that some resources change frequently. Some of the materials described in this chapter may not be available in certain geographical areas, activities may be discontinued, or brochures or other pieces of literature may be out of print. The World Wide Web, especially, is a rapidly evolving resource, and it is not unusual for an organization to change the information available through its home page weekly. The organizations, brochure titles, and other resources listed in the tables in this manuscript were available when this book went to press.

Since there is a wide diversity of services, this chapter will cover those resources primarily of interest to occupational therapists and physical therapists including exercise programs, self-help programs, support groups, and educational materials. It is intended to give therapists information about specific resources that are available both nationally and in most communities and also to provide guidance to help them locate other appropriate services. Therapists will need to research the available services in their own communities. Community organizations exist to provide services and usually will respond quickly to requests for information. If you are unfamiliar with the local organizations, national organizations often are an excellent place to begin as their resources generally are more uniform and widely available than the more idiosyncratic local ones. The chapter also includes information about rheumatology-specific professional resources to enhance therapists' professional skills and knowledge about arthritis and other rheumatic diseases.

Volunteering is an an excellent way to become familiar with community organizations. They usually depend on volunteers to deliver many of their programs, and volunteering provides an outstanding opportunity to offer organizations much-needed help while learning more about their valuable work. Volunteers are frequently needed to lead support groups, exercise programs, and distribute literature. Becoming part of a community activity enriches both our lives and the lives of the people for whom we care.

ORGANIZATIONS

The following is a representative list of health organizations, but it is not all-inclusive. Consult the local telephone directory, National Arthritis Musculoskeletal and Skin Diseases Information Clearinghouse (see Table 5), or listings on the Internet for additional organizations.

ARTHRITIS FOUNDATION
1330 West Peachtree Street
Atlanta, Georgia 30309
(404) 872-7100
(800) 283-7800
http://www.arthritis.org

AMERICAN JUVENILE ARTHRITIS ORGANIZATION
Same address and phone number as AF above.

ARTHRITIS SOCIETY (CANADA)
250 Bloor Street East, Suite 901
Toronto, Ontario, M4W 3P2
(416) 967-5679
Fax: (416) 967-7171

SPONDYLITIS ASSOCIATION OF AMERICA
PO Box 5872
Sherman Oaks, CA 91413
(818) 981-1616
(800) 777-8189
http://www.usa.net/welcomesaapage.html

NATIONAL OSTEOPOROSIS FOUNDATION
1150 17th Street, NW, Suite 500
Washington, DC 20036
(800) 223-9994
http://www.nof.org/

LUPUS FOUNDATION OF AMERICA
4 Research Place, Suite 180
Rockville, MD 20850-3226
(301) 670-9292

THE AMERICAN LUPUS SOCIETY
260 Maple Court, Suite 123
Ventura, CA 93003
(805) 339-0443
(800) 331-1802

FIBROMYALGIA ALLIANCE OF AMERICA
PO Box 21990
Columbia, OH 43221-0988
(614) 457-4222

NATIONAL FIBROMYALGIA RESEARCH ASSOCIATION
PO Box 500
Salem, OR 97302

UNITED SCLERODERMA FOUNDATION
PO Box 399
Watsonville, CA 95077-0399
(408) 728-2202

SJOGREN'S SYNDROME FOUNDATION, INC.
333 N. Broadway
Jerico, NY 11753
(516) 933-6365

NATIONAL SJOGREN'S ASSOCIATION
3201 West Evans Drive
Phoenix, AZ 85023
(602) 516-0787

LYME DISEASE FOUNDATION
I Financial Plaza
Hartford, CT 06103
(203) 525-2000

Table 1: Organizations

HEALTH ORGANIZATIONS

National nonprofit health organizations usually provide literature, programs, and other services that generally have been professionally developed and reviewed. The materials and programs may be of a higher quality than those developed locally, but they may not fit unique local needs. It is wise, especially when referring patients to an unfamiliar source, to preview the materials and services that the patient will be receiving.

Several organizations target the specific needs of people with arthritis, and others target a specific age group, for example, seniors or children. Table 1 lists several of the major rheumatic disease organizations, including the current address, telephone number, and web address, if available. The following section briefly describes a few of these rheumatic disease organizations.

ALL RHEUMATIC DISEASES
THE ARTHRITIS FOUNDATION

The Arthritis Foundation (AF) is the only nationwide organization that provides information and services for most of the rheumatic diseases. A network of 65 chapters throughout the United States offers information and referral, educational materials and programs, group exercise classes (both aquatic and nonaquatic), exercise and educational videos, loan closets for adaptive equipment, home study educational programs, and support groups. Much of the information and programs is sufficiently generic to be relevant and applicable to most individuals with arthritis. Nevertheless, many of the materials and services are adapted specifically for certain diseases—for example, there are brochures for many specific rheumatic diseases, there is an educational program specifically for people with systemic lupus erythematosus, and there are support groups specifically for people with fibromyalgia.

An extensive list of print materials is available. Brochures cover topics such as pain management, exercise, travel tips, and insurance questions. *The Arthritis Helpbook* (Lorig & Fries, 1990) is the companion text for The Self-Help Course and is an extremely useful text for both professional and patient use. It provides detailed information on numerous topics including symptomatology, pathology, medications, surgery, nutrition, joint protection principles, and exercise. Other materials include a catalog of assistive devices and suggestions for adapting activities of daily living.

Through its chapters the Arthritis Foundation offers programs that primarily are for adults in their middle years or older adults. Programs for children, young adults, and families of children with arthritis are offered through the American Juvenile Arthritis Organization, a council of the Arthritis Foundation.

Those services and materials that therapists probably would find most helpful include the individual disease brochures and those on selected topics including exercise, joint protection, fatigue, and pain management (see Table 2 for a list of brochures). Aquatic and "land" group exercise programs are offered in a variety of settings in many communities. The Self-Help Courses (general arthritis, systemic lupus erythematosus, and

ARTHRITIS FOUNDATION PAMPHLETS, BROCHURES, AND FACT SHEETS

Arthritis Answers	Marfan Syndrome
Diet	Myositis
Managing Your Health	Osteoarthritis
Unproven Remedies	Osteoporosis
Arthritis and Employment	Paget's Disease
Arthritis and Pregnancy	Polymyalgia Rheumatica
Managing Your Fatigue	Psoriatic Arthritis
Managing Your Pain	Raynaud's Phenomenon
Managing Stress	Reiter's Syndrome
The Family	Rheumatoid Arthritis
Arthritis Foundation Services	Scleroderma
Exercise and Your Arthritis	Sjogren's Syndrome
Surgery	Living and Loving—Fact Sheet
Managing Your Activities	Behcet's Disease—Fact Sheet
Ankylosing Spondylitis	Reflex Sympathetic Dystrophy Syndrome—Fact Sheet
Arthritis in Children	Aspirin and Other Nonsteroidal Anti-inflammatory Drugs (NSAIDS)
Back Pain	
Bursitis, Tendonitis and Localized Pain Syndromes	Corticosteroid Medications
Carpal Tunnel Syndrome	Gold Treatment
Fibromyalgia	*Arthritis Today* Drug Guide
Gout	Methotrexate
Lupus	
Lyme Disease	

Table 2: Arthritis Foundation Pamphlets, Brochures, and Fact Sheets

---

BROCHURES AVAILABLE FROM THE LUPUS FOUNDATION OF AMERICA

Facts About Lupus Series
What is Lupus?
Living Well with Lupus
Blood Disorders in SLE
Lupus and Vasculitis
Laboratory Tests Used in the Diagnosis of Lupus
Kidney Disease and Lupus
Depression in Lupus
Joint and Muscle Pain in Lupus
Pregnancy and Lupus
Medications
Lupus in Men
Lupus and Infections and Immunizations
Skin Disease in Lupus
Cardiopulmanary Disease and Lupus
Systemic Lupus and the Nervous System
Photosensitivity and Lupus Erythematosus
Antiphospholipid Antibodies and SLE
Steroids in the Treatment of Lupus
Imuran, Cytoxan, and Related Drugs
Anti-Malarials in the Treatment of Lupus
Nonsteroidal Anti-Inflammatory Drugs (NSAIDS)

Table 3: Brochures Available from the Lupus Foundation of America

fibromyalgia) emphasize the importance of rehabilitation for persons with arthritis and muscle pain and supply information on a variety of related topics including an overview of exercise, joint protection, energy conservation, and assistive devices. It is important to note that none of the programs or materials are designed to replace clinical care but rather to supplement or enhance it. Therapists have been involved extensively in the writing and review of all programs and materials. Certified instructors who have completed specialized training courses teach the programs (see chapter 15, Patient Education, for a review of the research outcomes from these groups).

Not all materials and services listed above are available in every chapter area. It would be advisable to call the local chapter or branch office and request a list of the services that it offers. Call the national organization local telephone number or the toll-free number in Table 1 for the local chapter or branch in your area.

DISEASE-SPECIFIC HEALTH ORGANIZATIONS

Many organizations provide services and materials for specific diseases and often more than one organization may target the same rheumatic disease. The number and quality of their national materials and programs can vary widely, as will the extent of their local presence. If a therapist treats many patients with a similar rheumatic disease, it is wise to be familiar with the materials and services of the rheumatic disease organization that specifically address the needs of this patient population.

National organizations that offer educational materials and services and also have a local presence in some communities include:

SPONDYLITIS ASSOCIATION OF AMERICA (SAA)

This organization provides materials and services for people with ankylosing spondylitis and the related spondyloarthropathies such as Reiter's syndrome. It publishes a variety of print materials including books and brochures and the quarterly newsletter, *Spondylitis Plus*. Local activities include several regional educational and support groups. Exercise materials include exercise videos and an audiotape. The information distributed by the SAA strongly emphasizes the importance of exercise and has been reviewed for accuracy by physical and occupational therapists who specialize in treating AS.

LUPUS FOUNDATION OF AMERICA (LFA)

The LFA has over 100 chapters nationwide. Services and materials vary among chapters but usually include educational brochures and books, support groups, and public forums (see Table 3 for a list of brochures in the Facts About Lupus series). National and local chapter newsletters and other educational materials are available also.

NATIONAL OSTEOPOROSIS FOUNDATION (NOF)

The NOF publishes numerous educational materials, including brochures on subjects such as bone health, medications, osteoporosis facts, and physician communication issues (Table 4 includes a list of brochures available through the NOF). It also distributes two newsletters, *Osteoporosis Clinical Updates* and *Osteoporosis Report*, an educational materials catalog, and a limited list of materials in large print and in Spanish. Health professionals can order a Patient Education Sample Pack that contains one each of educational brochures and a catalog.

FIBROMYALGIA ALLIANCE OF AMERICA (FAA)

The Fibromyalgia Alliance of America publishes a quarterly newsletter, *The Fibromyalgia Times*, and other materials including an information packet on disability. It also makes available support group resources.

NATIONAL FIBROMYALGIA RESEARCH FOUNDATION (NFRF)

The National Fibromyalgia Research Foundation supports research into fibromyalgia syndrome (FMS) but also serves as a clearinghouse for materials on fibromyalgia. Books

---

BROCHURES AVAILABLE THROUGH THE NATIONAL OSTEOPOROSIS FOUNDATION

Stand Up to Osteoporosis
How Strong are Your Bones
Medications and Bone Loss
Menopause and Osteoporosis
Men with Osteoporosis: In Their Own Words
Can It Happen to You
Talking with Your Doctor about Osteoporosis
Osteoporosis: A Woman's Guide
Facts about Osteoporosis, Arthritis and Osteoarthritis
Living with Osteoporosis
The Older Person's Guide to Osteoporosis
Strategies for People with Osteoporosis

Table 4: Brochures Available Through the National Osteoporosis Foundation

and other publications, professional medical journals and magazines, videos, and fibromyalgia organizations are included on a resource list. Requesting this resource list is the best place to start gathering information on resources for people with FMS.

HEALTH ORGANIZATIONS FOR NONRHEUMATIC DISEASES

Health organizations that are not arthritis-specific may offer services that are appropriate and of benefit for persons with arthritis. For example, Easter Seals targets children and in some communities offers water classes for anyone with a disability. For persons with comorbid disease, organizations such as the American Heart Association, the American Cancer Society, The American Lung Association, and The Alzheimer's Association often provide excellent community resources. The American Red Cross also provides valuable materials and programs including water exercise classes in many communities.

PROFESSIONAL ORGANIZATIONS

Professional organizations produce educational materials and other resources for both health professionals and patients. The materials generally are of high quality and have been developed and reviewed by health professionals, often in conjunction with professional writers. National professional organizations frequently have local or state chapters that may also produce materials.

AMERICAN COLLEGE OF RHEUMATOLOGY (ACR)

The ACR is a professional organization that includes practicing physicians, research scientists, nurses, physical and occupational therapists, and other health professionals who are specialists in the care of patients with rheumatic diseases. The majority of the materials produced are for health professionals and include two scientific journals of which one, *Arthritis Care and Research*, is primarily for clinicians, and a clinical text, *Clinical Care in the Rheumatic Diseases* (Wegner, Belza, & Gall, 1996), which serves as a valuable resource for clinicians and schools of physical therapy and occupational therapy. Several patient brochures also are available. The Association of Rheumatology Health Professionals (ARHP) is a membership council of the ACR. Members include physical and occupational therapists, social workers, nurses, health educators, and health service researchers. A membership directory includes a comprehensive listing of all members and is a valuable resource for arthritis health professional specialists. Membership in the ARHP entitles one to receive the *Bulletin on the Rheumatic Diseases*, a publication of the Arthritis Foundation specifically for health professionals that provides concise, informative articles that describe the state of the art in various aspects of the rheumatic disease. The ACR and ARHP have an annual scientific meeting where state-of-the-art information on the rheumatic diseases is presented. The ACR has a home page on the World Wide Web; see Table 5 for addresses.

OTHER PROFESSIONAL ORGANIZATIONS

Many cities and states have local rheumatism associations that provide continuing education programming for their members. Usually they do not produce patient education materials or participate in community outreach activities but can serve as an excellent resource to locate local area rheumatologists.

The American Occupational Therapy Association (AOTA) and The American Physical Therapy Association (APTA) produce many professional and patient educational materials. A list of their resources may be obtained from the national organization headquarters. State chapters can provide names of area therapists; see Table 5.

FEDERAL AND STATE ORGANIZATIONS

Numerous federal and state organizations provide services for people with arthritis. The majority are not arthritis-specific, but their materials and programs may be appropriate or can easily be adapted for persons with rheumatic diseases. For example, most services for the elderly address the needs of most older individuals with arthritis, and many services for children with special needs are appropriate for those with juvenile arthritis.

The following is a brief overview of a few of the services. Federal services are often administered through the individual states and may be found in the state and/or federal resource pages of the local telephone book.

PROFESSIONAL, STATE, AND FEDERAL ORGANIZATIONS THAT OFFER ARTHRITIS-RELATED RESOURCES

AMERICAN COLLEGE OF RHEUMATOLOGY
60 Executive Park South
Suite 150
Atlanta, GA 30329
(404) 633-3777
http://www.rheumatology.org

AMERICAN OCCUPATIONAL THERAPY ASSOCIATION
4720 Montgomery Lane
PO Box 31220
Bethesda, MD 20824-1220
(301) 652-7711
http://www.aota.org

AMERICAN PHYSICAL THERAPY ASSOCIATION
1111 N. Fairfax St.
Alexandria, VA 22314
(800) 999-2782
http://www.apta.org

MISSOURI REGIONAL ARTHRITIS PROGRAM
BUREAU OF CHRONIC DISEASE CONTROL AND HEALTH PROMOTION
101 Park Deville Drive
Suite A
Columbia, MO 65203
http://www.hsc.missouri.edu/arthritis/

PRESIDENT'S COMMITTEE ON EMPLOYMENT OF PEOPLE WITH DISABILITIES
1331 F Street, NW
Suite 300
Washington, DC 20004
(202) 376-6200

NATIONAL INSTITUTE OF ARTHRITIS AND MUSCULOSKELETAL AND SKIN DISEASES
NATIONAL ARTHRITIS MUSCULOSKELETAL AND SKIN DISEASES INFORMATION CLEARINGHOUSE
1 AMS Circle
Bethesda, MD 20892-3675
(301) 495-4481
http://www.nih.gov/niams

Table 5: Professional, State, and Federal Organizations That Offer Arthritis-Related Resources

AREA AGENCIES ON AGING (AAA)

The United States is divided into several regions, and the telephone book lists the nearest local office. This office can provide the numbers and locations of offices for specific counties. Area Agencies on Aging, the "Triple-As," are funded by the Older Americans Act and state monies, and services vary from one state and county to another. Services can include Meals-on-Wheels, family support services, information regarding transportation, case management, home health services, social security, respite care, and long-term care. Many health organizations collaborate with them, and a call to the local AAA office opens the door to several other organizations.

Services specifically of interest to therapists include group exercise classes that are offered in some locations. The local Area Agency on Aging may be able to provide information regarding transportation for therapy treatments, group exercise classes for older age individuals, and exercise videos for seniors.

THE CENTERS FOR DISEASE CONTROL AND PREVENTION (CDC)

The CDC is a rich source of data about arthritis prevalence, prevention, and treatment. However, it currently is not a source of patient education materials.

DEPARTMENTS OF PUBLIC HEALTH

The state departments of public health offer services for individuals with chronic disease. All offer materials and services for the elderly and for children, and a few have specific services addressing the needs of people with arthritis. No two states provide exactly the same resources, and state public health departments have widely varying services for arthritis. State arthritis programs usually are administered through the department of public health, and two states, Missouri and Ohio, provide funding for education and services through state-supported arthritis centers. The Missouri Department of Public Health divides the state into seven regions to administer the state arthritis program, and each region offers a wide variety of services for people with arthritis, including extensive educational programming, aquatic and nonaquatic exercise classes, and literature dissemination. Information may be accessed through the Department of Public Health, and a home page on the internet includes limited information about the services offered by each Regional Arthritis Center (Table 5).

THE PRESIDENT'S COUNCIL ON EMPLOYMENT OF PEOPLE WITH DISABILITIES AND GOVERNORS' COMMITTEES ON EMPLOYMENT OF PEOPLE WITH DISABILITIES

The national President's Council on Employment of People with Disabilities and the State Governors' Committees on Employment of People with Disabilities address employment and accessibility issues. Activities vary from state to state. One of the most useful materials available in some states is a comprehensive directory of organizations that includes the name, address, and telephone number of the majority of organizations within the state that provide services to people with special needs. Similar directories are available for child-specific organizations (see Table 5).

NATIONAL INSTITUTE OF ARTHRITIS AND MUSCULOSKELETAL AND SKIN DISEASES (NIAMS)

NIAMS, one of the institutes of the National Institutes of Health, funds research to find the cause and cure for the over 100 rheumatic diseases and related conditions. It also supports the National Arthritis Musculoskeletal and Skin Disease Information Clearinghouse (NAMSIC), a clearinghouse of arthritis information. In response to requests, NAMSIC provides information packets on specific diseases including basic and state-of-the-art treatment information. The NIAMS page on the World Wide Web includes information regarding recent research and treatment findings. The NIAMS also funds Multipurpose Arthritis and Musculoskeletal Disease Centers that conduct biomedical and health-services research in rheumatology. Some of the arthritis community programs now available nationally such as The Self-Help Course were originally developed and evaluated at these centers. A list of the currently funded centers is available through the NIAMS (see Table 5).

COMMUNITY ORGANIZATIONS

Community organizations, including city/town and county organizations, often provide the most extensive and varied resources. They may not be highly visible, but even the smallest community usually offers a diversity of potential services.

COMMUNITY CENTERS

Depending on size, most communities have one or more community centers that frequently offer group exercise programs, meeting space for organizations such as the Arthritis Foundation to hold public forums, and other educational programs. Community centers may fund day care centers for the elderly, transportation services, and other similar programs. Settlement houses in inner-city neighborhoods frequently offer many services for the medically underserved and low-income populations, including exercise, education, and support programs. Many are targeted specifically for the elderly and are appropriate for older individuals with arthritis. Wellness programs usually address arthritis-related health needs including prevention, diet, and exercise.

RELIGIOUS ORGANIZATIONS

Many religious organizations offer programming for special groups. Churches, temples, synagogues, and other religious facilities provide programs or make space available for use by other organizations. Depending on the size of the facility and the extent of the outreach programming, services can potentially include senior social and support groups, day-care centers for seniors, exercise classes, educational and recreational activities, and lunch programs. Some organizations make their programs and services available throughout the community to individuals of other faiths.

YOUNG MEN'S (YMCA) AND YOUNG WOMEN'S (YWCA) CHRISTIAN ASSOCIATIONS

YMCAs and YWCAs often offer programs for seniors. The YMCA of America, in partnership with the Arthritis Foundation in many cities and smaller communities, offers AFYAP, the Arthritis Foundation–YMCA Aquatic Program. These adapted arthritis warm-water exercise classes are taught by trained water exercise instructors.

FITNESS CENTERS

Fitness centers occasionally include adapted exercise classes in their regular schedule. Usually these classes are appropriate for seniors, and arthritis-specific exercise classes may be offered if there is sufficient interest. The Arthritis Foundation collaborates with fitness organizations in many communities to offer PACE, People with Arthritis Can Exercise, an exercise class adapted for persons with arthritis.

HEALTH CARE PROVIDER ORGANIZATIONS

These organizations are an increasingly rich source of resources and services that extend far beyond their clinical care. Increased efforts of hospitals and managed-care organizations to reach their target populations frequently include many community outreach activities. Health care facilities often offer a broad diversity of programming including public education forums, health fairs, support groups, stress management programs, literature, and exercise classes. Programming frequently targets seniors and occasionally is designed specifically for people with arthritis and/or back pain. Prevention messages are emphasized and the local chapter of the Arthritis Foundation often collaborates on program offerings.

AGE-SPECIFIC COMMUNITY ORGANIZATIONS

Many community organizations target specific age groups. Programs for seniors and for children are especially common. Children's adapted water-exercise classes can be found in many communities as can classes for older age individuals. Many community organizations offer a wide diversity of programs for the elderly. Transportation services, day care centers, senior social and support groups, and many other resources are available in most communities. Usually they are sponsored by local churches, city and county public and community health departments, the Area Agency on Aging, or hospital outreach programs for seniors. Accessing one agency usually leads to information about others in the community.

AMERICAN ASSOCIATION OF RETIRED PERSONS (AARP)

The AARP is a membership organization for individuals over 50 years of age. It is an excellent source of programs, services, and informative publications about social security and other entitlement benefits, investment plans, medigap policies, and other benefits for seniors. Membership cost is low and includes *Modern Maturity* magazine.

The AARP Pharmacy Service fills prescriptions at low prices and includes information about the medication with each prescription.

SUMMARY

The above list of resources should provide the therapist with an introduction to many potential sources of materials, classes, and services that can augment rehabilitation of patients with a rheumatic disease. Appropriate referral requires the therapist to know the general quality of the services and materials offered. Recommending the patient to poor, inadequate, or medically unsound resources does the patient a disservice. However, the initial effort to familiarize oneself with the available resources will facilitate later referral. Most importantly, the benefits to the patients will far outweigh the time required to become familiar with, and to refer patients to, appropriate community organizations.

Most patients will benefit from referral to several resources. This may seem a daunting task but actually could take only a few minutes. For example: Mrs. Smith, a 67-year-old patient with a 10-year history of rheumatoid arthritis, has been experiencing increased pain, weakness, and decreased function. She was referred to physical therapy for exercise to improve gait and lower extremity strength, and occupational therapy for instruction in joint protection and energy conservation techniques. Community resource referral for Mrs. Smith would include providing her with the telephone number of the local chapter of the Arthritis Foundation and, if available in the rehab department, AF brochures including *Rheumatoid Arthritis* and *Arthritis Answers*. She should be encouraged to join the arthritis aquatic exercise class at her neighborhood YMCA and to consider taking the next Self-Help Course offered by the AF. As she lives alone and transportation is difficult for her, she should be given the telephone number of the local Area Agency on Aging office, since in her community it coordinates transportation services and day-care programs for older citizens. The marketing department of the hospital in which you work has scheduled a health fair the following month, and Mrs. Smith should be given the flyer for its community activities that includes the time and date of the health fair.

The few minutes required to provide Mrs. Smith with two telephone numbers and a flyer may have opened up a world that will offer her increased socialization as well as exercise and education. It also demonstrates to Mrs. Smith that you are interested in more than her gait pattern or joint status and that her function and quality of life beyond the clinic setting is important to you. If time allows, it obviously is preferable to talk with Mrs. Smith about the importance of following through with these recommendations and possibly even to make the first calls for her.

In conclusion, it is important to note again that community organizations frequently depend on volunteers to provide their programs and services. These organizations benefit greatly from the knowledge, talent, and commitment of health professionals. Occupational therapists and physical therapists make outstanding volunteers due to their unique awareness of the needs of people with a rheumatic disease. Volunteering also offers the opportunity to be a part of the truly comprehensive care that so often eludes us in the clinical setting.

REFERENCES

Danneskiold-Samsoe, B., Lynberg, K., Risum, T., & Teling, M. (1987). The effect of water exercise therapy given to patients with rheumatoid arthritis. *Scandinavian Journal of Rehabilitation Medicine, 19*, 31-35.

Hochberg, M. C., Altman, R. D., Brandt, K. D., Clark, B. M., Dieppe, P. A., Griffin, M. R., Moskowitz, R. W., & Schnitzer, T. J. (1995). Guidelines for the medical management of osteoarthritis. *Arthritis and Rheumatism 38*, 1535-1540.

Lorig, K., & Fries, J. F. (1990). *The arthritis helpbook* (3rd ed.). Addison-Wesley.

Lorig, K., Holman, H., O'Leary, A., & Shoor, F. (1986). Outcomes of an efficacy enhancing arthritis patient education experiment. *Arthritis and Rheumatism 29*, S145.

Lorig, K., Lubeck, D., Seleznick, M., Drqines, R. G., & Holman, H. R. (1985). Outcomes of self-help education for patients with arthritis. *Arthritis and Rheumatism 28*, 680-685.

Minor, M. A., Hewett, J. E., Webel, R. R., Anderson, S. K., & Kay, D. (1989). Efficacy of physical conditioning exercise in rheumatoid arthritis and osteoarthritis. *Arthritis and Rheumatism 32*, 1396-1405.

Mullen, P. D., Laville, E., Biddle, A. K., & Lorig, K. (1987). Efficacy of psycho-educational interventions on pain, depression, and disability with people with arthritis: A meta-analysis. *Journal of Rheumatology 14*, 33-39.

Moncur, C. (1988). Physical therapy competencies in physical therapy management of arthritis. In B. F. Banwell & V. Gall (Eds.), *Clinics in Physical Therapy* series, Churchill Livingstone.

Wegner, S., Belza, B., & Gall, E. (Eds.). (1996). *Clinical care in the rheumatic diseases*. Atlanta, GA: American College of Rheumatology.

Zischke, J. (1986). Physical and psychological effects of a community-based exercise program on adults with rheumatoid arthritis and osteoarthritis. *Arthritis and Rheumatism 29*, S144.

APPENDIX 1:
RECOMMENDING SHOES AND FOOT ORTHOTICS FOR PEOPLE WITH RHEUMATIC DISEASES

Jeanne Melvin, MS, OTR, FAOTA, and Dennis Janisse, CPed

There is an old saying: "When the feet hurt, everything hurts." Proper footwear is an important part of pain management for people with arthritis.

THE RIGHT FOOTWEAR FOR PEOPLE WITH ARTHRITIS

Ideally everyone who wants to prevent foot problems and reduce stress to the weight-bearing joints should wear comfortable shoes, ones with good arch support, cushion soles instead of leather soles, and adequate length, width, and toe depth (sufficient to allow curling of the toes). Many walking and casual lace shoes offer these features. If a nonathletic, sturdy shoe allows a person to walk pain-free for a couple of hours, it is probably sufficient for his or her needs. However, if a person using even a walking shoe finds that his or her feet hurt after several hours of walking, say at a mall, he or she should consider using an athletic running shoe or foot orthotics.

Most people with OA do well with a comfortable shoe or running shoe. When people have a stiff or painful 1st MTP joint, an extended steel shank and rocker sole (see below) may be helpful for reducing the amount of motion needed in the toes for push-off when walking. Hallux valgus requires a shoe with a wide toe box that does not cause pressure on the 1st MTP joint or push the toes laterally. Of course, all of the foot problems that affect the general population, e.g., flat feet, pes cavus, Morton's neuroma, can also affect people with arthritis.

People with RA, JRA, SLE, SSc, PA who are prone to developing dynamic foot deformities generally benefit from the extra support of a "running shoe." In the early stages those with active MTP joint synovitis generally need custom foot orthotics to support the arch and reduce weight-bearing pressure on the MTP joints. Patients with subtalar synovitis may need the support of a heel-cup orthotic to reduce inversion and eversion. Those with severe deformities may need in-depth shoes or custom-molded shoes.

Which shoe is best for a specific person? How do you find the best shoe out of the myriad of selections now available? When are athletic shoes not sufficient or the best choice? When are foot orthotics needed? The answers to these questions are discussed in this section.

ATHLETIC SHOES

Athletic shoes have become the most popular shoe in North America. This is fortunate for people with arthritis and foot pain, for these are generally the best shoes for support and reducing impact on joints. They are stylish, too. Even Velcro® closures and elastic shoe laces, which are easier for arthritic fingers, are mainstream today.

Of all the shoes commercially available, athletic shoes designed for running have the most heel support and sole cushion for reducing impact to the joints during walking. Many also have a mild rocker sole that facilitates push-off. Because of these features, athletic shoes are recommended over "walking" shoes. For people who need foot orthotics, most athletic shoes offer the advantage of a removeable insole to make space for the orthotic. (See Table 1 for Guidelines for self-fitting shoes.)

The elderly at risk for falling need some special consideration. Shoes with extra-soft crepe soles or athletic shoes with flared soles may increase their risk of tripping or falling. These patients may do best with a firm, non-skid rubber sole, perhaps even a leather shoe that is a little heavier than an athletic shoe.

LACES

The location of the laces, high or low, can make a big difference in the stability of the foot in the shoe and the ease or difficulty of putting on the shoe. Some shoes are made with Velcro® closures, and those that are not can have them added at a shoe repair shop. There are also elastic shoe laces that are curled like a corkscrew (Lastic Laces®) that eliminate the need for tying. See chapter 16 on Assistive Technology for information on the national Abledata database.)

FOOT ORTHOTICS AND SHOE ADAPTIONS TO REDUCE PAIN/STRESS ON THE FOOT AND IMPROVE GAIT

1. Internal shoe modifications and indications
Custom-made foot orthosis (CFO)

These insertable orthotics are made from a mold of the patient's foot. For people with inflammatory arthritis, the most well-tolerated type is one made of a combination of soft materials (e.g., polyethylene foams) and semi-flexible materials (leather and cork).

They can be designed to *accommodate* deformity by distributing pressure over the entire plantar surface and to be *functional* in that they alter the biomechanics of the foot to reduce deforming forces or improve stability and gait. The surface is referred to as the "shell," and the material between the shell and the shoe is referred to as the "posting." Corrections to the orthotic are also referred to as a "posting," for example, "the orthotic was 'posted' for valgus instability."

Some design features that are commonly used for people with arthritis are:

- a metatarsal pad that reduces weight-bearing stress to the MTP joint by shifting the pressure of weight-bearing proximal to the painful metatarsal heads

- a medial wedge in the posting to help correct valgus deformity or a lateral wedge to reduce varus deformity

- heel modifications to reduce pressure on heel spurs.

When subtalar pain and instability are a problem, a rigid polyethylene CFO with an extension that cups the heel is used to reduce subtalar motion (inversion and eversion). It can also be posted to correct for valgus or varus deformity.

HEEL LIFTS

When a person has a leg-length discrepancy greater than 1", an extension to *both* the heel and sole may be needed to restore balance to the pelvis and spine. Heel lifts less than 3/8" may be used in the shoe; lifts greater than that need to be added to the external sole and heel.

HEEL CUSHIONS

Sponge inserts with a hole cut to relieve pressure over heel spurs are helpful for many people, but they may require a shoe with extra depth (Clark, 1996).

HEEL CUPS

Prefabricated rubber or plastic heel cups can help reduce pain associated with Achilles enthesitis, plantar fasciitis, or subcalcaneal spurs. They mold the soft tissues to provide greater protection between the tender point and the shoe during weight-bearing (Clark, 1996).

2. External Shoe Modifications and Indications

ROCKER SOLE

The function of a rocker sole is literally to "rock" the foot from heel-strike to toe-off without bending the shoe. It reduces the amount of motion required in the ankle and MTP joints to accomplish push-off. Therefore, it is a very helpful adaptation for people with ankle synovitis or surgical fusions and for people with limited or painful MTP joints. There are six different styles depending on the foot problem being treated (Janisse, 1995, 1997). Many walking and running athletic shoes are made with a mild or generic rocker sole. (Nawoczenski, Birke, & Coleman, 1988)

EXTENDED STEEL SHANK

This is a strip of spring steel inserted between the layers of the sole, extending from the heel to the toe of the shoe. It is commonly used in combination with a rocker sole to further prevent the shoe from bending. This is helpful for people with limited MTP motion, for example, hallus rigidus.

METATARSAL BAR

This bar is an addition to the sole that shifts weight-bearing pressure proximal to the MTP joints instead of directly onto the metatarsal heads.

STABILIZATION FLARE

This is an addition to the heel, or to both heel and sole, to stabilize the hindfoot or midfoot. It can be either medial or lateral, but the most common use in arthritis is a medial flare to support a valgus heel deformity.

SOLID ANKLE CUSHION HEEL (SACH HEEL)

This is a wedge of shock-absorbing material that is added at the heel of the shoe. Its purpose is to provide a maximum amount of shock absorption under the heel. It is commonly used in conjunction with a rocker sole to improve gait for people with limited or fused ankles.

WEDGE

Sole material in a wedge shape is sometimes added to the heel or heel and sole to redirect the weight bearing position of the foot. It can be useful in accommodating a fixed deformity by essentially bringing the ground to the foot. A medial wedge is indicated in cases of extreme pronation, while a lateral wedge can be used for ankle instability or a varus heel deformity.

EXTENSIONS

Sole material added to increase the thickness of the sole and heel to accommodate leg length discrepancy or added to just the heel to accommodate a plantar-flexion contracture.

PRESCRIPTION SHOES

When a person has severe or fixed-toe deformities that cannot be accommodated comfortably in even adapted commercial shoes, there are three other options:

1) in-depth shoes that allow extra depth in the shoe to accommodate custom shoe orthoses.

2) in-depth shoes with uppers that can be heat molded to reduce pressure on specific toes or bony prominences. Moncur and Ward (1990) reported that 25 patients fitted with these shoes reported reduced pain and 80% reported "walking better."

3) in cases of extreme deformity custom-made shoes or sandals (Deland & Wood, 1993) can be constructed from a mold of the person's foot.

GUIDELINES FOR SELF-FITTING ATHLETIC SHOES IN THE STORE

- Shoes should be comfortable at the time of purchase, and people should be encouraged not to purchase shoes that need to be "broken in." After buying new shoes, people should be encouraged to wear them for gradually increasing periods of time and to check their feet after wearing to make sure there are no areas of redness, tenderness, or skin breakdown.
- The type of socks you wear can affect the fit of the shoe. When buying new shoes, take your socks with you.
- If you use orthotics, take them with you, too.
- Women sometimes find that men's shoes are wider and accommodate certain orthotics or swelling better than women's shoes.
- Request a pair of each brand in your size. (Typically there are three-six brands or styles from which to choose.).
- Systematically cross compare each shoe to the other. Try on the left shoe of brand A and the right shoe of brand B. Select the best fitting of the two. Then compare it to brand C, walking in one of each. Select the best fitting of the two. Continue this process with each brand in your size, comparing one against the previous best. Ultimately the last, best one wins the cross-comparison. However, since people's feet are not the same size and shape, try on both the left and right of the winning brand or style. Walk in the "best" pair and make sure they are comfortable on *both* feet. Be sure the shoe is long enough and that the arch and midfoot sections are comfortable and that the toes can curl and straighten.
- The first MTP joint (base of the large toe) should be at the widest part of the shoe.
- The shoe should be about 3/8" to 1" longer than your longest toe to allow the foot to slide forward during push-off.
- The heel should be snug.
- The top part of the shoe (the vamp) should be comfortable when laced securely.

Table 1: Guidelines for self-fitting athletic shoes in the store

REFERENCES

Clark, B. M. (1996). Foot Management and Ambulatory Aids. *Clinical care in rheumatic diseases.* Atlanta, GA: Arthritis Foundation.

Deland, J. T., & Wood, B. (1993). Foot pain. In W. N. Kelly, E. D. Harris, S. Ruddy, and C. B. Sledge (Eds.), *Textbook of rheumatology* (4th ed.,). Philadelphia: Saunders.

Moncur, C., & Ward, J.R. (1990). Heat-moldable shoes for management of forefoot problems in rheumatoid arthritis. *Arthritis Care and Research, 3,* 222-226.

Nawoczenski, D. A., Birke, J. A., & Coleman, W.C. (1988). Effect of rocker sole design on plantar forefoot pressures. *Journal American Podiatric Medical Association, 78,* 455.

Janisse, D. J. (1995). Prescription insoles and footwear. *The Diabetic Foot, Clinics in Podiatric Medicine and Surgery 12,* 41-61.

ADDITIONAL RESOURCES

Janisse, D. (1995). Pedorthics in the rehabilitation of the foot and ankle. In G. J. Sammarco (Ed.), *Rehabilitation of the foot and ankle.* St. Louis: Mosby.

Janisse, D. Wertsch, J. J., & DelToro, D. R., (1995). Foot orthoses and prescription shoes. In J. B. Redford, J. V. Basmajian, & P. Trautman (Eds.), *Orthotics: Clinical practice and rehabilitation technology.* New York: Churchill Livingstone.

Moncur, C. Characteristics of rheumatoid arthritis in the forefoot. In C. G. Hart & T. G. McPoil (Eds.), *Physical therapy of the foot and ankle* (2nd ed.). New York: Churchill Livingstone.

Moncur, C. Characteristics of rheumatoid arthritis in the midfoot. In C. G. Hart & T. G. McPoil (Eds.), *Physical therapy of the foot and ankle* (2nd ed.). New York: Churchill Livingstone.

Moncur, C. Characteristics of rheumatoid arthritis in the hindfoot. In C. G. Hart & T. G. McPoil (Eds.), *Physical therapy of the foot and ankle* (2nd ed.). New York: Churchill Livingstone.

Spiegel, T. M., & Spiegel, J. S. (1982). Rheumatoid arthritis in the foot and ankle: Diagnosis, pathology and treatment: The relationship between foot and ankle deformity and disease duration in 50 patients. *Foot Ankle International, 2,* 318-25.

APPENDIX 2:

PHYSICAL THERAPY COMPETENCIES IN RHEUMATOLOGY

Carolee Moncur, PT, PhD

Reprinted with permission of Banwell, B.F., Gail, V. (Eds.), *Physical Therapy Management of Arthritis*. New York: Churchill Livingston, 1988: 29-41.

COMPETENCY STATEMENTS

BASIC KNOWLEDGE

The entry-level physical therapist should be able to make decisions regarding screening and the need for specific evaluation techniques based on a basic knowledge of the following:

1. Pathophysiology of the common forms of rheumatic disease
2. Progression of the common forms of rheumatic disease
3. Medication regime, side effects, and speed of efficacy
4. Impact of rheumatic disease on all phases of the patient's life
5. Common types of surgery, precautions for treatment, and the process of tissue healing.

PATIENT EVALUATION

The entry-level physical therapist should be able to perform physical therapy assessment procedures on the patient with arthritis including an evaluation of the patient as follows:

1. Ambulation and transfer status
2. Skin and vascular condition
3. Neurologic signs
4. Knowledge of the disease and the treatment regimen
5. Ability to cope with the chronicity of the illness
6. Pain status
7. Swelling and/or synovitis of joints
8. Muscle strength
9. Deformity and joint stability
10. Respiratory functions
11. Fatigue and endurance levels
12. Morning stiffness and joint gelling
13. Dexterity
14. Personal care
15. Home conditions
16. Ability to participate in recreational activities
17. Ability to fulfill an occupational role
18. Work place conditions.

DESIGNING A PHYSICAL THERAPY PLAN OF CARE

The entry-level physical therapist should be able to design a plan of care based upon the results of the physical therapy evaluation including the following patient information:

1. History
2. Goals, expectations and motivation
3. Pain and/or tolerance for activity
4. Deficits in muscle strength
5. Status of joint deformities (fixed versus correctable)
6. Deficits in functional activities
7. Activity of the disease (flare versus remission)
8. Potential problems which could develop due to the disease or the patient's lifestyle
9. Ambulation status
10. Ability to rest
11. Tolerance for physical therapy modalities
12. Need for adaptive and orthotic equipment.

The entry-level physical therapist should also be able to do the following:

1. Recognize and respond in changes in the patient's physiologic status
2. Recognize and respond to changes in the patient's ability to cope with the disease
3. Continue, modify or discontinue the physical therapy treatment and/or goals when necessary
4. Design a discharge plan of care and home program based upon the results of periodic physical therapy reassessment.

IMPLEMENTING A PHYSICAL THERAPY PLAN OF CARE

The entry-level physical therapist should be able to implement these programs:

1. A therapeutic exercise program for the patient with arthritis-related problems
2. An ambulation program for the patient with arthritis-related problems
3. A pain management program
4. An activities for daily living program for the patient with arthritis related problems
5. A joint protection and energy conservation training program
6. Relate the hospital and/or clinic treatment program to a home management program
7. Recommend solutions for adapting the patient's home and work environment.

PATIENT COMPLIANCE

The entry-level physical therapist should be able to enhance the patient's compliance to the physical therapy regime as follows:

1. Determine the patient's expectations about the physical therapy treatment
2. Determine treatment goals of the patient and physical therapist
3. Design a treatment program that has simplicity in terms of numbers of exercises/tasks the patient must do and that transfers to the patient's life situation
4. Establish that the patient knows what is expected by having him or her repeat or demonstrate what has been instructed
5. Provide written instructions for home programs
6. Interpret and respond appropriately to the nonverbal message of patients.

PATIENT, FAMILY AND COMMUNITY EDUCATION

The entry-level physical therapist should be able to design and implement patient education strategies including the following:

1. Lectures
2. Leading discussions
3. Individualizing instruction
4. Programmed learning programs
5. Leading practice skills and activities
6. Role-playing techniques
7. Imitating correct behavior.

The entry-level physical therapist should be able to instruct the patient and family in the proper use of the following:
1. Therapeutic exercise and activity
2. Joint protection
3. Energy conservation
4. Therapeutic electrical equipment (transcutaneous electrical nerve stimulation [TENS], biofeedback, etc.)

Table 1: Competency Statements (continued)

5. Traction
6. Therapeutic massage
7. Therapeutic heat and cold
8. Orthotic devices and supports.

The therapist should be able to instruct the patient
1. And the family about the nature and progression of the type of arthritis the patient has
2. And the family about community resources available to them
3. And the family about the hazards of unproven remedies
4. Appropriately about physical/sexual problems related to contracture, deformities, and postoperative joint replacement.

The entry-level physical therapist should be able to
1. Design and implement a community education program about physical therapy and arthritis
2. Select and refer the patient to other health professionals for treatment, education, and/or utilization of community resources.

RESEARCH ACTIVITIES
The entry-level physical therapist should be able to
1. Interpret the results of a research project
2. Apply the results of the research to patient care
3. Participate in an on-going project designed by another investigator
4. Design and carry out an independent clinical investigation to answer a frequently arising question in physical therapy treatment of rheumatic disease.

Table 1: Competency Statements (continued)

STANDARDS OF PRACTICE

OCCUPATIONAL THERAPY COMPETENCIES IN RHEUMATOLOGY

Task Force Members:

Gloria Purst, OTR, MPH
Mary J. Bridle, MA, OTR
Jill A. Noaker, OTR, CHT
Pamela B. Harrell, OTR, CHT
Bonnie C. Thornton, OT
Y. Lynn Yasuda, MSEd, OTR, OTCCMCL-DOC

BASIC KNOWLEDGE

The occupational therapist involved in care of the individual with rheumatic disease should be able to:

A. Discuss the pathophysiology of the following rheumatic diseases from a multisystem focus, including etiology, epidemiology, course, and pathogenesis.
    1. Most commonly seen rheumatic diseases
        a. Rheumatoid arthritis
        b. Degenerative joint disease/osteoarthritis
        c. Systemic lupus erythematosus
        d. Fibromyalgia
    2. Additional rheumatic diseases
        a. Spondylarthropathies
        b. Juvenile rheumatoid arthritis
        c. Reflex sympathetic dystrophy
        d. Systemic sclerosis
        e. Polymyositis/dermatomyositis
        f. Psoriatic arthritis
        g. Gout

B. Discuss medications commonly used with rheumatic diseases.
    1. Purpose of medication
    2. Side effects that may alter function
    3. Timing of administration to affect function

C. Describe the pathomechanics of deformity, including the nature of periarticular and articular destruction.

D. Define the following surgical interventions for patients with rheumatic disease, including the process of healing, precautions, and postoperative treatment.
    1. Synovectomy
    2. Joint replacement
    3. Arthrodesis
    4. Arthroscopy
    5. Osteotomy
    6. Resection

E. Explain basic diagnostic techniques, such as laboratory tests and X-rays, and their purpose.

F. Describe the process of activity analysis for purposes of treatment and/or adaptation.

G. Describe the following occupational therapy modalities.
   1. Functional adaptation, such as adaptive procedures for activities of daily living, work, and leisure
   2. Therapeutic activities
   3. Availability and uses for a wide range of activity of daily living equipment
   4. Orthotics
   5. Psychosocial interventions

H. Describe joint protection and energy conservation techniques related to rheumatic diseases.

I. Discuss the impact of rheumatic disease.
   1. Interrelationship between the patient's motivation, daily routines, roles, and performance
   2. Environment and family interaction
   3. Common emotional reactions to chronic disease
   4. Factors that influence adaptation

J. Describe the influence of cultural differences and values in approach to health care for common daily living activities.

K. Explain how the following factors are associated with patient adherence to treatment programs.
   1. Depression
   2. Fatigue
   3. Powerlessness (perception of external control)
   4. Secondary gains
   5. Responsibility for self
   6. Relationship with and role in family
   7. Knowledge and acceptance of disease

L. Describe the roles of other health professionals who treat patients with rheumatic disease.

PATIENT EVALUATION

A.   Evaluate the patient's knowledge of his or her rheumatic disease, treatment regimen, and goals for treatment through verbal interaction and observation.

B.   Evaluate and interpret the patient's functional status through interview, assessment procedures, and/or skilled observation in the following areas.
   1. Physical abilities
      a. Self-care tasks, such as dressing, household activities, and transfers
      b. Strength and range of motion
      c. Dexterity
      d. Pain
      e. Sensation
      f. Fatigue and endurance
      g. Stiffness in the morning or following periods of inactivity
      h. Cognitive screening
      i. Leisure activities, such as sports and hobbies
   2. Occupational behaviors
      a. Habits and routines
      b. Value sand priorities
      c. Occupational history
      d. Home, work, school, and community environment

C.   Perform a physical evaluation and assessment, including recognition and assessment of the following items.
   1.   Swelling/synovitis
   2.   Tendon integrity
   3.   Joint stability
   4.   Ligamentous laxity
   5.   Soft tissue involvement
      a. tenosynovitis
      b. Tendinitis
      c. Bursitis
      d. Subcutaneous nodules
      e. Trigger finger
   6.   Common hand deformities
      a. Swan neck
      b. Boutonniere
      c. Malleet

      d. Ulnar deviation

      e. Thumb deformity

      f. Subluxation

      g. Dislocation

      h. Wrist/hand zigzag deformity

      i. Flexion/extension contracture

      j. Mutilans

      k. Heberden's nodes

      l. Bouchard's nodes

      m. Carpometacarpal squaring

7. Intrinsic/extrinsic tightness

8. Range of motion lag

9. Crepitus

10. Ankylosis

11. Skin integrity

12. Vascular involvement

13. Sensory involvement

14. Muscle strength

15. Ambulation

16. Transfers

17. Posture and positioning

DEVELOP A TREATMENT PLAN

A. Consolidate information from the evaluations and prioritize intervention strategies by considering patients' priorities and addressing problems identified.

   1. Short- and long-term goals, including vocational and avocational considerations

   2. Need for adaptive and orthotic equipment

   3. Realistic consideration of available resources to the patient; including, but not limited to the following areas

      a. Physical and psychological capacities to benefit from rehabilitation

      b. Family, community, and other environmental support

   4. Information from other health care providers working with the patient to enhance understanding of all problems that will affect setting functional goals

   5. Financial abilities/insurance

   6. Inpatient/outpatient options

B. Select functional activities and exercise appropriate to the patient's roles, interests, stage of disease, and activity level.

C. Design a splinting program to address problems identified on the evaluations, including patient's goals and willingness to wear splints. Identify realistic splinting outcomes. Identify and apply pathomechanics, select appropriate splint designs, prioritize splinting needs, select custom versus commercial splints, and train patient in use and care.

D. Design an individualized education plan to provide training in energy conservation and joint protection principles.

    1. Appropriate for the patient's psychological readiness and acceptance level

    2. Appropriate to the educational and cognitive levels of the patient and family members

    3. Sensitive to and understanding of sociocultural issues

       a. Cultural background

       b. Level of education

       c. Methods of learning to which the patient is responsive

E. Ability to evaluate architectural barriers and recommend changes to modify the environment.

IMPLEMENT A TREATMENT PLAN

A. Demonstrate the ability to perform activities of daily living training.

    1. Select appropriate equipment with regard to patient's abilities/disabilities, needs, and resources

    2. Practice of daily activities using appropriate joint protection, energy conservation techniques, and adaptive equipment

B. Provide effective patient education, including the following areas.

    1. Joint protection, energy conservation, and home exercise techniques

    2. Basic treatment principles

    3. Practice of specific techniques

    4. Use of audiovisual aids

    5. Follow-up to assess learning

    6. Instruction in posture and body positioning

C. Implement functional activities designed to facilitate role activities and to improve strength, range of motion, dexterity, and endurance.

D. Implement a graded activity program appropriate for rheumatic diseases that will facilitate occupational therapy interventions.

    1. Select exercises appropriate to the problems identified on initial evaluation

       a. Range of motion (passive or active)

       b. Stretching exercises

       c. Strengthening

    2. Identify boundaries of exercise program

      a. repetitions

      b. Modification of program in response to changes in joint and disease status

    3. Select appropriate setting for exercise program to be carried out

      a. Home exercise program

      b. Outpatient, therapist-assisted exercise/treatment program

E. Correctly fabricate the following splints.

    1. Resting hand

    2. Wrist cock-up

    3. Finger and thumb splints

    4. Ulnar deviation

    5. Dynamic outrigger

    6. Elbow extension

F. Place treatment program appropriately for patient's cognitive and fatigue levels and degree of disease activity.

G. Provide consultation and training for mobility aids, including wheelchairs and power scooters.

H. Provide assistance in modifying/redefining daily role involvement, environment, and exploring new interests in keeping with functional limitations, patient's goals, and joint protection and energy conservation requirements.

I. Demonstrate skills in postoperative management of related rheumatic diseases, including the spine and upper and lower extremities.

    1. Adaptation during recovery

    2. Graded return to productive role activities

MODIFY A TREATMENT PLAN

A. Recognize and respond to changes in the patient's status by making appropriate modifications in the plan of care.

    1. Continuing/discontinuing treatment

    2. Modifying goals of treatment

B. Refer patients to other healthcare professionals and community resources as appropriate.

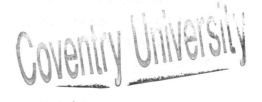

PATIENT EDUCATION

A. Write measurable learning objectives and evaluate the outcome of educational interventions.

B. Use educational materials relevant to the patient's social environment, taking into consideration family, work, school, and leisure activities.

C. Identify arthritis resources for patient education, including printed materials, commercially available audiovisual aids, and facility and community resources.

RESEARCH

A. Demonstrate knowledge of occupational therapy research literature selected to rheumatology and patient care; also show ability to search that literature for relevant information.

B. Apply research results and knowledge gained through continuing education to patient care.

C. Collect and analyze outcome measures.

REFERENCES

The American Occupational Therapy Association has an Arthritis Resource Guide that includes

- Names of resource personnel
- Organizational resources
- Databases/information centers/directories
- Journals and newsletters
- Key references
- An extensive topic-specific bibliography
- Audiovisual references
- Sample forms.

The resource guide is available from:

American Occupational Therapy Association
Product Department
4720 Montgomery Lane
PO Box 31220
Bethesda, MD 20824-1220
(301) 652-AOTA.

OCCUPATIONAL THERAPY COMPETENCIES IN RHEUMATOLOGY

This document is designed to provide arthritis health professionals, educators, and potential employers of health care providers with guidelines for the competent practice of occupational therapy for persons with rheumatologic disorders. The competencies are intended for all registered occupational therapists (OTR) inexperienced in rheumatology. They do not apply to certified occupational therapy assistants (COTA).

These competencies are considered to be the minimum necessary for a therapist working without supervision.

Index

A